MANAGEMENT IN HEALTH CARE

A Theoretical and Experiential Approach

Elaine Lynne La Monica EdD FAAN

Professor of Nursing Education
Teachers College, Columbia University, New York
and
Consultant in Management for Health Care

Additional material for the Macmillan adaptation by

Philip Ian Morgan, BA Hons MA PhD

Lecturer in Human Resource Management
Cardiff Business School,
University of Wales College of Cardiff

MACMIL

© Springer Publishing Company, Inc. 1990
Adaptations for Macmillan edition © Philip I. Morgan 1994

First published 1990 by
Springer Publishing Company, Inc.
536 Broadway
New York, NY 10012
under the title
Management in Nursing:
An Experiential Approach That Makes Theory Work For You
Written by Elaine Lynne La Monica

This edition first published 1994 by
THE MACMILLAN PRESS LTD
Houndmills, Basingstoke, Hampshire RG21 2XS
and London
Companies and representatives
throughout the world

ISBN 0–333–56385–9 hardcover
ISBN 0–333–56386–7 paperback

A catalogue record for this book is available
from the British Library

Printed and bound in Great Britain by
Mackays of Chatham PLC, Chatham, Kent

Dedicated to

My best friend,
Robert S. Rigolosi

For feeling without saying
And
For saying with feeling. . .

Always. . . .

Elaine Lynne La Monica

Elaine L. La Monica, EdD, FAAN, is Professor of Nursing Education at Teachers College, Columbia University, New York. Currently, she is also Director of the Institute of Research and Service in Nursing Education. Her formal education includes a Doctor of Education degree in human relations and counseling from the School of Education, University of Massachusetts, Amherst; a Masters of Nursing in medical and surgical nursing administration from the College of Nursing, University of Florida, Gainesville; and a Bachelor of Science in nursing from Columbia Union College, Takoma Park, Maryland.

In addition to administrative and academic responsibilities at Teachers College, Dr La Monica maintains a private consulting practice in management for health care organizations and other public and private industries throughout the US, Canada and overseas. She also conducts training programmes on organizational behaviour both nationally and internationally.

Scholarly activities included serving as the Management Briefs Editor for *The Journal of Nursing Administration* and as a frequent author on management, empathy, and related topics in professional journals. Dr La Monica's most recent books are *Nursing Leadership and Management: An Experiential Approach,* 1986, and *The Humanistic Nursing Process,* 1985; both are published by Jones and Bartlett, Boston, Massachusetts. *The La Monica Empathy Profile,* 1986, published by XICOM, Inc., Sterling Forest, Tuxedo, New York, is an instrument for measuring empathy in helpers—teachers, nurses, managers, and other care givers.

Dr La Monica maintains membership in the following professional organizations: American Academy of Nursing, American Nurses Association, American Psychological Association, New York State Nurses Association, and Sigma Theta Tau–Alpha Theta Chapter, an honour society for nurses.

This book is an adaptation of *Management in Nursing: An Experiential Approach That Makes Theory Work For You,* solely authored by Dr Elaine La Monica, and published by Springer Publishing Company, New York, 1990.

Philip I. Morgan, PhD, MA, BA(Hons), is a lecturer in Human Resource Management at Cardiff Business School, University of Wales. His formal education included a BA with Honours in Business Administration from Strathclyde University and doctoral studies at The Ohio State University.

Dr Morgan has taught management subjects at universities in the US and the UK at postgraduate and undergraduate levels. In addition to teaching and academic responsibilities, he researches, lectures, and consults for various public and private organizations, including various hospitals in the UK. His research interests include Organisational Development and Total Quality Management issues related to the National Health Service.

Dr Morgan's additions to Dr Elaine L. La Monica's book are identified by footnotes, as are the chapters of which he is the sole author.

Acknowledgments

Even though the author first imagined and then created this book, the theory, exercises, and philosophy represented have been derived from many personal and professional resources. Some materials are original, and some are from established sources to whom credit is most gratefully given; others have evolved from an interchange with professionals and learners whose commitment has been to quality. I would like particularly to thank Donald Carew, Kenneth Blanchard, and Paul Hersey, whose teachings and writings were the foundation of my doctoral education and are the cornerstones of my current professional activities; Frederic Finch for sharing his knowledge; Phil Graf for his reinforcement and assistance—for believing many years ago that I had something to offer future managers; and my colleagues in education and practice for the constant interchange that has shaped today.

To all who have moulded my beliefs, to all from whom I have received, I express my sincere gratitude.

Elaine Lynne La Monica

Preface

It is widely recognized that health care professionals must become effective managers and leaders in order to fulfil their responsibilities to themselves, to their clients, and to the professions. Practice environments, roles, and educational programmes are expanding. There is an actual and projected decline in the numbers entering the professions; there is an actual and projected need for increased professional services due to changing demographics of the population and crises emanating from disease states.

Other trends in health care include (a) changing emphases imposed by federal and state cost-containment regulations; (b) changing and alternative methods for health care delivery; (c) increasing focus on health maintenance—primary care—in addition to the ever-present foci on secondary care and tertiary care; and (d) greater quantities of data to support the mind/body relationship in health and disease, suggesting that not only is cure important, but altering behaviours is crucial so that the need to cure may be unnecessary or less frequent.

Wherever their placement in the health care arena, health care managers will be leaders of themselves; of colleagues and peers in interdisciplinary clinical teams, of technicians and other health care providers; of colleagues in various management levels within formal health care organizations; of the public sector through media; of the individual clients, in city, state, national, and international political entities, and so forth. In these placements, they will be called upon for creative strategies, disciplined and cost-contained programmes, and the abilities to research and analyse systems critically and chart growth—all in response to rapid health care changes. It is therefore mandatory that professionals perceive themselves in the roles of managers and leaders and increase their knowledge and application of theory and research in practice so that quality, comprehensive, efficient care is provided to clients in any setting.

Leadership and management involve processes that are essential in making any health care role, in any environment, alive. Disciplines and professions such as organizational behaviour, educational administration, and business have developed theories that assist managers in increasing the probability of achieving specified goals. Managers must apply these theories into leadership and management, and then extend them into theory through research. Responsibility and authority granted by a practice act, an institution, an individual's unique experience and personality, and one's personal philosophy on the constituents of quality care and effective management, must be integrated with knowledge and an ability to apply existing theories of management in health care practice.

This book covers the processes of management and leadership in health care practices. It evolves from my experience in teaching future managers of health care personnel in the delivery of care. Content focuses on increasing organizational effectiveness in service and practice. Theories and concepts from the professions of business, organizational psychology, and educational administration are applied to topics in each chapter.

Sections of the book include simulations (for example, case presentations and multimedia activities) to provide practice experiences that illustrate the content of the chapters, as well as to expand the learner's range of experience. The simulations comprise the experiential approach; they provide learners with an opportunity to observe, experience, and carry out new behaviours in a safe, low-risk practice environment. Careful explanations are provided for each simulation. The textbook and exercises are designed for use both in self-learning and classroom environments, in both individual and group learning experiences. It is suggested that study be weighted so that more time is devoted to the experiential elements, since enriched learning in management is derived more from actual and vicarious experiences than from reading and studying the printed word.

This book is written primarily for undergraduate students in health care management and leadership courses. It is also intended as a resource for graduate administration students, practitioners, learners in inservice and continuing education programmes, and faculty.

It is a pleasure to have Dr Morgan's additions in the Macmillan version of this book and to have had the opportunity to work with Dr Morgan on the adaptation.

Elaine Lynne La Monica

Introduction

Management and leadership in health care involve an individual's efforts to influence the behaviour of others in providing direct, individualized, professional care. The basic premise of management is that managers set goals that represent some level of growth for a particular group in a particular environment. Managers then develop strategies for reaching these goals. Results are evaluated and altered or new directions are set. There is no value of good or bad to the actual state of the group, the group's goals, or the outcomes. Managers simply and constantly design strategies for moving groups of personnel to more efficient and more qualitative levels of functioning. The actual beginning points and the end points are of lesser importance than is the process of constantly developing strategies that result in identifiable, effective, and positive growth. In conducting these processes, managers plan, organize, motivate, and control the work of other allied health care personnel in the delivery of professional care.

The processes of management and leadership are based on a scientific approach called the problem-solving method. The function of this scientific method is to increase the probability of success for a manager's actions, given the particulars of a unique environment. In a typical health care environment, there are staff members, clients, managers, situational variables such as policies and norms, and material resources; these are unique since it would be impossible to find this exact environment in another place or time. The goal of the manager is to identify the environment's resources and to put them to work as a whole system in accomplishing goals and facilitating growth. Use of the scientific method in management simply assists the manager in assessing many needs of the system and in choosing the priorities, identifying the people and situational elements that are important in carrying out specified goals, critically assessing the strengths of those people, and developing strategies that put those strengths to work.

A manager can be functional in the role without using the problem-solving method. This alternative, called "seat-of-the-pants" management, evolves from following only impulses and personal beliefs about self and others. Such management comes from involuntary behaviours that do not involve thinking about what a group needs from the manager in order to accomplish its goals. It is possible for seat-of-the-pants management to be successful. That is, by some stroke of luck, the impulses, beliefs, and behaviours of this manager are exactly what the system requires. Though possible, however, such success is unlikely.

Use of a scientific approach brings no guarantee of success; there is no way to predict the behaviour of others with complete accuracy. An effective manager analyses an environment and chooses the best strategy for achieving a specified goal, given the particular strengths and weaknesses of the employees who will be working to carry out that goal. There is always some unknown that cannot be controlled—the risk factor. Because all managers desire success, their goal in choosing the best strategy should be to identify the strategy that balances the lowest risk factor with the highest rate of return. This automatically increases the probability for success. A manager who uses seat-of-the-pants thinking will have a higher risk factor in every undertaking than will the manager who applies a scientific approach. The scientific management method forces the manager to plan, organize, motivate, and control logically and analytically. Further, it allows the manager to build contingency plans for all possible outcomes rather than to face problems unprepared.

Why does use of the scientific method offer so much? It is derived from methodologically sound research within the disciplines and professions of business, educational administration, and psychology—the purists in management. Given the numerous investigations that allow the label *theory* to be attached to a process or belief, the results suggest that this theory, applied in a particular way, produces these outcomes at least 95% of the time. A person who simply or randomly guesses in all decisions has an equal chance of being right or wrong. Managers, however, should not be satisfied with such a ratio—this is mediocrity. The use of intuition is appropriate and necessary only after the application of theory. It is the à la mode on home-made apple pie.

Parts I and II, "Conceptual Framework" and "Manager Responsibilities", present the process steps of health care management and leadership. Each chapter has its own conceptual and theoretical discussions with health care applications. In Chapter 7, the whole process of health care management and leadership is presented through a case study. Part III, "Management Skills", takes a close look at the specific skills that managers must use to implement the management process effectively in a variety of health care environments. Part IV studies management processes that increase understanding of health care structure.

An experiential approach in learning management and leadership sets the book into motion for the learner. The simulations at the end of Parts II and III present specific ways to learn the chapter contents. These simulations are designed to provide experience in applying theory in a low-risk setting. It is known that as anxiety increases, perception decreases. When perception decreases, people most often do not think; they merely function intuitively. These intuitive behaviours are derived from practices and experiences earlier in life—from behaviours previously learned. It is also known that in a real management environment, a person's anxiety is generally greater than it is in a classroom or laboratory. This is due to tensions increasing when others are really looking to a person for guidance or are expecting something from that person. Because it takes time for learners to incorporate theory into practice, to think while doing instead of doing and then thinking, the use of simulations provides added experience so that the likelihood of a manager effectively applying theory while in any state of anxiety increases. This experiential model, the group dynamics laboratory, has been widely used in management training and this author has adapted it to health care simulations.

The exercises in Part I of this book are ice-breaking, getting-acquainted activities. They are designed to help in the formation of effective groups and are most appropriately used at the beginning of study in a management and leadership course or programme.

The ultimate goal of this book is identical to the ultimate goal of health care: to assist the client to reach full health potential. In achieving this goal, an intermediate goal of assisting the manager to achieve optimal effectiveness is emphasized. The educational process attends to the unique individual learner. A satisfied manager has a high probability of having staff members who are also satisfied; satisfied staff members have a high probability of having satisfied clients; a satisfied client has a high probability of reaching full health potential.

Elaine Lynne La Monica

Preface to the Macmillan Edition

I am pleased to introduce the Macmillan edition of *Management in Health Care* to a British audience. Previously the book was printed and published in the US under the title *Management in Nursing* by Dr Elaine Lynne La Monica. The new edition, entitled *Management in Health Care*, has an additional section, Part IV, with six new chapters specially written for it.

The change in title reflects a more general orientation to health care management and was intended to increase the book's appeal to a wider audience of health care professionals and other generalists, in addition to nurses. This was done since it was felt that the recent changes in the National Health Service (NHS) affect everyone working in health care and require them to display more managerial and leadership abilities than ever before.

The present edition of this book is, therefore, intended for health care professionals who have managerial responsibilities in health care or allied health care at supervisory level or above, e.g. staff nurses, ward sister or heads of departments of radiography, physiotherapy, chiropody, medical records, theatre, etc. Included in this group are both purchasers and providers of health care, including staff in directly Managed Units, NHS Trusts, Independent Hospitals, Local Authorities and Voluntary Agencies.

The book is especially intended for those who may be undertaking a management course in higher education at a university or polytechnic. However, it is possible to use the book for private study also.

Although the general focus and structure remain the same, spelling and nomenclature have been altered to reflect British usage. For example, where "nurses" or "nurse managers" have been used in the original "health care manager" or "manager" have been substituted where appropriate.

Some minor additions have also been made to certain chapters. For example, in Chapter 1 Mintzberg's research on managerial roles has been added.

Philip Ian Morgan

Introduction to the Macmillan Edition

Health care in the 1990s is still in a period of transition, following the major government NHS management reforms of the 1980s. These reforms together with the recommendations of the National Health Service Management have considerable implications for the organization of health care throughout the UK. In addition, the NHS and Community Care Bill, which makes provision for the establishment of NHS Trusts, introduces new arrangements for provision of local health services, including contracts between NHS bodies, and new frameworks for the provision of community care. All of this means that now, more than ever, there is a greater need for effective leaders and managers with vision in the health service to implement and effectively manage these changes. To do this, health care professionals require a sound understanding of leadership and management principles together with a sound understanding of the system in which they operate.

This is why I am pleased to join with Dr La Monica in bringing this book to the attention of a British audience. Anyone who diligently studies the theories and principles contained within these pages and who is willing to make the effort to translate the principles into their own practice will be well rewarded with an overall improvement in their managerial performance.

The present volume has been expanded to include a new section, "Management Processes" (Part IV), while in Part III, "Management Responsibilities", two additional chapters have been added: Chapter 19, which covers research related to stress and its management, together with suggested strategies managers might adopt in coping with the negative effects of stress in themselves and others, and Chapter 20, which covers total quality management issues in the delivery of quality health care.

In Part IV, "Management Processes", Chapter 21 covers the historical development of the NHS since its inception and provides an overview of how it has evolved managerially and structurally to the present day, while Chapters 22 and 23 complement the previous chapters by providing a review of the various organizational theories as well as the "nuts and bolts" involved in structuring an organization. Chapter 24 discusses organizational culture—a topic which is assuming increasing importance in management literature—and relates it to the NHS. Additional experiential exercises have also been added to complement some of the added chapters.

Philip Ian Morgan

Contents

PART III   MANAGEMENT SKILLS

PART IV   MANAGEMENT STRUCTURE
AND PROCESSES

Part I

A CONCEPTUAL FRAMEWORK

Part I provides a discussion of the theories and concepts on which management processes are based. These theories are derived from research in organizational psychology, business, and educational leadership; the theories are applied to a health care environment.

Chapter 1 defines leadership and management, differentiating the roles of managers and leaders from the processes of managing and leading. The management process and the problem-solving method are the foci of this chapter.

Chapter 2 involves a discussion of the conceptual roots on which contemporary management practices are built—nonclassical organization theory. General system theory forms the basis for leader behaviour, and the group dynamics laboratory is the mode used in this book for learning leadership and management content as well as process. The theory of motivation is then explained as it relates to management and leadership responsibilities.

CHAPTER 1

The Management Process and the Problem-Solving Method

This chapter provides a definition of management and leadership and discusses the general process of management. Management processes and roles frame all leadership activities. Broad areas of management skills and roles are then presented; the chapter concludes with a discussion of the problem-solving method (the scientific method for a leadership role). The content in this chapter forms the foundation for specific leadership responsibilities that are addressed in Part II of this book.

MANAGEMENT AND LEADERSHIP

Many definitions of management and leadership can be identified when surveying the literature (Brooten, Hayman, & Naylor, 1988; Koontz & O'Donnell, 1986; Lucio & McNeil, 1979; Marriner-Tomey, 1988; Newman & Warren, 1982; Sayles, 1979; Stevens, 1978). Themes, however, are evident. Hersey and Blanchard (1988) provided a comprehensive definition of management as "working with and through individuals and groups and other resources to accomplish organizational goals" (p. 3). Leadership also involves working through individuals and groups to accomplish goals, but these goals may be different from organizational goals, or they may involve one segment of the organizational goals. In a sense, the key difference between the concepts of management and leadership is the phrase "organizational goals". A manager works for an organization (for example, a hospital administrator) and carries the responsibility of accomplishing the organization's goals through specific professional services. Leadership is a much broader concept because all health care professionals are leaders. Anytime a person is a recognized authority and has followers who count on this person's expertise to carry out their objectives, the person is a leader. Furthermore, anyone who is responsible for giving assistance to others is also a leader. The staff nurse is a leader to clients; the student nurse also is a leader to clients; the head nurse is a leader to all team followers; and parents are leaders to children.

It is necessary to define management and leadership in order to understand the differences between the roles of managers and leaders; to reiterate, the key difference is that managers are responsible for organizational goals while leaders may only be responsible for one segment of the overall goals. When management and leadership theory are applied to leader activities, however, the theory serves roles of both managers and leaders. What changes is the system that the leader influences. Obviously, the system that the primary care nurse manages is much smaller than that of the nursing sister. For clarity, therefore, there are both leader and manager roles in health care. The theory that people in these roles apply, however, is called management and leadership theory and should be the foundation upon which all influencing activities are based.

THE MANAGEMENT PROCESS

The process of management is relevant to all people who seek to influence the behaviour of others. Many authors who discuss management and leadership consider the process germane even though authors often differ semantically when identifying the process components (Brooten *et al.*, 1988; Haynes, Massie, & Wallace, 1975; Longest, 1984; Marriner-Tomey,

1988). Hersey and Blanchard (1988) cited four managerial functions; planning, organizing, motivating, and controlling. Their definitions of these components are expanded here and combined with applications in health care.

Planning

This involves identifying problems, setting and specifying both long-term and short-term goals, developing objectives, and then mapping how these goals and objectives will be accomplished. Longest (1984) asserted that planning involves a means to blend the actions of all participants in a system so that the group's members function together toward an identified goal. Planning greatly reduces the chance of being caught unprepared. Planning, according to Marriner-Tomey (1988), is the first and most important step of the management process.

Organizing

This part of the management process involves bringing all of the system's resources—people, capital, and equipment—into action toward goal accomplishment. Hersey and Blanchard (1988) discussed it as integrating resources. A leader's desire is to include all people and situational elements into the system that will be carrying out a particular goal and to organize them so that the group is working together toward goal accomplishment.

Motivating

Motivation is a large factor in determining the performance level of employees and the quality of goal accomplishment (Hersey & Blanchard, 1988). William James of Harvard, conducting research on motivation, concluded that hourly employees could maintain their jobs by only working to 20 to 30% of their capacity. When properly motivated by their leader, however, they could work to 80 to 90% of their ability (Hersey & Blanchard, 1988). James felt that approximately 60% of employee performance can be affected by motivation. There is never a zero point or top level (100%) in employee performance because one should not say that people are at the maximum absolute level in their motivation to attain a goal. There are no limits on what human beings can accomplish, which is why Olympic records, for example, are broken. One must always strive to do a little bit better. Managers must always set goals that are higher than what employees had accomplished previously, based on the assessment that the goals are not beyond the capabilities of the people trying to attain them. That is the unidirectional process of growth.

Controlling

This last component in the management process involves setting up mechanisms for ongoing evaluation. Hersey and Blanchard (1988) said that controlling is obtaining feedback of results and periodically following up in order to compare results with plans. Adjustments in plans can be made accordingly. Quality-control systems, client-care audits, and client census and acuity information are examples of this aspect of the process.

Controlling is one aspect of management that is subject to myths and misinterpretations. When students are asked to share the first adjective or emotion that comes to mind when the term *controlling* is presented, responses include "manipulation", "rigid", "tight", "autocratic", and "oppressed". Controlling need not be any of these things; it is an essential aspect of managerial functions because a manager is ultimately responsible for followers' actions, given that a manager energizes the resources of a group to accomplish a goal. An effective health care manager does not do everything. Rather, the manager leads the group to accomplish, and keeps track of what is happening at given points in time. Misinterpretations of controlling stem from the leader's verbal and nonverbal communications in the management process. It is possible to say, for example, that you as a manager would like to meet every week with your group in order to discuss progress and problems on a particular goal without being called autocratic, rigid, or tight. This is an area that should be role-played in a practice environment so that one's intent is perceived accurately.

Even though the four aspects of the management process are distinct, they are interrelated. When a leader plans, the plan also contains strategies for organizing, controlling, and motivating resources. Hence, all parts of the management process are connected. The case study in Chapter 7 illustrates this point further.

MANAGERIAL SKILLS

There are three general categories of skills that managers and leaders must possess: technical skills, human skills, and conceptual skills. Katz (1955) first classified these skills, and Hersey and Blanchard (1988) adapted them to the field of behavioural science.

> *Technical Skill*—Ability to use knowledge, methods, techniques, and equipment necessary for the performance of specific tasks acquired from experience, education, and training.
>
> *Human Skill*—Ability and judgment in working with and through people, including an understanding of motivation and an application of effective leadership.

Conceptual Skill—Ability to understand the complexities of the overall organization and where one's own operation fits in the organization. This knowledge permits one to act according to the objectives of the total organization rather than only on the basis of the goals and needs of one's own immediate group (Hersey & Blanchard, 1988, p. 7).

For example, suppose a nurse leader has the goal of increasing the quality of nursing care. Technical skill is the leader's ability to perform the comprehensive individualized nursing care that is expected from staff nurses and from nursing practice standards. Human skill involves ability to influence others by teaching, role modelling, and so forth in order to accomplish the goal. Conceptual skill involves seeing how the goal that is being accomplished fits into the overall organizational goals of client service in the agency—how it affects the entire health care facility.

Research has shown that managers at different levels require varying amounts of technical and conceptual skills in order to carry out their responsibilities effectively. Human skills are a constant in all levels and occupy the greater part of the management function, as Figure 1.1 illustrates.

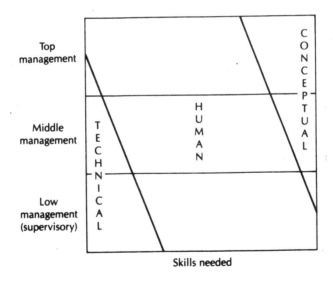

FIGURE 1.1 Management skills by levels of management.

Source: Reprinted by permission of the *Harvard Business Review*. From "Skills of an Effective Administrator", by R. Katz (January/February 1955). Copyright © 1955 by the President and Fellows of Harvard College; all rights reserved; and from Paul Hersey and Kenneth H. Blanchard, *Management of Organizational Behavior: Utilizing Human Resources*, 5th ed., © 1988, p. 8. Reprinted by permission of Prentice-Hall, Inc., Englewood Cliffs, NJ.

ROLE THEORY*

Mintzberg (1973) summarized much of the evidence on how managers spend their time and concluded that executive work is characterized by fragmentation, brevity, and superficiality. Many of the tasks lasted on average only nine minutes or less. Based on his research, Mintzberg suggested de-emphasizing the manager as formal decision maker and, instead, proposed that a new emphasis be given to the kinds of roles a manager performs. Mintzberg identified three roles: interpersonal, informational, and decisional.

Interpersonal Roles

The interpersonal roles managers perform are based on the formal authority they enjoy which facilitates interpersonal relationships. There are three types of interpersonal roles:

1. Figurehead—involving taking visitors to dinner, conducting and attending ceremonies, etc.
2. Leader—involving hiring, training, and motivating employees by providing a model for others to follow, e.g. performing under pressure.
3. Liaison-person—involving dealing with people outside the organization on a continuing basis, e.g. maintaining good working relations with key suppliers so that in times of scarcity supplies may be obtained based on good working relationships.

Informational Roles

These flow from the interpersonal roles, e.g. in the process of fulfilling the roles as figurehead, leader, and liaison-person, managers are in a unique position to gather and disseminate information. Information roles can be subdivided into three types:

1. Monitoring—involving seeking information that may be of value, e.g. querying subordinates who are receptive to information and attempting to be well informed.
2. Disseminating information—involving transmitting relevant information to subordinates in the workplace.

---

*"Role theory" written by Dr Philip Morgan.

3. Spokesperson—involving dealing with people external to the organization, e.g. speaking to representative organizations at professional meetings and making presentations to interested bodies.

Decisional Roles

Informational roles lead naturally to the decisional roles, i.e. managers acquire information as a result of various kinds of decisions they make. There are four kinds of decisional role:

1. Entrepreneur—a person who is the voluntary initiator of change or risk-taker, e.g. in this role managers identify problems and opportunities and initiate a change of strategy to deal with the new situation.
2. Disturbance handler—involving dealing with strikes and disputes. This role is usually initiated by others.
3. Resource allocator—involving deciding who will be allocated various parts of a company's limited resources.
4. Negotiator—involving negotiating on behalf of the company, e.g. negotiating the union contract, agreements with consultants, or long-term relationship with a supplier.

Using the concept of "role" as a framework to understand what managers actually do enables us to conceptualize as Mintzberg has shown, that managers tend to fulfil many different roles in the course of their work. Identifying and defining these roles provides us with a greater understanding of the management process.

THE PROBLEM-SOLVING METHOD*

Effective management and leadership are not based on seat-of-the-pants thinking. The roles mandate methodical thinking that draws first from theory (what has been shown to be effective in a significant number of research incidents) and then intuition (what has been shown to be effective in one's own experience, given application of research principles). The priority goal of a manager is to accomplish goals (commonly referred to as growing) by activating a system. Everything that a manager

---

*This section is an adaptation of the method presented by Hersey and Blanchard (1988) in their book and in their classes at the University of Massachusetts, 1973–1975.

or leader does toward goal accomplishment should be based on a conscious, identified strategy that has the highest probability for success. Again, there are no absolute points because human behaviour cannot be predicted with complete accuracy. Rather, the manager seeks awareness of all in a system to mobilize forces toward goal accomplishment. Fortunately, a scientific method for doing this is available, just as one is available for giving nursing care. The latter is called the nursing process and the former is called the problem-solving method. Both are adapted from the scientific method, as is evident in Table 1.1.

The problem-solving method is presented theoretically in this chapter. It is the framework upon which all management practices are built. Part II of this book is devoted to the process of carrying out this method; examples for making the process alive are provided.

Problem Identification

This is the first step in the problem-solving method. A problem is identified by the difference between what is actually happening (the actual) in

TABLE 1.1   Comparison of the Problem-Solving Method, the Scientific Method, and the Nursing Process*

Problem-Solving Method	Scientific Method	The Nursing Process
		Problem Finding
1. Problem identification	1. Gathering information	Data collection
Point of view	2. Examining information	Data processing
	3. Interpreting information	
2. Problem definition and/or goal statement	4. Identifying problem(s)	Diagnosis
	5. Stating the problem(s)	
3. Problem analysis		
		Problem Solving
4. Alternative solutions	1. Developing alternatives	Care plans
	2. Making a decision	
5. Recommended action	3. Deciding on a plan of action	
	4. Executing the plan of action	Implementation
	5. Evaluating the results	Evaluation
	6. Redefining problem and change	

*Source: La Monica, E. (1985). *The humanistic nursing process.* Boston: Jones and Bartlett.

a situation and what one wishes to have occur (the optimal). Figure 1.2 illustrates this point. To determine a problem area, it is necessary to gather, examine, and interpret information from all sources available— primary and secondary—and to decide whether the problem area warrants attention. Primary sources are your followers, and secondary sources are all other people from whom information can be collected— clients, doctors, associates, superiors, and so forth. Data can be gathered from these sources on one-to-one or group bases. The manager's own point of view should be identified by being conscious of individual self-perceptions and beliefs. These data should be shared with members of the problem-solving group.

Problem Definition

After a situation has been assessed to determine a priority need area, to identify where a group is in relation to this need (the actual), and to identify where one wishes to go relative to this need (the optimal), then a problem can be stated as shown in Figure 1.2. This procedure represents the difference between real and optimal and should be specific and tractable. Managers who identify problems may be comforted by the knowledge that problems are indicative of growth. A manager should always be identifying problems—specifying where a group is and delineating where it can go. This is the process of growth. Once the optimal is attained, it becomes the actual or the real situation and the whole process of identifying problems should begin again.

Problems should be specific and tractable. For example, if performance is the focal point, it is necessary to determine the aspects of performance that one wishes to change. Is it that care plans are not routinely written? Or do employees spend too much time with administrative tasks? A clearly stated problem structures the whole problem-solving process because what has to be done to solve the problem and evaluate outcomes becomes apparent only when the problem statement is clear and specific. Further, Goode and Fowler (1949) demonstrated early that a clear state-

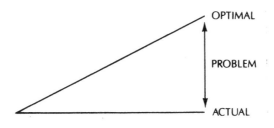

FIGURE 1.2 Identifying the problem.

ment of problems contributed to follower support in solving the problem because followers were aware of the focus of their efforts. Locke, Saari, Shaw, and Latham (1981) asserted that designating problems and setting goals "affect performance by directing attention, mobilizing effort, increasing persistence, and motivating strategy development" (p. 125).

A goal is simply a restated problem. Hence, goals flow from the problem statement. If a problem is that nursing care plans are not written routinely, then the goal would be to have nursing care plans written for all clients. A problem statement can be thought of as a negative statement— that is, something one wishes to eradicate or get rid of. A goal is something one wishes to attain; it is a positive statement. Obviously, problems and goals comprise different ends of the same continuum. It is individual choice whether a manager wishes to work with problems or goals or both. This author's preference is to accentuate always positive thinking by working with goals rather than problems.

The specification of the optimal can be a long-term or a short-term goal. Even though it is essential that a manager identify both types of goals, one should be aware that research in motivation suggests that people are more highly motivated at the beginning of task accomplishment and when the goal is almost accomplished (Atkinson, 1957). Since increased employee motivation usually results in an increase in productivity, with follower job satisfaction as a by-product, the manager should set goals with followers that can be accomplished in a reasonable amount of time. The success and rewards that follow goal achievement serve as both a reinforcement and a stimulus in further endeavours. Shorter-term goals may also be viewed by followers as more realistic and achievable. Livingston (1969) aptly stated that subordinates must consider goals as realistic in order to be motivated to reach high levels of productivity. For example, if care plans are never written for clients (the actual) and a leader desires that they be written for all clients (the optimal), an intermediate short-term goal might be to write care plans on clients who have chronic health problems. There are many rungs in the ladder toward accomplishment of the long-term goal. Each should be accomplished in stepwise progression toward a long-range goal.

Problem Analysis

After the problem is identified, it must be analyzed. Analysis entails four steps: (1) to determine why the problem exists; (2) to identify the unique group who will participate in solving the problem/achieving the goal; (3) to analyse the ability of a group to accomplish the goal (level of maturity); and (4) to specify an appropriate leader behaviour style, indicated by the group's level of maturity, that is required in order to meet the needs of a group as it accomplishes the goal. It is in this fourth phase that

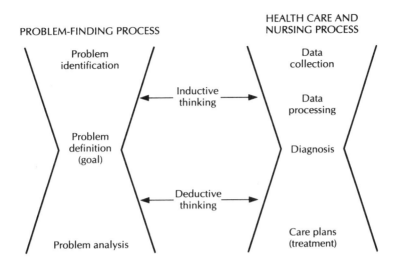

FIGURE 1.3 Comparison of the problem-finding process with the health care and nursing process.

leader behaviour theories are brought into focus. By applying theory in each of these four steps, one increases the probability that analysis will be comprehensive and that the decision on the appropriate leader behaviour style will be based on what works according to research findings.

The problem-finding process that was previously discussed can be compared with the health care and nursing process (La Monica, 1985), as portrayed in Figure 1.3. It is evident that vast information is boiled down in both methods to focus on a specific problem. Once the problem is specified, then analysis broadens in order to solve it. Problem identification and data collection and processing involve inductive thinking in order to make a conclusion about the problem; all information in these processes is used to identify a problem. Problem analysis and care plans, however, are examples of deductive reasoning; a focal area exists and all that follows relates to solving the problem.

Alternative Solutions

Based on analysis, the next step is to brainstorm various alternative solutions or strategies that have the potential to solve the problem or achieve the goal. Brainstorming, a step in the creative process (McNeil, 1973), can be used to foster creativity and to develop alternatives that reflect the individuality of a unique system—people, environment, and time. This process is a way to expand possibilities by answering the question. "If I could achieve this goal with this identified system, ideally doing anything I wished, reflecting my knowledge and experience, what would I want done and how should I get it done?" All ideas are important and during the process of brainstorming, no value judgments of good or bad operate.

After the ideas are listed, then each solution should be studied for anticipated positive results and anticipated negative results. In other words, it is necessary to play out behaviour and attempt to predict reactions of followers; these reactions should include both the negative and the positive.

Recommended Action

Following analysis of alternative solutions, one strategy must be chosen. Unfortunately, it is rare when a strategy played out has no negative consequences. The recommended action, therefore, usually has the highest probability for reducing the discrepancy between real and optimal and the lowest probability for resulting in negative consequences, given that there are most often some negative consequences in all strategies. It should be noted that solution phases are too frequently hurried. A good analysis in these steps is important since it most often results in the recommended action becoming obvious.

SUMMARY

Management and leadership are different concepts when they are defined in terms of roles; managers are responsible for organizational goals while leaders are such because people look to them for guidance. In leader/ manager activities, however, management and leadership theory is applied in both roles.

The management process contains four interrelated elements: planning, organizing, motivating, and controlling. Technical, human, and conceptual skills are required in order to carry out this process. Different levels of management require lesser or greater amounts of technical and conceptual skills; human skills are constant in all levels of management.

The problem-solving process is the manager's scientific method. It is the foundation on which all manager activity should be based. A problem must first be identified inductively, resulting in a specific problem statement. Deductive processes are then employed to analyse the problem and identify alternative solutions. A recommended action is the final outcome of the problem-solving method.

REFERENCES

Atkinson, J. (1957). Motivational determinants of risk-taking behavior. *Psychological Review, 64*, 365.

Brooten, D., Hayman, L., & Naylor, M. (1988). *Leadership for change: An action guide for nurses* (2nd ed.). Philadelphia: Lippincott.

Goode, W., & Fowler, I. (1949). Incentive factors in a low morale plant. *American Sociological Review, 14*, 618–624.

Haynes, W., Massie, J., & Wallace, M. Jr. (1975). *Management: Analysis, concepts, and cases.* Englewood Cliffs, NJ: Prentice-Hall.

Hersey, P., & Blanchard, K. (1988). *Management of organizational behavior: Utilizing human resources* (5th ed.). Englewood Cliffs, NJ: Prentice Hall.

Katz, R. (1955). Skills of an effective administrator. *Harvard Business Review, 33*, 33–42.

Koontz, H., & O'Donnell, C. (1986). *Essentials of management.* New York: McGraw-Hill.

La Monica, E. (1985). *The humanistic nursing process.* Boston: Jones and Bartlett.

Livingston, J. (1969). Pygmalion in management. *Harvard Business Review, 47*, 81–89.

Locke, E., Saari, L., Shaw, K., & Latham, G. (1981). Goal setting and task performance: 1969–1980. *Psychological Bulletin, 90*, 125–152.

Longest, B. (1984). *Management practices for health professionals* (3rd ed.). Norwalk, CT: Appleton-Lang.

Lucio, W., & McNeil, J. (1979). *Supervision in thought and action* (3rd ed.). New York: McGraw-Hill.

Marriner-Tomey, A. (1988). *Guide to nursing management* (3rd ed.). St. Louis: Mosby.

McNeil, J. (1973). The creative process. Unpublished paper, University of Massachusetts, Center for the Study of Aesthetics in Education, Amherst.

Mintzberg, H. (1973). *The nature of management work.* New York: Harper & Row.

Newman, W., & Warren, E. (1982). *The process of management: Strategy, action, results* (5th ed.). Englewood Cliffs, NJ: Prentice-Hall.

Sayles, L. (1979). *Leadership: What effective managers really do . . . and how they do it.* New York: McGraw-Hill.

Stevens, W. (1978). *Management and leadership in nursing.* New York: McGraw-Hill.

CHAPTER **2**

Management and Leadership Theory

CLASSICAL AND NONCLASSICAL
ORGANIZATION THEORY
   Classical Organization Theory
   Nonclassical Organization Theory
GENERAL SYSTEM THEORY
GROUP DYNAMICS LABORATORY
MOTIVATION
   Motivation Factors
   Applying Motivation Theory
SUMMARY

The management process and the problem-solving method are the procedures for all management responsibilities. These procedures outline how managers should function. Chapter 2 discusses the concepts and theories explaining why managers function in particular ways. This chapter also provides the rationale for the educational design of the book, the intent of which is to enable learners to grow and therefore change; change is synonymous with growing or learning. The goal of this book parallels the goal of health care managers and leaders, that leaders also facilitate change and growth in their personnel. The conceptual framework presented in this chapter applies to learning how to become a manager as well as to the role of being a manager. The conceptual framework, therefore, holds together the education of future leaders and managers as well as the process of management and leadership.

This chapter includes discussions of classical and nonclassical organization theory, general system theory, and the group dynamics laboratory as an educational mode. It concludes with the theory of motivation, which is an essential concept in understanding management and leadership processes.

CLASSICAL AND NONCLASSICAL ORGANIZATION THEORY

The literature reflects two categories of leadership: classical organization theory (COT) and nonclassical organization theory (NCOT). Prior to 1950, COT was the rule in organizations. NCOT, which has evolved from criticisms of COT, is the basis for contemporary management practices.

Classical Organization Theory

COT has a list of assumptions, delineated by McGregor (1966, 1960/1985), called Theory X assumptions about human nature. These are as follows:

1. People find work distasteful;
2. People are not ambitious and prefer direction;
3. People do not solve organizational problems creatively;
4. People are motivated only by physiological and safety factors; and
5. People require close control and coercion to achieve goals.

Given these assumptions, organizations designed the leadership structure to counteract these traits of people so that organizational goals would be accomplished. The traditional organization therefore had centralized decision making and a pyramid form of superior-follower control. In essence, workers were told what to do and were not required to think. The leadership style used with the employees was autocratic (Davis & Newstrom, 1985; Hersey & Blanchard, 1988).

Severely criticizing classical organizations, which were built on Theory X assumptions, McGregor (1966, 1960/1985) asserted that people had those traits because the organization or past experience made them that way. When leaders treat workers as if workers have no thinking power or are robots, workers soon start behaving as if these traits are real. What motivation would one have to do otherwise?

Nonclassical Organization Theory

In contrast to Theory X assumptions about human nature, McGregor (1966, 1960/1985) further proposed the following Theory Y assumptions about people:

1. People regard work to be as natural as play, when conditions are favourable;

2. People are self-directed in achieving organizational goals;

3. People are creative in solving problems;

4. People are motivated at all levels of Maslow's (1970) hierarchy of needs—physiological, safety, social, esteem, and self-actualization; and

5. People are self-controlled if properly motivated.

Nonclassical organizations, which have Theory Y assumptions about people, design the leadership structure so that workers will be able to grow within the organization; the aim is to have people fulfill the Theory Y assumptions.

Obviously, people are neither good nor bad, and it must be pointed out that McGregor had no intent of portraying them as good or bad when delineating Theory X and Theory Y. Theory Y assumptions allow managers in an organization to find out what motivates people and then give the appropriate leadership style that enables workers to grow within an organization. Some people may in fact need close control, for example; then the autocratic style of leadership is appropriate. Others may need support from the leaders and a democratic leader behaviour style may be indicated. There may be those who are completely self-motivated and are committed to the growth of the organization. These people are usually best if left alone—the laissez-faire leadership style. Theory Y assumptions, therefore, permit the organization's leaders to respond to the needs of the people who make up the organization as these people work to achieve the organization's goals. Leader behaviour reflects the needs of a group given a particular problem or goal. If the group changes or the goal changes, the appropriate leader behaviour style must be reassessed and designated again.

GENERAL SYSTEM THEORY

All contemporary management practices are based on nonclassical organization theory. NCOT employs a situational approach to leadership. It assumes that all people can be helped and educated to achieve organizational goals, that people vary as to what motivates them, and that the styles of leadership used in organizations must respond to the needs of the organization's constituency (Argyris, 1971; Herzberg, 1966; Likert, 1967; McGregor, 1966, 1960/1985). The situational approach to leadership is based on an understanding of general system theory, which provides a construct for studying people within their environment and as builders of their environment.

General system theory is a model developed by von Bertalanffy

(1968, 1975) and applied to nursing practice by Putt (1978). It mandates analysis of all the system's parts, the relationship between and among those parts, as well as the system's purposes, beliefs, and tasks. Yura and Walsh (1987) simplified general system theory by saying that it includes purpose, content, and process.

Von Bertalanffy (1968) designated two main types of systems, closed systems and open systems, as means of conceptualizing the world and the universe. Closed systems end when a quantity needed for fulfillment is obtained. Further, results are exactly predictable in closed systems. An example of a closed system is a chemical equation. If water (H_2O) is added to salt (NaCl), a chemist (or a manager) can predict and quantify exactly what will occur—water plus the breakup of sodium and chloride ions. Hence, the balanced equation:

$$NaCl + H_2O = H_2O + Na^+ + Cl^-$$

Open systems have no designated quantity and are not exactly predictable. Human beings are open systems because even though one can spend great amounts of time finding out the properties, personality, wishes, and desires of people, there is and will always be the unknown. Open systems are the only concern for study, therefore, when general system theory is applied in management.

Von Bertalanffy (1968) identified four assumptions of open systems:

1. *A system is more than a sum of its parts.* In other words, a system is composed of all people and things within it, but the composite system contains more than its constituents. This composite has a character of its own, made up of the parts, but different from those parts. The system or group becomes the "I" or first person, not the individuals and things within the system.

Another example of the first assumption involves taking ten people in a group and giving each person an energy range that moves from 1 (lowest amount of energy) to 10 (highest amount of energy). If the assignment were given to one person in the group to use 10 units of energy and go out on a motorway and stop traffic in both directions from 8:00 A.M. to 8.30 A.M. one morning, would that person be successful? Maybe, but success is doubtful. Suppose the assignment were given to all ten people to do the same in the same spot but work independently. Then there would be 100 units of energy working on a goal. The ten people would have more chances of being successful than the single person. Give the same assignment to ten people, but instruct them jointly to plan a strategy for accomplishing the task—that is, to work together as a group on the goal. The chances of the group being successful would be far greater than the chances for success in either the single assignment or the task in which ten individuals worked alone.

Given a perfectly functioning group, the amount of energy contained within the group is not simply 10 times 10 or 100 units. The amount of energy is 10 to the tenth power (10^{10}) or 100,000,000,000 units of energy because the interaction between and among every combination of people in the group elicits energy toward goal accomplishment. So, a group of people working together toward a common goal is the manager's best bet, even though groups rarely function perfectly. The greater the amount of energy a group has working toward a goal, the higher the probability for effective goal completion. This is the principle behind collective bargaining units. The challenge for management, however, is to keep the groups working *for* the organization rather than against the organization.

2. *A system is ever-changing.* The absence of a member or part of a system or the inclusion of a new member or piece of equipment changes the system. On a smaller scale, the passage of time changes a system. Since humans are constantly learning from and therefore changing with the environment, people are different at every point in time. Even though a group may be composed of the same constituents, the group is always changing because the constituents are always changing. An effective leader must allow for the group's growth (or regression) to be reflected in the group's goals and the strategies that will best enable the goals to be attained. This process involves constant assessment of the group.

3. *A system has boundaries* that are defined by the system's purpose. Community care can be considered as one system. All of the human and the material resources in this unit are part of the system. In fact, the community in which the unit is located can be conceptualized as the supra-system. The universe is our absolute outer system, given the limits of human knowledge. All that occurs in the world falls into subsystems. One system is always related to or is part of a larger whole. Figure 2.1 provides one example of how this principle works.

Problem solving requires that boundaries be designated. In increasing the quality of health care, for example, the subsystem of the community is important but not as important as the health care team. Boundaries are circumscribed by responding to the question: "What and who are the important components of the larger system that will have the most direct effect on solving a given problem?" The answer becomes the system for that problem. It follows that each system is unique for each problem, given the available human and material resources in a specified time and place. The system that

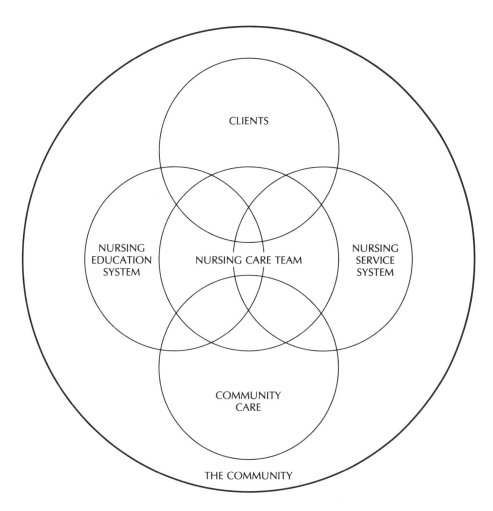

FIGURE 2.1 The nursing system viewed from a health-care service perspective.

has a goal of increasing the quality of care in a given unit may not be the same system in another unit or at another time in the same unit. Part II will discuss designating systems in greater detail than is presented here.

4. *Systems are goal-directed.* This assumption flows directly from the previous one. Once the problem or goal is specified, the boundaries of a system can be specified. A system with no goal has no reason to exist, no motivation to function, and no drive to succeed. A system with no goals has nothing to evaluate because evaluation requires measurement points—a beginning point and an end point.

Without goals, one can easily feel a lack of accomplishment and a feeling of "never getting anything done". Behaviourally, this can become a self-reinforcing negative cycle. Principles of time management, discussed in Chapter 17, are built on this goal-setting principle.

These four assumptions guide the manager to state problems/goals, to designate the system that will be primarily responsible for goal attainment, and to understand how the group working as a single, integrated unit of one becomes foremost in effective goal accomplishment.

GROUP DYNAMICS LABORATORY

The group dynamics laboratory, the most widely used method for management training, has experiential learning as its focus (Fiedler, Chemers, & Mahar, 1984; Finch, Jones, & Litterer, 1976; Stogdill, 1974). Various group exercises form the laboratory experience: case studies, films, role playing, business games, and other media that involve group problem-solving projects.

The laboratory group is actually a microcosm of the real work world. Participants have an opportunity to apply and use the skills and behaviours that a manager must possess: how to lead, follow, draw out opinions, use power, resolve conflicts, be assertive, give and receive feedback, and so forth. Because the role of a manager always involves working with people in groups, the group dynamics laboratory serves to enable both learning the required content in management and leadership and the actual process of being a manager.

The group dynamics laboratory, developed by the National Training Laboratories in Bethel, Maine, grew from the sensitivity and T-group movement (Benne, 1969; Berne, 1978; Bradford, Gibb, & Benne, 1964; Perls, 1969; Schein & Bennis, 1965; Schutz, 1967). Several underlying assumptions about the learning process distinguish T-groups and the group dynamics laboratory from other modes of instruction. According to Seashore (1970, pp. 15–16), these assumptions are:

> *Learning Responsibility.* Participants are responsible for their own learning. What is learned depends upon style, readiness, and the relationships developed with other members of the group.
>
> *Staff Role.* The staff person's role is to facilitate the examination and understanding of the experiences in the group by helping participants to focus on the way the group is working, the style

of an individual's participation, or the issues that are facing the group.

Experience and Conceptualization. Most learning is a combination of experience and conceptualization. A major T-group aim is to provide a setting in which individuals are encouraged to examine their experiences together in enough detail so that valid generalizations can be drawn.

Authentic Relationships and Learning. A person is most free to learn when authentic relationships are established with other people, thereby increasing one's sense of self-esteem and decreasing defensiveness. In authentic relationships, persons can be open, honest, and direct with one another so that they are communicating what they are actually feeling rather than masking their feelings.

Skill Acquisition and Values. The development of new skills in working with people is maximized as a person examines the basic values underlying behaviour, as appropriate concepts and theory are acquired, and as one is able to practise new behaviour and obtain feedback on the degree to which that behaviour produces the intended impact.

The intent of the group dynamics laboratory is to accomplish one or more of the following changes in attitude or behaviour on the part of the leader trainees (Stogdill, 1974, p.182):

1. Greater sensitivity to follower needs and desires;
2. Greater openness and sharing of information;
3. Greater sharing of decision-making responsibilities with followers;
4. More intimate, friendly, and egalitarian interaction with followers; and
5. Less structuring, personal dominance, and pushing for productive output.

Studies by Gibb (1971), Harrison and Lubin (1965), Callahan and Wall (1987), Wright (1983), and Miles (1965) have all found the laboratory method to increase effective interpersonal communication among members; members can test and learn trust, risk-taking, openness, and interdependence. Further, outcome studies on the effects of the group dynamics laboratory approach in leadership training have been widespread and positive. Stogdill (1974) presented and discussed an extensive review of this body of literature.

Blumberg (1977, pp. 15–16) asserted that in order for training goals in laboratory education to be realized, certain conditions in the laboratory must be met. These are:

> *Presentation of Self.* Until an individual has an opportunity to reveal the way one sees things and does things, there is little basis for improvement and change.

> *Feedback.* Individuals do not learn from their experiences. They learn from bringing out the essential patterns of purposes, motives, and behaviour in a situation where they can receive back clear and accurate information about the relevancy and effectiveness of their behaviour. They need a feedback system which continuously operates so that they can change and correct what is inappropriate.

> *Atmosphere.* An atmosphere of trust and nondefensiveness is necessary for people both to be willing to expose their behaviour and purposes, and to accept feedback.

> *Cognitive Map.* Knowledge from research, theory, and experience is important to enable the individual both to understand experiences and to generalize from them. But normally, information is most effective when it follows experience and feedback.

> *Experimentation.* Unless there is opportunity to try out new patterns of thought and behaviour, they never become a part of the individual. Without experimental efforts, relevant change is difficult to make.

> *Practice.* Equally important is the need to practise new approaches so that the individual gains security in being different.

> *Application.* Unless learning and change can be applied to back-home situations, they are not likely to be effective or lasting. Attention needs to be given to helping individuals plan application.

> *Relearning How to Learn.* Because much of our academic experience has led us to believe that we learn from listening to authorities, there is frequently need to learn from presentation-feedback-experimentation.

Regarding the group mode of instruction in training, Carkhuff (1969) concluded that this model is goal- and action-directed in its work-oriented structure. Emphasis is on behaviour one wishes to effect, leaving the trainee with tangible and usable skills. Longer retention of learned skills results because learning is an outcome of actual experience. Further, the nature of the systematic training involves steps that lead to measurable outcomes, thereby making evaluation explicit. "In summary, what can be accomplished individually can be accomplished in groups—and more!" (p. 184).

MOTIVATION

The theory of motivation is the last area to be discussed in the conceptual framework of management and leadership. Motivation, as stated in Chapter 1, comprises the largest area of a manager's responsibilities; its major importance in management activities remains constant regardless of one's management level.

In comparing motivated and unmotivated personnel generally, the more followers are motivated to accomplish a goal, the shorter time will be required to succeed. In addition, quality will increase, costs will decrease, and personnel will have a positive experience, which serves as a stimulus for motivating them to accomplish again. In short, as motivation increases, time and costs decrease while quality and satisfaction increase. Motivating personnel is the responsibility of managers. Theories are available that guide the leader to find out what motivates individuals and then to apply the appropriate leader behaviour style that will increase the probability of motivating people to get the task done while enabling them to grow in their positions. Applications of these theories will be discussed and applied in Part II of this book. This section will present the theory of motivation, which is essential in understanding the applied motivation theory that is explained later.

Motivation Factors

The following definitions provide keys to understand motivation (Davis & Newstrom, 1985; Hersey & Blanchard, 1988):

> *Motives*—Needs, wants, drives, or impulses within an individual that prompt behaviour; motives may be conscious or unconscious.
>
> *Motive Strength*—A means for categorizing the strength of a motive or need. Since people normally have a variety of motives all competing for fulfilment, the highest-strength motive is satisfied through behaviour first. Once a need is satisfied, it decreases in motive strength and the need next in priority receives attention.

Goals—"Hoped for" rewards, incentives, and external desires. Goals are outside an individual; they are what one wishes to attain.

Behaviour—What a person does and what others perceive. Behaviour is observable, measurable action.

If a need is present within an individual, the need (internal) is attached to a goal in the environment (external) and causes the individual to work toward attaining that goal, thereby satisfying the need. Davis and Newstrom (1985) discussed external goals as intrinsic and extrinsic factors. Intrinsic factors occur at the time work is performed, an example of which is positive reinforcement from a supervisor immediately following task completion. Extrinsic factors occur away from work, for example, fringe benefits and days off.

People work on satisfying needs in an orderly fashion. Those needs that have the highest motive strength receive attention first. Maslow (1970) presented a theory that designates categories of needs and their strength when unsatisfied. The theory is called Maslow's hierarchy of needs and is shown in Figure 2.2. According to Maslow's widely accepted theory of motivation, the physiological needs (shown at the bottom of the pyramid in Figure 2.2) are top priority in motive strength when unsatisfied. Physiological needs have the highest priority until satisfied. Once physiological needs become less important or are in balance, safety needs take

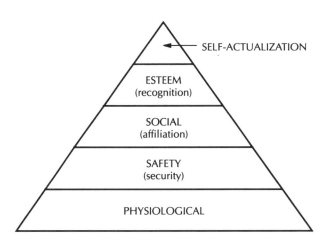

FIGURE 2.2 Maslow's hierarchy of needs.

Source: "Hierarchy of Needs" from *Motivation and Personality*, 2nd ed., by Abraham H. Maslow. Copyright 1954 by Harper & Row Publishers, Inc. Copyright © 1970 by Abraham H. Maslow. Reprinted by permission of the publisher.

priority. This format follows as the pyramid climbs to self-actualization, which is a priority only when the other four needs are satisfied. It must be noted that all needs are present within an individual; the priority of the needs, however, shifts. A person may be functioning at a physiological level at 12:00 noon and then be at an esteem level after lunch. Hersey and Blanchard (1988) diagrammed this movement as shown in Figure 2.3. Theorists such as Argyris (1971), Herzberg (1966), Hersey and Blanchard (1988), and McGregor (1966) presented variations on motivation factors. These theories are discussed and compared in Part II of this book.

In order to understand motivation fully, another concept requires discussion. This concept involves the difference between internal and external motivation. Internal motivation comes from within a person; external motivation is outside a person. The old saying, "You can lead a horse to water but you cannot make it drink", is true. A leader cannot

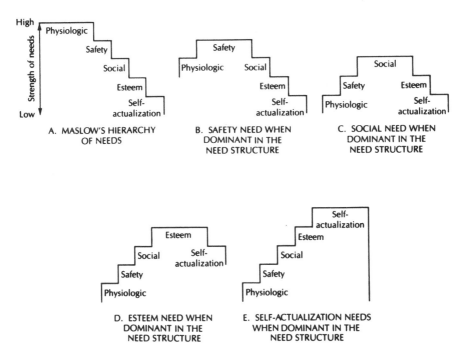

FIGURE 2.3 Movement of Maslow's hierarchy of needs.

Source: Paul Hersey & Kenneth H. Blanchard, *Management of Organizational Behavior: Utilizing Human Resources*, 5th ed., pp. 33–35, © 1988. Reprinted by permission of Prentice-Hall, Inc., Englewood Cliffs, NJ. "Hierarchy of Needs" from *Motivation and Personality*, 2nd ed., by Abraham H. Maslow. Copyright 1954 by Harper & Row Publishers, Inc. Copyright © 1970 by Abraham H. Maslow. Reprinted by permission of the publisher.

make someone behave in a certain way. If someone has an internal need, the sight of an external goal increases the probability that behaviour aimed at goal attainment will follow; no guarantee, however, exists. For example, if a person is hungry and food is in sight at a nearby restaurant, it is probable that the person will be motivated to travel to get the food but one cannot be absolutely sure.

Applying Motivation Theory

A manager is responsible for motivating personnel to accomplish organizational goals. Using motivation theory toward this end, the leader must first assess the highest motive strength of the employee and then designate a goal having a reward that directly meets the need of the worker. The leader uses intrinsic and extrinsic factors in the goal. The route to obtaining the goal and thereby satisfying the need is through a journey that accomplishes the organizational goal.

The process just described is theoretically how people are externally motivated. Since a manager can only attempt to motivate someone externally, it follows that the external motivational process may not work; it may fail to lead a person to act or behave. It is the manager's responsibility to try again by delineating another strategy to motivate the employee externally. It may be necessary to reassess or to rediagnose the needs of the follower. Obviously, if the first assessment was not on target, the chances increase that the external motivational strategy will not work. Also, different things work for different people. In a sense, being a manager or leader is a commitment to struggle—constantly to develop ways of motivating people to get the work done. If a strategy for accomplishing an immediate organizational goal does not work, another strategy must be developed or the goal may be adjusted. Once the immediate goal is attained, another goal should be designated and new strategies must then be built on the needs of workers at that particular point in time.

The motivation process previously described was applied to motivating one person. Since a leader is most often trying to motivate a group to accomplish a task, motivation theory is applied to individual people in the group first. Individual needs are assessed and then the need that is the group mode is used by the leader in planning a strategy for externally motivating the group to accomplish an organizational goal. It is logical to conclude that the strategy may not be best for all people in the group; however, it should be best for the majority of people in the group. A leader may not be all things to everyone. A leader should be on target for the majority (mode) of people in a group and then try to work on a person-to-person basis with those individuals who are not directly satisfied. Application of the theory of motivation is extended in Chapter 4.

SUMMARY

Two categories of leadership style are discussed in this chapter: classical organization theory and nonclassical organization theory. NCOT forms the basis of contemporary leadership models and assumes that people must be motivated to fulfil themselves within the organization. Because people are different, leaders must diagnose what people need and then provide the appropriate leader behaviour style that will enable a goal to be accomplished and enable workers to grow while in their positions. NCOT employs a situational approach to leadership and sees an organization as a system that is composed of human and material resources working as one unit toward goal accomplishment.

Von Bertalanffy's (1968, 1975) general system theory is the framework that explains how systems work. The group dynamics laboratory is the educational mode that enables experiential learning of management and leadership content. The group dynamics laboratory enables future leaders to experience the process of being a manager through an application of theory. A manager's primary responsibility is externally motivating followers to achieve organizational goals. This is accomplished by diagnosing the internal need of a person, specifying an external goal and reward, using intrinsic and extrinsic factors that fulfil the follower's need, and setting a path through which the follower can attain the goal and reward through behaviour that accomplishes the particular goal of the organization at a given point in time.

REFERENCES

Argyris, C. (1971). *Management and organizational development: The path from XA to YB.* New York: McGraw-Hill.

Benne, K. (1969, January). The self, the group or the task: Differences among growth groups. Paper presented at the Ninth Annual Conference on Personality Theory and Counseling Practice, University of Florida, Gainesville.

Berne, E. (1978). *Games people play.* New York: Ballantine.

Blumberg, A. (1977). Laboratory education and sensitivity training. In R. Golembiewski, & A. Blumberg (Eds.). *Sensitivity training and the laboratory approach: Readings about concepts and applications.* Itasca, IL: Peacock.

Bradford, L., Gibb, J., & Benne, K. (Eds.). (1964). *T-Group theory and laboratory methods: An innovation in re-education.* New York: Wiley.

Callahan, C., & Wall, L. (1987). Participative management: A contingency approach. *Journal of Nursing Administration, 17*(9), 9–15.

Carkhuff, R. (1969). *Helping and human relations: A primer for lay and professional helpers* (Vol. 2). Amherst, MA: Human Resource Development Press.

Davis, K., & Newstrom, J. (1985). *Human behavior at work: Organizational behavior* (7th ed.). New York: McGraw-Hill.

Fiedler, F., Chemers, M., & Mahar, L. (1984). *Improving leader effectiveness: The leader match concept.* New York: Wiley.

Finch, F., Jones, H., & Litterer, J. (1976). *Managing for organizational effectiveness: An experiential approach.* New York: McGraw-Hill.

Gibb, J. (1971). The effects of human relations training. In A. Bergin, & S. Garfield (Eds.). *Handbook of psychotherapy and behavior change.* New York: Wiley.

Harrison, R., & Lubin, B. (1965). Personal style, group composition and learning. *Journal of Applied Behavioral Science, 3,* 286–301.

Hersey, P., & Blanchard, K. (1988). *Management of organizational behavior: Utilizing human resources* (5th ed.). Englewood Cliffs, NJ: Prentice-Hall.

Herzberg, F. (1966). *Work and the nature of man.* Cleveland: World Publishing.

Likert, R. (1967). *The human organization.* New York: McGraw-Hill.

McGregor, D. (1966). *Leadership and motivation.* Boston: MIT Press.

McGregor, D. (1985). *The human side of enterprise: 25th anniversary printing.* (Original work published 1960). New York: McGraw-Hill.

Maslow, A. (1970). *Motivation and Personality* (2nd ed.). New York: Harper & Row.

Miles, M. (1965). Changes during and following laboratory training: A clinical experimental study. *Journal of Applied Behavioral Science, 1,* 215–242.

Perls, F. (1969). *Gestalt therapy verbatim.* Lafayette, CA: Real People Press.

Putt, A. (1978). *General system theory applied to nursing.* Boston: Little, Brown.

Schein, E., & Bennis, W. (Eds.). (1965). *Personal and organizational change through group methods: The laboratory approach.* New York: Wiley.

Schutz, W. (1967). *Expanding human awareness.* New York: Grove Press.

Seashore, C. (1970). What is sensitivity training? In R. Golembiewski, & A. Blumberg (Eds.). *Sensitivity training and the laboratory approach: Readings about concepts and applications.* Itasca, IL: Peacock.

Stogdill, R. (1974). *Handbook of leadership.* New York: Free Press.

von Bertalanffy, L. (1968). *General system theory.* New York: Braziller.

von Bertalanffy, L. (1975). *Perspectives on general system theory: Scientific-philosophical studies.* New York: Braziller.

Wright, M. (1983). The humanistic side of management. *Nursing & Health Care, 4,* 178–180.

Yura, H., & Walsh, M. (1987). *The nursing process* (5th ed.). Norwalk, CT: Appleton-Lang.

Part I

Ice-Breaking and Getting Acquainted: Experiential Exercises

EXERCISE 1   Group Formation

Purposes
1. To divide the group into subgroups of six to eight members.

2. To increase group members' awareness of their self-perceptions concerning the roles assumed in group activities.

Facility
Large comfortable room in which participants can mill around.

Materials
Magic markers or crayons, 5" × 7" index cards, scotch tape, paper, and pencils.

Time required
Thirty to 45 minutes.

Group Size
Unlimited.

Design
1. Participants should choose one word from each of the following three pairs of words. The word chosen should describe what they believe their behaviour is when they are working on a group activity.

    A. Leader/follower

    B. Obsessive/carefree

    C. Rigid/flexible

2. Have members use a magic marker or a crayon to write their three chosen words in large print on the index card.

3. Tape the index card to their clothes, back or front.

4. Instruct members to mill around the room, talk with each other, and form into groups of six to eight people. These small groups will stay the same throughout the course and will work as one unit on all small-group exercises. Explain that a group should be composed of all kinds of people—leaders, followers, obsessive, carefree, rigid, and flexible—in order

for the group to be balanced. Balance plays a large part in the effective outcomes of group activities (15 to 30 minutes).

5. When groups have been formed, ask that each group record the names, addresses, and phone numbers of the members. These records should be duplicated and given to every member of the smaller group.

Discussion

The formation of groups early in a class is necessary to encourage a group identity to begin. The groups will further develop throughout the course as they do the experiential exercises that require small groups. If possible, do not add any members to the groups once they have been formed.

Variation

The word pairs can be expanded to include other areas that might be important. Examples are: smoker/nonsmoker; likes to write/hates to write; enjoys presenting to a large group/hates presenting to a large group; and needs to talk/needs to listen. The longer the list of word pairs, the longer time is required to decide on group membership. Having more than seven word pairs should be avoided because arriving at a balance in the group is too complicated and time-consuming.

EXERCISE 2   Member Introductions

Purposes
1. To introduce members of the small group to each other.

2. To begin formation of the team.

3. To establish an atmosphere that is conducive to experiential learning.

Facility
Large room with tables so that the members of the small group can sit facing one another.

Materials
None.

Time Required
Thirty minutes.

Group Size
Six to eight.

Design
1. Have small group members form into pairs or triads (if there is an odd number in the group).

2. Request that each pair (triad) share information about themselves—thoughts, experiences, backgrounds, goals, hobbies, likes, dislikes, and so forth (15 minutes). Discussion should avoid labels such as age, class level, and marital status. Labels do not tell others about the true self—what is inside.

3. Form into a group of the whole, which is composed of the six to eight members.

4. Ask each member of the pair (triad) to introduce the other(s) to the rest of the group.

Discussion
This exercise should be done after the small groups have been formed in Exercise 1. It does not matter if members of the pairs or triads know one another. If they do, instruct them to introduce themselves by telling their partner(s) something they know is unknown to the partner(s).

Variations
1. Have members wear name tags on which they have only drawn a picture. Then proceed with

the design and have them relate to the picture in introducing themselves.

2. Use adjectives or animals in the above variation instead of a picture.

EXERCISE 3   Self—My Management Shield*

Purposes

1. To look at the thoughts, feelings, and experiences that develop one's desire to become a manager.

2. To become aware of one's personal values or philosophy of management.

3. To explore one's desires and beliefs about ideal management practice.

4. To probe into the ways one actually practices while in a management position.

5. To identify personal goals in management.

Facility

Large room with tables so that the members of the small group can sit facing one another.

Materials

Construction paper and felt-tipped pens or crayons.

Time Required

One hour.

Group Size

Six to eight.

Design

1. Working individually, have participants draw a large shield on construction paper and divide it into six parts as shown.

2. Have them place their names at the top of the shield. Explain that this is their personal management shield, symbolizing various aspects of themselves as managers.

3. Request that the areas in the shield be numbered from 1 to 6, as shown.

4. Ask that members draw in each designated area a picture or symbol that answers one of the following six questions:

---

*This exercise is based on the PELLEM Pentagram, a model of self developed by Elaine L. La Monica and Eunice M. Parisi. It is an adaptation of an exercise published in: La Monica, E. (1985). *The humanistic nursing process.* Boston: Jones and Bartlett.

NAME

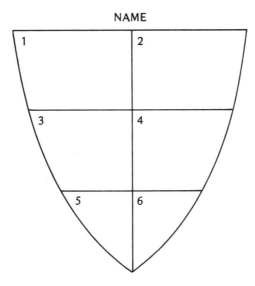

A. What or who has been significant to me in developing a desire to become a manager?

B. What describes the "best" manager I have known?

C. What do I believe the essence of management to be?

D. What signifies my personal practice in management?

E. How do I feel as a manager?

F. In five years, if all were ideal, how would I be as a manager?

5. After completing the shield, ask the small group members to discuss their shields with each other. Suggest that they explore the reasons, thoughts, and feelings that went into each picture or symbol.

6. Discuss the experience.

Discussion   It is necessary for a person to explore globally the various feelings and experiences that form the

(*continued*)

EXERCISE 3   *(continued)*

person today. From this point, the person can begin to conceptualize the ideal versus reality. Goals can then be identified and strategies set up to meet them.

Variation

The questions to be answered and pictured in the shield can be changed according to the needs of the group. The questions stated in the exercise can be made future-oriented if the exercise is used with students who have had no management experience.

EXERCISE 4   Beginnings

Purposes	1. To begin information and group interchange.
	2. To assist with group introductions.
	3. To assist participants to identify personal goals relative to the experience.
Facility	Large room with tables so that the members of the small groups can sit facing one another.
Materials	Worksheet A, pencils or pens, a blackboard, and chalk.
Time Required	Thirty to 45 minutes.
Group Size	Six to eight.
Design	1. Each participant should sit alone and complete the questions on Worksheet A. This should take approximately 15 minutes.
	2. After participants complete the questions on Worksheet A independently, they should share their responses with each other in the small groups. Someone should record the list of major goals that the participants in the small group identified for the course/experience/ workshop.
	3. In the large group, the facilitator should list the major goals from all of the groups on the blackboard and themes should be identified. These themes can be woven into the course content or can be achieved in course assignments or extra activities.
Discussion	Participants should have the opportunity to see that they can achieve their personal objectives by moving through an organized experience. By combining a participant's needs with the course objectives, motivation can be increased.

(continued)

EXERCISE 4 *(continued)*
WORKSHEET A

1. What is your name, where do you attend college/university/work, and what do you do?

2. What is your major goal while attending this course/workshop/ experience?

3. What do you like most about your current educational programme/ position?

4. What is the most difficult aspect of your current programme/ position?

5. What is the easiest aspect of your current programme/position?

6. Describe one of your recent achievements.

7. Write some words you would use to describe yourself.

EXERCISE 5   Role Analysis*

Purposes	1. To clarify role expectations of both role senders and role receivers.
	2. To identify problems derived from the formal organization, job structure, policy and/or procedures.
Facility	Large room—individual meetings with groups or individuals.
Materials	Worksheet B and pen and paper or flipchart.
Time Required	Can be done in a few hours but it is better to allow a week for people to reflect on the questionnaire.
Design	1. An individual regarded as occupying a focal role identifies all other role senders with whom he or she interacts during the course of his or

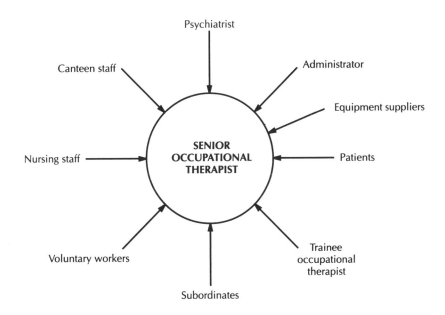

(*continued*)

---

*Exercise 5 written by Dr Philip Morgan using the format set by Dr Elaine La Monica.

EXERCISE 5   *(continued)*

her work (see diagram for senior occupational therapist).

2. Having identified the major role senders, distribute questionnaires to them and have them fill them in.

3. Clarify any discrepancies and share expectations.

Variations   Face-to-face interviews can be conducted with individuals or groups.

WORKSHEET A: Role Analysis—Main Points

1. The end product of role analysis is threefold:

   i. The activity itself may stimulate the learning required to cover some of the original problems.

   ii. It may identify situations where further learning about the situation is required and provide information on what form that learning might take.

   iii. It may identify problems that derive previously from formal organization, job structure, systems, and procedures, and provide information against which decisions in these areas may be taken.

2. Role analysis implies a great deal more than job analysis leading to written job descriptions but may contain this activity or identify a need for it.

3. Role analysis derives from the observation of problems in a role situation that seems to be concerned with relationships at either a procedural or personal level. It is an activity to be carried out selectively.

4. It is carried out for the benefit of the organization in that the organization will benefit if the people in it have a clearer understanding of their roles.

5. It is aimed primarily at helping the individual in the role resolve his or her own conflicts and recommendations, although it may also throw up information that will demand further action by others in the organization.

6. It may sometimes be difficult to identify where role analysis ends and subsequent action begins, e.g. a meeting between the main parties concerned with the role may be part of role analysis or it may be part of the factor being identified.

7. The best person to be role analysed is the job holder. He or she may need help from a specialist. It may also be initiated and encouraged by the manager.

(*continued*)

WORKSHEET A   *(continued)*

8. Role analysis usefulness is not confined to roles at the top of the organization but may be appropriate for any level with up, down and sideways relationships.

9. It is particularly useful for people moving into a newly created or changed role.

WORKSHEET B: Role Analysis Questionnaire

1. What do you think is the main purpose of my job?

2. A. In your view, what do you think are the main activities of my job? Please number in order of priority.

   B. Which of these do I fulfil?

   C. Which of these affect you directly?

3. How could I do my job differently in a way that would help you?

4. How do you see my role/job developing in the future?

5. Will this cause you any difficulties?

(continued)

EXERCISE 5
WORKSHEET B   *(continued)*

6. What do you think are the problems/obstacles which prevent me from developing/improving my job?

7. Which areas identified in question 6 do you share?

8. Do you have any difficulty in your relationship with me?

9. Is there anything I do that causes you difficulty (what do I do that annoys you)?

10. A. Should my relationship with you be:
    (please circle appropriate rating)

    Informal   Formal
       1   2   3   4   5

    Comment

    B. How do you see it at the present time?

    Informal   Formal
       1   2   3   4   5

    Comment

11. How would you describe my behaviour/attitudes to the following:

   A. Work

   B. Colleagues

   C. Clients (*patients*)

Thank you for your help. Would you, if required, be willing to discuss these points further?

YES ☐   NO ☐

Part II

MANAGER RESPONSIBILITIES

Part II contains a discussion of a manager's responsibilities in motivating followers to accomplish goals. Motivating followers is the most important aspect of management and leadership. As has already been discussed, properly motivated employees, in comparison with unmotivated employees, accomplish tasks more quickly, thereby costing the organization less money. Also, quality of outcomes increases and employees have a greater chance for being satisfied. Employee satisfaction is a built-in positive reinforcer for accomplishing again.

Chapter 1 emphasized that effective management and leadership begins with the identification of a problem/goal. The system must then be filled in with material and human resources that are important in carrying out the goal or solving the problem. People and things that are essential and/or helpful in order to get the task done should be included in a system. Every system, therefore, is unique given the particular problem. System boundaries should be methodically identified so that important parts are not omitted, and nonessential parts are not included. One wishes to create a group that contains as much energy as possible working toward goal accomplishment. Nonessential parts of a system tend to detract from the group because energy can shift elsewhere. Remember that a group working together is affected by all parts of the group so you want to build a system that has as much positive energy as is possible.

It is helpful to consider the followers' human and material resources when identifying a system for a particular problem:

1. *Superiors*—those above the leader in the organizational chart. If a problem is not delegated to the manager to solve in any way deemed appropriate, superiors maintain varying amounts of control in how a problem is solved. Therefore, they may have to be included in the planning process.

2. *Associates*—those on the same level as the manager in the organizational chart. If associates have roles in the problem, they must be part of the system. If associates do not have roles in the problem but have had positive experiences in solving a similar problem, they should be included in the system if they are willing to participate.

3. *Followers*—those below the manager in the organizational chart. Followers usually comprise the largest part of the system.

4. *Situational Variables*—time demands, budget allocations, and the nature of the task.

5. *Material Resources*—technical equipment and other things that are available for use in solving a problem.

After the problem and the system for solving the problem have been designated, members of the system must be effectively motivated and educated to solve the problem and accomplish the goal. The manager behaves with the goal of influencing and motivating others. Leader behaviour thereby responds to the needs of the environment and can be expressed in the following equation:

The manager behaviour that results from following this equation becomes the pivot on which alternative solutions and the ultimate recommended action for solving a problem through the system are based. The appropriate manager behaviour can be thought of as an umbrella, guiding leaders in the strategy for goal accomplishment with ways that have the highest probability for success, given a unique problem and a unique system.

This equation forms the focus of Part II. Chapter 3 provides a discussion of how to diagnose self. Diagnosing the system is explained in Chapter 4. Given the system diagnosis, an appropriate leader behaviour is identified in Chapter 5. Chapter 6 discusses how to diagnose the task, Chapter 7 applies the theories and processes by presenting and discussing a case study, and Chapter 8 contains a discussion of a foundation for management—ethics. Experiential exercises conclude Part II.

Diagnosing Self

Chapter 3 focuses on diagnosing self since the manager is an important part of the environment, and diagnosing self is the first step of the equation for diagnosing the organizational environment. This diagnosis involves identifying the manager's view of the problem/goal and of the unique environment, a viewpoint that will be influenced by the manager's values and perceptions. The manager must also diagnose the behaviour style that is part of his or her leader personality—how the manager behaves involuntarily without cognitively thinking about actions. A discussion of the conceptual framework for diagnosing self begins this chapter.

CONCEPTUAL FRAMEWORK

The PELLEM Pentagram (named for its originators, Elaine L. La Monica and Eunice M. Parisi) is a model of self, comprised of five interrelated yet separate parts (La Monica, 1985):

- Thoughts, feelings
- Philosophy, values
- Desires
- Behaviours
- Experiences

Figure 3.1 depicts the five-pointed star. While each point of the star represents one aspect of self, the aspects merge in the centre to form the total self. The body is represented by a circular line running through each point. It is symbolized in this way because the body affects how and what one experiences, feels, and thinks, as well as how one behaves.

The points of the model represent what theorists believe to be operating within a person's total experience. The body is the vehicle for self-expression—it is one's language—and therefore crosses all facets of the pentagram. Self, portrayed in the centre of the model, is the blending of all.

The influence of psychic powers and mystical phenomena that may have a part in total experience is absent from the model. These energies are neither denied nor claimed as fact even though their influence is undetermined and looked upon by pure scientists as based on superstition or at least unknown.

The PELLEM Pentagram provides a way to study self holistically. The interplay of all parts produces the unique individual. It is all of the components acting in unison that determine experience at any given moment. Denying the significance of any one part denies an important aspect of being. This model provides one simple though comprehensive way to view the complexities of a person. It stems from personal and professional struggles to know and understand self, to direct self.

The areas of the PELLEM Pentagram should be explored in analysing why problems and goals are considered important, why people are perceived in certain positions, and why self and others behave in certain

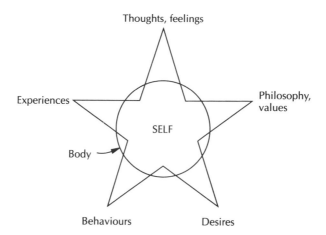

FIGURE 3.1 PELLEM Pentagram.

Source: Based on the PELLEM Pentagram, a model of self developed by Elaine L. La Monica and Eunice M. Parisi. La Monica, E. (1985). *The Nursing Humanistic Process.* Boston: Jones and Bartlett.

ways. Self-exploration will provide the manager with insight, thereby raising self-awareness so that the environment being studied is looked at as objectively as is possible. Finch, Jones, and Litterer (1976) asserted that "accurate self-perception increases the likelihood of accurate interpersonal perception, and realistic perceptions of others are key elements in our ability to communicate, engage in joint problem-solving, and otherwise work with others" (p. 167).

POINT OF VIEW

Identifying the leader's point of view means starting honestly with one's perceptions of the problem/goal, feelings about followers in the system, past experiences relating to the problem/goal, personal desires, and so forth. Frieze and Bar-Tal (1979) and Kelley (1967) studied attribution theory, which is concerned with understanding perceptions of the causes of an event. They explain that people first form an idea about something or somebody and then collect data to support that idea. Krech, Crutchfield, and Ballachey (1962) posited that the first step in responding to another is to form an impression. This impression influences the interpersonal behaviour in the event; it steers reactions.

Based on the previously cited theories, therefore, leaders' and managers' points of view affect the outcomes of a problem-solving process. Hersey and Blanchard (1988), Livingston (1969), and Likert (1961) discussed this concept in terms of an effective cycle and an ineffective cycle. In an effective cycle, people respond to a manager's high expectations with high performance. In an ineffective cycle, a manager's low expectations of employees generally result in low performance. Even though it is human nature to form impressions, a manager can reduce the impact his or her own perceptions may have on others by being conscious of them and then controlling them. A manager cannot control impressions if not aware of them. Cognitively thinking about personal perceptions increases the probability that the manager will not behave solely on the basis of those perceptions—at the very least not to the same degree that one would behave given no consciousness of the perceptions.

It is also important to note that even though high expectations generally result in high performance, set goals should be within the reach (with some stretching) of the people who are to be involved in accomplishing the goal. Setting expectations or goals that are unattainable results in high follower anxiety that becomes counterproductive and results in decreased motivation and maybe even "giving up" (Livingston, 1969). Managers should always examine goals carefully and then set reasonable expectations that can incrementally move a group to a much better level of performance over a period of time. Major change can then be charted and visualized by looking backward and adding all of

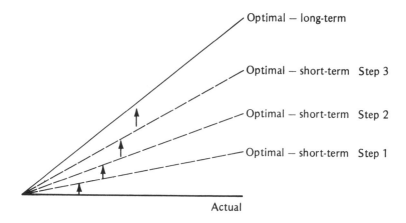

FIGURE 3.2 Progressive setting of attainable goals.

the smaller accomplishments that were made. Figure 3.2 portrays this principle.

Finch, Jones, and Litterer (1976) and Krech, Crutchfield, and Ballachey (1962) have documented three persistent human tendencies that influence a manager's point of view: stereotyping, the halo-horn effect, and implicit personality theory.

Stereotyping

Stereotyping occurs when an individual attributes characteristics to someone that are assumed, given the individual's past experience, to typify a particular group (Finch, Jones, & Litterer, 1976). Racial, ethnic, and sexual stereotyping are most common, but stereotyping is seen in other areas as well. There are stereotypes about clinical instructors, doctors, nurses, and hospital administrators who have been in the same position for 40 years, and so forth. These stereotypes can blind a manager to the unique characteristics of an individual filling any of these roles. Further, stereotypes can cause the manager to respond inappropriately to another person based on past values and assumptions about people in those roles. It does not matter whether the stereotypes are negative or positive; behaviour based on a stereotype has a high chance of being inappropriate.

Halo-Horn Effect

The halo-horn effect is another human tendency that must be checked. The halo effect refers to a favourable impression of one characteristic in an individual that the manager sees as important. This favourable impression becomes generalized to all of that individual's traits or characteristics. The horn effect is the same principle applied to an unfavourable impression of a characteristic the manager deems important. For example, if an employee is efficient in organizing responsibilities, and the evaluating manager loves organized people, then the manager assumes the employee must be good in carrying out all of those responsibilities. Conversely, if an employee cannot organize work properly, the chances of being perceived as effective overall are slim. Such thinking is not discriminating; rather, it is biased and generally results in ineffective management.

Implicit Personality Theory

Implicit personality theory refers to grouping personality traits together (Finch, Jones, & Litterer, 1976). If a person is observed to be inflexible, is that person also demanding, cold, and hostile? Maybe and maybe not. Managers should always try to separate traits from one another in order to diagnose each unique individual objectively. Otherwise, misperceptions, misunderstandings, and inaccurate communication may result.

Informal group discussions with associates and superiors are effective means for uncovering biases such as those presented. Exploring why a problem is considered personally important and why one reacts negatively and/or positively to certain people and traits is an excellent consciousness-raising activity that reaps rewards in management and leadership. A trusting relationship among those discussing is essential for positive outcomes to this process.

LEADER BEHAVIOUR STYLE

A manager behaves first as a human being with unique personality characteristics and second in the role of manager. Some managers enjoy working with people who are unskilled, training the unskilled worker every step of the way. Other managers most enjoy working with skilled people who are socially inclined—those who work together and also socialize together. Still other managers are inclined to lead people who need little on-site direction and reinforcement. All such inclinations are normal and expected given the humanness of an individual.

If a manager's system for solving a problem requires the behaviour style that is the leader's forte, leading that system toward accomplishing a goal will be natural and will require only moderate cognitive thinking about leader actions. A perfect match is not often the case, however, especially in every problem situation. Since the system is always changing and the manager's goal is to facilitate growth so that followers are both willing and able to carry out their responsibilities, using only one leader behaviour style is rarely enough. A manager must be able to function appropriately using different leader behaviour styles.

Since all the styles of leadership are seldom the forte of the leader, the manager must know one's inclinations (that which comes involuntarily) and then cognitively think about how to behave in order to meet the requirements of followers for other leader behaviour styles. This requires diagnosing one's personal leader behaviour style. The experiential exercises at the end of Part II contain an instrument that is valid for this purpose—the Leader Behaviour (Self) Questionnaire, developed by staff members of the Ohio State Leadership Studies, Center for Business and Economic Research (see Exercise 1: Worksheet A).

SUMMARY

Identifying the manager's view of a problem/goal, as well as the unique environment, are aspects of diagnosing self. The PELLEM Pentagram (La Monica, 1985), a model of self, is the conceptual basis for the process of diagnosing self. A manager must be aware of personal beliefs such as stereotypes, halo-horn effects, and implicit personality groupings. Only with such insight can the manager reduce the impact of self-perceptions on others. This is necessary in management so that leader behaviour responds to the unique characteristics of people and things in a system rather than to the effects of past experience, which may not be present reality. A manager must also be aware of personal inclinations toward a specific leader behaviour style. Because followers require all styles of leadership at different points in time, the manager must know his or her own inclination and then plan to meet the followers' needs for other leader behaviour styles.

REFERENCES

Finch, F., Jones, H., & Litterer, J. (1976). *Managing for organizational effectiveness: An experiential approach.* New York: McGraw-Hill.

Frieze, I., & Bar-Tal, D. (1979). Attribution theory: Past and present. In I. Freize, D. Bar-Tal, & J. Carroll, (Eds.). *New approaches to social problems: Applications of attribution theory.* San Francisco: Jossey-Bass.

Hersey, P., & Blanchard, K. (1988). *Management of organizational behavior: Utilizing human resources* (5th ed.). Englewood Cliffs, NJ: Prentice-Hall.

Kelley, M. (1967). Attribution theory in social psychology. In D. Levine (Ed.). *Nebraska Symposium on Motivation* (Vol. 15). Lincoln: University of Nebraska Press.

Krech, D., Crutchfield, R., & Ballachey, E. (1962) *The individual in society.* New York: McGraw-Hill.

La Monica, E. (1985). *The humanistic nursing process.* Boston: Jones and Bartlett.
Likert, R. (1961). *New patterns of management.* New York: McGraw-Hill.
Livingston, J. (1969). Pygmalion in management. *Harvard Business Review, 47,* 81–89.

Diagnosing the System

The introduction to Part II contained a discussion of the human and material resources that must be considered when designating the system that will carry out a goal or solve a problem. Once a system is identified, it must be diagnosed. This system diagnosis is part of the equation that was introduced in Part II:

Five theories that can be used to diagnose a system are presented, discussed, and applied in this chapter. These theories are: Maslow's (1970) hierarchy of needs, Hersey and Blanchard's (1988) levels of readiness, McGregor's (1966, 1960/1985) Theory X and Theory Y, Argyris's (1971) maturity–immaturity continuum, and Herzberg's (1966) motivation–

hygiene theory.* Maslow's theory can best be used to diagnose the motivational needs of the system, as previously introduced in Chapter 2, while the balance of theories are best used to diagnose the educational needs of the system. Building a strategy for goal accomplishment, therefore, involves a focus on (a) what the system needs in order to be motivated and willing to achieve and (b) what the system needs in order to be educated and able to achieve, thereby accomplishing the stated goal within an acceptable range of that identified as optimal. The strategy is implemented by the manager using the most appropriate leader behaviour indicated, given the maturity level of the majority of people in the unique system.

The general purpose of diagnosing a system is to determine the maturity level of the system regarding the system's ability to carry out the goal or to solve the problem; this is commonly referred to as diagnosing the maturity of the system. Maturity has nothing to do with chronologic years. Rather, its only concern is discriminating the system's ability to solve a problem or accomplish a goal. Leader behaviour rests predominantly on this diagnosis. The system's diagnosis, therefore, is the most important assessment that managers make. Accurate assessment results in appropriate leader behaviour, which increases the probability for success in solving the problem. Unfortunately, the converse—that inaccurate assessment results in inappropriate leader behaviour and a decreased probability for success— is also true. The case called Urban City Hospital at the end of Part II is designed to enable learners to sharpen their diagnostic skills.

The theories provide various clues to managers concerning different behaviours and/or concepts that may be studied in the system. Each theory offers a different perspective, and the assessor should choose a theory or a combination of theories that best fits the system and seems most appropriate in a particular situation. The leader first assesses the individual parts of a system and then combines data on the system to determine the level of maturity of the system as a whole. Because leader behaviour must respond to the majority in the group, the group mode (majority) of maturity is then used to determine the appropriate leader behaviour style for solving a specific problem. If only one individual is in the system, then the manager can base leader behaviour specifically on the individual's level of maturity. It is also essential to point out that leader behaviour varies according to the needs of the system in solving a particular problem. Even though the leader may be the same person for two

---

*The integration of theories into maturity levels and their comparisons is an adaptation of that presented by Hersey and Blanchard (1988).

systems and even though the systems may be the same for two problems, the level of maturity of the system may be different as that system is diagnosed for its ability to solve different problems. Diagnosis is always done in response to a unique system's needs regarding a specified goal/ problem.

MASLOW'S HIERARCHY OF NEEDS

The first theory to be discussed in diagnosing a system belongs to Maslow (1970), who developed a hierarchy of human needs that contains five categories. In order of priority, these needs are: physiological, safety, social, esteem, and self-actualization. All of these needs are vital parts of a person's system but physiological needs are top priority when unsatisfied. When physiological needs are satisfied or are in balance, then safety needs become top priority. This ladder effect follows to self-actualization, which is top priority only when all other needs are satisfied. All needs are present within an individual, but the priority shifts according to the time, the place, and the activity of an individual. Maslow's (1970) hierarchy of needs is diagrammed and discussed in Chapter 2. A manager can use Maslow's theory to diagnose the system's level of maturity, specifically its motivational needs, for accomplishing a particular problem. How the theory is applied for this purpose is discussed in the next section of this chapter; how this assessment leads to the decision of the appropriate leader behaviour style that should be used to get the problem solved is the focus of Chapter 5. Remember, in order to diagnose a system, diagnose the individual parts of the system first and then decide the group's (system's) modal level of maturity.

Physiological Needs

Physiological needs are those that sustain life. They are biological and personal in nature and include air, water, food, clothing, and shelter. Assurance of income in order to meet physiological needs is an essential aspect in this area. Since most people can always use more money, assurance of income only becomes a need priority when basic needs are threatened or when a lower standard of living would occur due to decreased income.

Adults are usually able to satisfy their own physiological needs when these are a priority. A wise manager, however, tries to make easy fulfillment of these needs possible. For example, if a leader plans a 9 A.M. meeting and the system contains coffee drinkers, provide coffee for the group at the beginning of the meeting. Do not expect that people will be so dedicated to hearing about the agenda that they will forget about their physiological needs or that the people will bring their own coffee—these chances are risky. Rather, most people during the meeting will start thinking about how nice it would be to have a cup of coffee. This means that participants will not be thinking about business.

Another example is that nurses are often accused of spending much of their time in the staffroom eating and/or smoking. If a leader knows that such behaviour is prevalent in a group, to say that these nurses are remiss or not dedicated is foolish; it will only make the nurses resentful of authority and increase the need, which will in turn decrease the amount and the quality of time spent with clients. Rather, keep the coffee pot going, set up a system so that coffee is easily available, and tell the members of the system that even though they are on the unit to give nursing care, it is recognized that they need frequent breaks—give people what they need. At the same time, tell followers that management's hopes are that frequent breaks will increase the quality of nursing care provided because the nurses will be more satisfied. By giving system members what they need, thereby satisfying their need, a manager moves them to the next need level. Ideally, the manager wishes to move the system to esteem and self-actualization levels because motivation to solve a problem is highest at these levels. Physiological needs are also the easiest to satisfy.

Safety Needs

Hersey and Blanchard (1988) defined safety needs as involved with self-preservation. Protection from physical injury in the environment is a safety need. Douglass (1988) further included stability and predictability in life, freedom from constant stressful situations, familiar surroundings, and provision for job security.

A leader can conclude that a member of a system is at a safety level of maturity when the physical environment is potentially harmful, when the member's position or status quo is threatened, when someone is new in a position, or when the problem involves a noticeable change from normal service. Suppose that new cardiac monitors were installed in the Intensive Care Unit (ICU). The goal is to orient the ICU staff to these new monitors. Even though the ICU staff members were mature in ICU nursing care, they would be at a safety level regarding the new monitors until they become proficient in running the new equipment.

A new nurse beginning a first position is at a safety level of maturity; so is a 20-year veteran taking a position in a new unit. Given the goal of orienting new staff, the new nurse is most probably in a stressful state, not knowing the environment, the expectations others will have for the role, and whether the ability to fulfill the role is present. The 20-year nurse veteran will most likely be concerned with the new environment and the expectations of others. Because the veteran has a library of experience, however, this person may move out of the safety level of maturity more quickly than will the new nurse. Nevertheless, at the outset, both can be diagnosed as at a safety level of maturity.

Social Needs

Hersey and Blanchard (1988) cogently expressed social needs as meaningful interpersonal relationships. Social needs involve a concern for others in the environment with focus of attention moving from self to others. Since the client should be the primary focus in health care agencies, health care personnel ideally should be at the social need level at the minimum whenever they are interacting with clients. If not, personnel will be more concerned with self—this is not the intent of any helping relationship. Even though the ideal just stated is not always possible, the manager should work toward this goal.

Examples of people who are functioning at a social level are those who enjoy working together in groups or in teams, sharing warm relationships, viewing the work environment as a social situation (Douglass, 1988), encouraging people to feel a part of the work group, and generally expressing concern for others in the environment. People who come to work primarily because they need the stimulation from and affiliation with others are at a social level of maturity. Social needs are a priority only when safety and physiological needs are in balance or are satisfied.

Esteem Needs

Maslow (1970) identified two types of esteem needs: (1) the desire for achievement, competency, and mastery of one's personal and professional activities and (2) the desire for prestige, status, importance, and recognition.

People who have esteem needs seek fulfilment by overtly and covertly asking to be noticed. They may want to be told that they are super nurses, that they always follow through on their responsibilities, that they are accountable, and so forth.

Overt esteem needs of people are obvious because a person asks for what is wanted—"What is your reaction to my ability?" Covert esteem needs must be diagnosed. For example, if a person comes back after having been asked to do something and shares that it was necessary to shorten lunch in order to get the task done, take this as a covert request for praise. Tell this person how much you appreciate what was done and how good it is to be so accountable and dependable. Maslow (1970) cautioned against being superficial when giving praise and reinforcement because a person motivated at the esteem level wants respect, not phoniness.

Therefore, be clear about your own positive feelings about what was done and then share those feelings.

Self-Actualization Needs

This need structure is of the highest order, becoming prominent when all other needs are satisfied. It involves one's desire to reach fullest potential (Hersey & Blanchard, 1988). Furthermore, this potential is reality-based on awareness of one's own strengths and weaknesses.

Douglass (1988) characterized self-actualized employees as those finding meaning and personal growth in work; they actively seek new responsibilities, and work becomes play. Further, these people reinforce self (intrinsic reinforcement) rather than seeking reinforcement from others (extrinsic reinforcement). Extrinsic reinforcement characterizes people at the esteem level. Self-actualized people will accomplish, tell the manager what is required, and then go on with responsibilities. They are dependent, interdependent, and independent according to their own direction and as the situation demands. A manager at this level strives to help self and others in the environment without being told to do so.

HERSEY AND BLANCHARD'S LEVELS OF READINESS

The second theory that is considered to be appropriate in diagnosing health care environments is Hersey and Blanchard's (1988) levels of readiness, which has two major components: ability and willingness. The first component involves one's ability to solve a problem, including knowledge and experience. The second component refers to one's willingness to carry out a task with self-confidence, commitment, and self-respect (Hersey & Blanchard, 1988).

Using the variables ability, willingness, and confidence, Hersey and Blanchard (1988, p. 176) designated four benchmarks in readiness levels:

Readiness level:	Follower is:
R1—Low maturity	Unwilling and unable or insecure
R2—Moderate maturity	Unable but willing or confident
R3—Moderate maturity	Able but unwilling or insecure
R4—High maturity	Able and willing or confident

Suppose that the middle managers in an acute-care hospital decided to change from team nursing to primary care nursing as the nursing-care delivery model. Further assume that one nursing unit was chosen as the pilot group for this goal. All of the nurses for all shifts on this unit, plus the sister, nurse manager, and assistant director in charge of the unit, became the system. The assistant director was the manager for solving the problem. This director was involved as a middle manager in making the decision to change from team nursing to primary care nursing.

The system would be at the R1 (unwilling and unable) level of readiness if the majority of its members neither knew about the primary nursing concept nor had experience with primary care nursing and if the members verbally and nonverbally expressed no desire for change. If the members were excited about the change, wanting to gain the knowledge even though primary care nursing was new, the system would be diagnosed as R2 (unable but willing or confident). Using the same hypothetical example, the system would be at the R3 level of readiness (able but not willing or confident) if the majority of the system's members had knowledge of primary care nursing and had previously experienced it but did not have a positive experience with the model and felt that team nursing was what they wanted. If the majority of members had knowledge about and experience with primary care nursing, liked it, and were eager to put it to work on their unit, this system would be at the R4 level of readiness (able and willing).

This hypothetical example illustrates how to diagnose a system using all of the levels in Hersey and Blanchard's (1988) theory of readiness. If the problem of the example were real, a manager would choose the unit with the highest readiness level as the target for the pilot project. This unit would provide the best chance for initial success, which is especially important when attempting a major change.

Another factor to remember when applying this theory is that a person is either willing or unwilling and able or not able. There are no gray areas. For example, if a person is willing to try something even though doubting its usefulness, then for the purpose of applying the theory, consider the person to be unwilling. People are able only when able to be left completely on their own—when they have the knowledge, the experience, and they understand the job requirements. People are willing or confident when they are willing to take responsibility, when they are secure in their abilities to perform effectively and when they need to achieve.

McGREGOR'S THEORY X AND THEORY Y

The third theory that can be used to diagnose a system is McGregor's (1966, 1960/1985) Theory X and Theory Y. It was introduced in Chapter 2 in a discussion of classical and nonclassical organization theory. Although McGregor's theory was intended for the purpose used in Chapter 2, it can be used appropriately for diagnosing the system. Table 4.1 lists the assumptions about human nature that underlie McGregor's theory.

TABLE 4.1 Assumptions About Human Nature That Underlie McGregor's (1966, 1960/1985) Theory X and Theory Y

Theory X Immature	Trait	Theory Y Mature
1. People find work distasteful	Work attitude	1. People regard work as natural as play, given favourable conditions.
2. People are not ambitious and prefer direction.	Ambition	2. People are self-directed in achieving organizational goals.
3. People do not solve organizational problems creatively.	Creativity	3. People are creative in solving problems.
4. People are motivated only by physiological and safety factors.	Motivation	4. People are motivated at all levels of Maslow's (1970) hierarchy of needs.
5. People require close control and coercion to achieve goals.	Control	5. People are self-controlled if properly motivated.

Table 4.1 lists five traits and opposite statements for each trait. The statements are explicit descriptions of how the traits can be observed in people. Since most people, however, may not fit totally into an either/or category, the manager should use McGregor's (1966, 1969/1985) theory as a continuum for diagnosing a system. Table 4.2 is one example of how this continuum can be established. The manager can indicate on Table 4.2 an assessment of where a system member is for each particular trait. These individual assessments can then be tallied according to the number of people in each category of the trait. The category with the highest number of people (the modal category) should be used to determine the appropriate leader behaviour style. The reader is cautioned against averaging the assessments because the average (or mean) is affected by extremes and is not a purely representative figure of the majority of people. A manager should base leader behaviour on the modal level of maturity.

ARGYRIS'S IMMATURITY–MATURITY CONTINUUM

The fourth theory that can be used to diagnose a system, developed by Argyris (1971), is called the immaturity–maturity continuum. Argyris depicted seven changes that take place in the personality of healthy people as they develop from immaturity to maturity.

TABLE 4.2 McGregor's (1966, 1960/1985) Theory X and Theory Y: A Continuum for Diagnosing a System

1. *Work Attitude*

Immature   Mature

├─────────────┼─────────────┼─────────────┤
        1   2   3   4
Finds work   Finds work like
distasteful   play

2. *Ambition*

Immature   Mature

├─────────────┼─────────────┼─────────────┤
        1   2   3   4
Has no ambition   Is ambitious and
and prefers   self-directed
direction

3. *Creativity*

Immature   Mature

├─────────────┼─────────────┼─────────────┤
        1   2   3   4
Is not creative   Uses widespread
in solving   creativity in
problems   solving problems

4. *Motivation*

Immature   Mature

├─────────────┼─────────────┼─────────────┤
        1   2   3   4
Is motivated only   Is motivated at all
by physiological   levels of Maslow's
and safety factors   (1970) hierarchy of
                                                                  needs

4. *Control*

Immature   Mature

├─────────────┼─────────────┼─────────────┤
        1   2   3   4
Requires close   Is self-controlled
control

First, people move from a passive state to a state of activity. Second, people are dependent on others and grow to an independent state. Third, immature people possess few behaviours, but when mature they can behave in many ways. Fourth, immature people have erratic and shallow interests while mature people have deep and intense interests. Fifth, people move from a concern only for the here and now (a short time perspective) to a concern for the past, present, and future (a long time perspective). Sixth, people move from a subordinate position to an equal or superordinate position. Seventh, a lack of self-awareness characterizes the immature whereas awareness and control over self characterizes the mature. Table 4.3 lists these changes. Like McGregor's (1966, 1960/1985) Theory X and Theory Y, Argyris's (1971) immaturity–maturity continuum (Table 4.4) can be used to assess individual people in a system.

TABLE 4.3 Argyris's (1971) Immaturity–Maturity Continuum

Immature	Trait	Mature
1. Passive	Work attitude	1. Active
2. Dependent	Dependence	2. Independent
3. Behaves in a few ways	Behaviour	3. Behaves in many ways
4. Erratic, shallow interests	Interests	4. Deep, strong interests
5. Short time perspective	Concern	5. Long time perspective (past and future)
6. Subordinate position	Position	6. Equal or superordinate position
7. Lack of self-awareness	Self-awareness	7. Awareness and self-control

HERZBERG'S MOTIVATION–HYGIENE THEORY

The last theory to be discussed for diagnosing a system is Herzberg's (1966) motivation–hygiene theory, commonly referred to as his two-factor theory. Herzberg identified higher-order needs relating to job content that can raise performance and increase one's total work output—motivators, such as achievement, recognition, challenging work, responsibility, advancement, and growth. Herzberg also delineated lower-order needs that referred to the job environment and context—hygiene factors, such as organizational policies, working conditions, interpersonal relations, money, status, security, and personal life. Herzberg found that employees who were dissatisfied with hygiene factors had lower performance. Claus and Bailey (1977) conceptualized this theory, as shown in Figure 4.1 (Herzberg, Mausner, & Snyderman, 1959).

Herzberg's theory is useful for the manager in identifying insights to the goals and incentives that may satisfy needs according to Maslow's (1970) hierarchy. For this purpose, Davis and Newstrom (1985) compared Maslow's need-priority model with Herzberg's (1966) motivation–hygiene model, as shown in Table 4.5. Herzberg's theory, therefore, can be used to

TABLE 4.4 Argyris's (1971) Immaturity–Maturity Continuum: A Continuum for Diagnosing a System

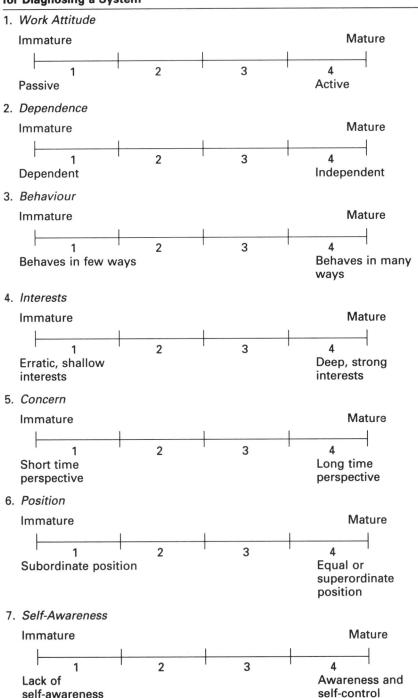

1. *Work Attitude*

   Immature   Mature

   ├────┼────┼────┼────┤
      1   2   3   4

   Passive   Active

2. *Dependence*

   Immature   Mature

   ├────┼────┼────┼────┤
      1   2   3   4

   Dependent   Independent

3. *Behaviour*

   Immature   Mature

   ├────┼────┼────┼────┤
      1   2   3   4

   Behaves in few ways   Behaves in many ways

4. *Interests*

   Immature   Mature

   ├────┼────┼────┼────┤
      1   2   3   4

   Erratic, shallow interests   Deep, strong interests

5. *Concern*

   Immature   Mature

   ├────┼────┼────┼────┤
      1   2   3   4

   Short time perspective   Long time perspective

6. *Position*

   Immature   Mature

   ├────┼────┼────┼────┤
      1   2   3   4

   Subordinate position   Equal or superordinate position

7. *Self-Awareness*

   Immature   Mature

   ├────┼────┼────┼────┤
      1   2   3   4

   Lack of self-awareness   Awareness and self-control

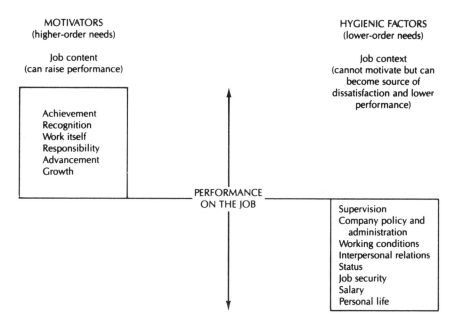

FIGURE 4.1 Herzberg's motivation-hygiene (maintenance) theory.
Source: Herzberg F., Mausner B., & Snyderman B. (1959). *The Motivation to Work* (2nd ed.). New York: Wiley. Reproduced by permission.

amplify the diagnosis made using Maslow's theory and to provide greater insight into the reasons for the diagnosis and strategies for motivating.

Herzberg (1966) is often credited with the concept of job enrichment—the Herzberg Solution. According to Herzberg, the way to enrich a job is to enlarge the responsibility, scope, and the challenge in the position. In this way, the motivators of achievement, recognition, responsibility, and advancement would be amplified, thereby giving employees what they value in the position.

SUMMARY

Diagnosing the maturity level of a system in terms of the system's ability to solve a problem is the most important aspect of the environmental diagnosis. Leader behaviour is based on the system's diagnosis. A manager diagnoses the individuals in a system first and then uses the modal level of maturity to determine leader behaviour. This leader behaviour is then used to begin implementation of the strategy for goal accomplishment.

Five theories for diagnosing a system were presented and discussed in this chapter. The manager may use one or more theories to diagnose a system, depending on what seems to be appropriate in a given context. Table 4.6 provides a concise summary and comparison of the theories presented.

TABLE 4.5 Parallels Between Maslow's Hierarchy of Needs and Herzberg's Motivation–Hygiene (Maintenance) Theory

Maslow's Need-Priority Model		Herzberg's Motivation–Maintenance Model
Self-actualization and fulfillment	*Motivational factors*	Work itself Achievement Possibility of growth Responsibility
Esteem and status		Advancement Recognition
		Status
Belonging and social needs	*Maintenance factors*	Relations with supervisors Peer relations Relations with subordinates Quality of supervision
Safety and security		Company policy and administration Job security Working conditions
Physiological needs		Pay

Source: Davis, K., & Newstrom, J. (1985). *Human Behavior at Work: Organizational Behavior* (7th ed.) New York: McGraw-Hill. p. 77. Reproduced by permission.

TABLE 4.6 Comparison of Five Theories for Diagnosing a System

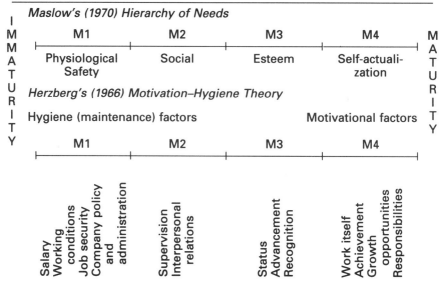

	Maslow's (1970) Hierarchy of Needs				
I M M A T U R I T Y	M1	M2	M3	M4	M A T U R I T Y
	Physiological Safety	Social	Esteem	Self-actuali- zation	
	Herzberg's (1966) Motivation–Hygiene Theory				
	Hygiene (maintenance) factors			Motivational factors	
	M1	M2	M3	M4	

Salary / Working conditions / Job security / Company policy and administration — Supervision / Interpersonal relations — Status / Advancement / Recognition — Work itself / Achievement / Growth opportunities / Responsibilities

TABLE 4.6 (*continued*)

Hersey and Blanchard's (1988) Levels of Readiness

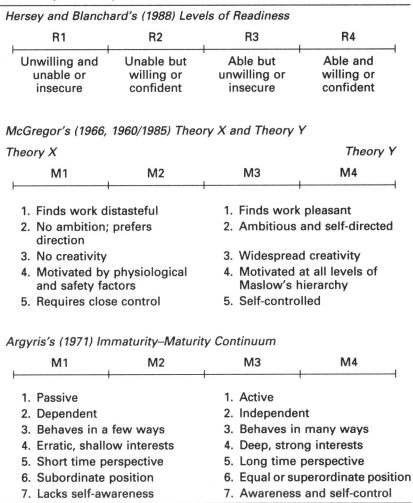

R1	R2	R3	R4
Unwilling and unable or insecure	Unable but willing or confident	Able but unwilling or insecure	Able and willing or confident

McGregor's (1966, 1960/1985) Theory X and Theory Y

Theory X   Theory Y

M1	M2	M3	M4

1. Finds work distasteful
2. No ambition; prefers direction
3. No creativity
4. Motivated by physiological and safety factors
5. Requires close control

1. Finds work pleasant
2. Ambitious and self-directed
3. Widespread creativity
4. Motivated at all levels of Maslow's hierarchy
5. Self-controlled

Argyris's (1971) Immaturity–Maturity Continuum

M1	M2	M3	M4

1. Passive
2. Dependent
3. Behaves in a few ways
4. Erratic, shallow interests
5. Short time perspective
6. Subordinate position
7. Lacks self-awareness

1. Active
2. Independent
3. Behaves in many ways
4. Deep, strong interests
5. Long time perspective
6. Equal or superordinate position
7. Awareness and self-control

REFERENCES

Argyris, C. (1971). *Management and organizational development: The path from XA to YB.* New York: McGraw-Hill.

Claus, K., & Bailey, J. (1977). *Power and influence in health care.* St. Louis: Mosby.

Davis, K., & Newstrom, J. (1985). *Human behavior at work: Organizational behavior* (7th ed.). New York: McGraw-Hill.

Douglass, L. (1988). *The effective nurse: Leader and manager* (3rd ed.). St. Louis: Mosby.

Hersey, P., & Blanchard, K. (1988). *Management of organizational behavior: Utilizing human resources* (5th ed.). Englewood Cliffs, NJ: Prentice-Hall.

Herzberg, F. (1966). *Work and the nature of man*. Cleveland: World Publishing.

Herzberg, F., Mausner, B., & Snyderman, B. (1959). *The motivation to work* (2nd ed.). New York: Wiley.

Maslow, A. (1970). *Motivation and Personality* (2nd ed.). New York: Harper & Row.

McGregor, D. (1966). *Leadership and motivation*. Boston: MIT Press.

McGregor, D. (1985). *The human side of enterprise: 25th anniversary printing*. New York: McGraw-Hill. (Original work published 1960.)

Leader Behaviour

This chapter contains a discussion of leader behaviour theory with an application of theory to the system diagnosis in order to determine the appropriate leader behaviour for a unique system that will achieve a goal.

Leader behaviour will be defined, followed by a discussion of the common leader behaviour styles. Theoretical components of leader behaviour and leadership styles will then be discussed. A leader behaviour model will be applied in determining the appropriate leader behaviour style, given a system's diagnosis. An examination of the components of leader effectiveness concludes this chapter.

DEFINITION OF LEADERSHIP

Stogdill (1974) aptly noted that "there are almost as many different definitions of leadership as there are persons who have attempted to define the concept" (p. 7). He does, however, provide a rough scheme of classification and a thorough review of the literature in this area. Highlights of Stogdill's discussion are presented in the following paragraph.

In early literature (Cooley, 1902; Knickerbocker, 1948), leadership was thought of as a focus of group processes. The idea that leadership was a personality trait also appealed to early theorists (Bingham, 1927/1973; Kilbourne, 1935). Allport (1924) and Bennis (1959) viewed leadership as the art of inducing compliance, and Shartle (1951) and Tannenbaum, Weschler, and Massarik (1961) similarly saw it as the exercise of influence. Fiedler (1967) suggested that leadership was an act or a behaviour, and Koontz and O'Donnell (1986) regarded it as a form of persuasion. Numerous theorists have suggested that leaders are instruments of goal achievement (Cattell, 1951; Urwick, 1953). Other organizational behaviourists have viewed leadership as an interactive effect (Merton, 1969), a differentiated role (Sherif & Sherif, 1956), and the initiation of structure (Homans, 1950).

The definitions of leadership developed by Fleishman (1973) and Hersey and Blanchard (1988) will be combined. For the purpose of this book, leadership is using communication processes to influence the activities of an individual or of a group toward the attainment of a goal or goals in a unique and given situation; leader behaviour is how a manager acts toward members of the system. Fleishman (1973) pointed out that leadership always involves attempts to influence; further, he stated that all interpersonal relationships can involve elements of leadership. This latter remark affirms the statement, which was made in Chapter 1, that all people in the health care system who influence others are leaders.

COMMON LEADER BEHAVIOUR STYLES

There are three common labels for leader behaviour: autocratic, democratic, and laissez-faire. Autocratic leaders are often described as authoritarian, firm leaders who make unilateral decisions, whereas democratic leaders involve the group in decision making, giving responsibilities to followers. Laissez-faire leaders generally maintain loose control over their followers.

An informal survey of leaders' and followers' opinions of the best leader behaviour style usually results in the democratic style obtaining the most votes. But imagine the following scene:

> You are in a car with two of your associates driving home on a country road after work. The car in front of you is sideswiped; you and your associates are the only people at the scene. The driver in the accident has a severely lacerated hand and is semi-conscious. You must do something. The bleeding must be stopped, and an ambulance must be called.
>
> Being a democratic leader, you say to your associates, "Listen, the bleeding must be stopped, and someone has to walk through the woods to a house in order to call an ambulance. It does not matter who does what . . . both of you jointly decide and let me know your decision."

The beauty of the democratic style is that participants have choice, but is choice appropriate in the situation just described? No! An autocratic statement is quickly needed to tell your associates what each must do. It is important to point out that autocratic statements are frequently perceived as hostile, mean, and unfriendly. Remember that any statement can be hostile or warm, depending on the verbal and nonverbal communication patterns that are used by the speaker.

Changing the scene slightly, suppose that you and your associates were emergency room nurses and had worked together for five years. Would it be necessary for anyone to say what should be done? No! In this example, laissez-faire leader behaviour would be appropriate.

Each leader behaviour style can be appropriate, depending on the situation. Determining the appropriate leader behaviour style is often more complex than in the previously cited example. For this reason, theorists have broken leader behaviour into components and then used models to determine scientifically the appropriate behaviour for a specific situation.

COMPONENTS OF LEADER BEHAVIOUR

Management theorists designate two basic components of leader behaviour, even though the theorists name the components differently. One component deals with getting the job done, and the other is concerned with interpersonal behaviour. Hersey and Blanchard (1988) referred to *task behaviour* and *relationship behaviour*. The Ohio State Leadership Studies staff call the components *initiating structure* and *consideration* (Kerr & Schriesheim, 1974). Tannenbaum and Schmidt (1958) labelled the components as *use of authority by the leader* and *area of freedom for subordinates* and Blake and Mouton (1964, 1978, 1984) said it is *concern for production* and *concern for people.*

A leader's behaviour style is never one component or the other. Rather, one's leader behaviour is a composite of both components with

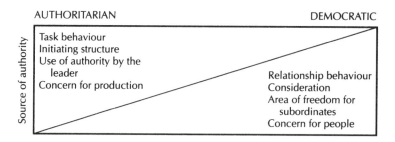

FIGURE 5.1 The balance of leader behaviour components.

Source: Adapted and reprinted by permission of the *Harvard Business Review*. An exhibit from "How to Choose a Leadership Pattern" by Robert Tannenbaum and Warren H. Schmidt (March/April, 1958). Copyright © 1958 by the President and Fellows of Harvard College; all rights reserved.

the weight of each varying, given the whole. Figure 5.1 portrays this balance.

In the figure, leader behaviour is conceptualized as filling the rectangle. As task behaviour decreases, relationship behaviour increases. There is always an element of job-related behaviour and relationship behaviour in any style.

LEADERSHIP MODELS

There are several theories that delineate leadership styles. Authors differ on the style labels, as with the components of leader behaviour, even though the framework and meaning of the models remain the same. Three prominent leader behaviour models will be discussed and compared. The Ohio State model has been used to diagnose leaders' personal behaviour styles in Chapter 3 and will be used predominantly in later sections of this chapter and in Chapter 7.

Ohio State Model of Leader Behaviour

The Ohio State model for leadership styles contains the following two components of leader behaviour:

Initiating structure refers to a leader's attempt to organize and define the roles and activities of group members. It is stating a goal and delineating what is to be done, how it will be done, when it will be done, where it will be done, and who is responsible for specific tasks. Structure involves one-way communication; the leader tells followers what to do in order to accomplish a goal.

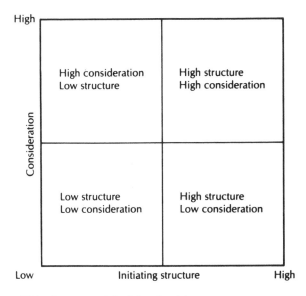

FIGURE 5.2 Oh⌐ State model of leadership.

Source: Paul Hersey and Kenneth H. Blanchard, *Management of Organizational Behavior: Utilizing Human Resources* (5th ed.), © 1988, p. 92. Reprinted by permission of Prentice-Hall, Inc., Englewood Cliffs, NJ.

Consideration involves two-way communication, responding to the group's needs by requesting opinions, beliefs, desires, and so forth. Group activities and discussions are consideration interventions. Further, consideration refers to establishing mutual trust between and among group members, showing respect and warmth. Establishing effective interpersonal relationships is part of consideration.

The Ohio State model can be seen in Figure 5.2 (Stogdill & Coons, 1957). When the two components of leadership are placed on separate axes and the window boxes are filled in, four leader behaviour styles result.

Situational Leadership Theory

Situational leadership theory (Hersey & Blanchard, 1988) grew out of the Ohio State model and can be seen in Figure 5.3. This theory looks exactly like the Ohio State model except that the names of the leader behaviour components are different. Task parallels structure, and relationship parallels consideration.

The four quadrants in the Ohio State model and in situational leadership theory can be explained as follows:

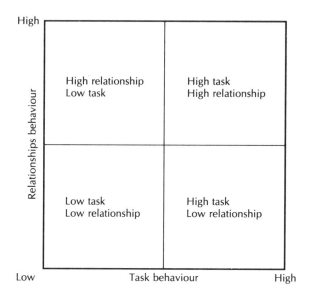

FIGURE 5.3 Situational Leadership Theory.
Source: Paul Hersey and Kenneth H. Blanchard, *Management of Organizational Behavior: Utilizing Human Resources* (5th ed.), © 1988, p. 117. Reprinted by permission of Prentice-Hall, Inc., Englewood Cliffs, NJ.

1. *High structure/task and low consideration/relationship.* A leader primarily defines the task, explains to the group each person's responsibility, and states when tasks should be done. One-way communication characterizes the leader's behaviour even though the low relationship behaviour should be observable. The low relationship behaviour is simply respect and warmth toward another and positive reinforcement after a goal is completed. No group decision making is included in this style.

2. *High structure/task and high consideration/relationship.* A leader balances concern for the intricacies of getting a task accomplished with a concern for the beliefs, desires, and needs of the group. The leader might define a goal, designate what needs to be done and who has specific responsibilities, and invite questions or reactions. The leader's original plan might be altered given the followers' reactions. In this style of leadership, the leader is still in full control but group interaction is begun.

3. *High consideration/relationship and low structure/task.* In this style, the leader's primary concern is not the task and its various intricacies. Rather, concern is for the process, for getting the group to work together effectively to accomplish the task. The leader still has some control over how the group accomplishes the task. In this style, for example, a leader might define the problem and ask the group members to make further decisions about how they will work together to accomplish the task.

4. *Low structure/task and low consideration/relationship.* The leader maintains a low profile in this style, permitting followers to function within previously defined limits. At times, the leader may be available for consultation, to give direction, or for positive reinforcement. Such interaction is not planned on a regular basis but rather occurs as the need arises. This leader behaviour style is delegation because control is shifted from the leader to the follower(s).

Managerial Grid®

Blake and Mouton (1964, 1978, 1984) developed the Managerial Grid (see Figure 5.4) and recently applied it to nursing leadership (Blake, Mouton, & Tapper, 1981). The grid has five styles of leadership based on a combination of concern for production and concern for people. The scale for each component moves from one (low) to nine (high). The five leadership styles are described as follows (Blake & Mouton, 1964):

> *Authority-Obedience (Task)* (9,1). The leader assumes a position of power by arranging work conditions efficiently and in such a way that human elements interfere minimally.
>
> *Team* (9,9).* People are committed to accomplishing a task; group members are interdependent, and everyone holds a "common stake". Relationships of trust, respect, and equality characterize the work climate.
>
> *Country Club* (1,9). The leader pays thoughtful attention to the needs of group members and fosters a comfortable, friendly atmosphere and work tempo.
>
> *Impoverished* (1,1). The leader extends minimal effort in accomplishing the required work.
>
> *Organization Man (Middle-of-the-Road)* (5,5). The leader balances the behaviour that is task-related while maintaining the morale of group members at a satisfactory level.

Comparison of Theories of Leadership

The three models of leadership discussed earlier are conceptually similar. Figure 5.5 merges the Ohio State model, Situational Leadership Theory, the Managerial Grid, and the three common styles of leadership.

---

* Recent research by Blake and Mouton (1981) determined that managers prefer the team (9,9) style.

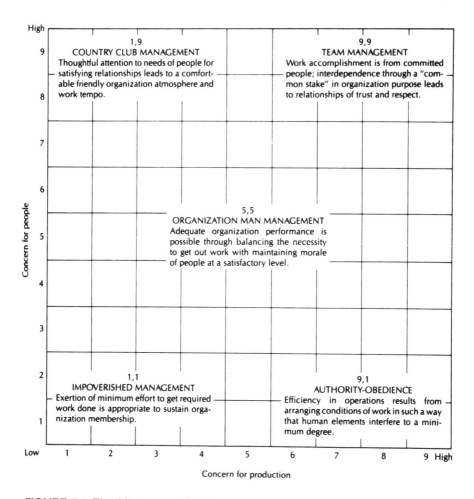

FIGURE 5.4 The Managerial Grid®.

Source: The Managerial Grid figure from *The New Managerial Grid III: The Key to Leadership Excellence*, by Robert R. Blake and Jane Srygley Mouton. Houston: Gulf Publishing Company, copyright © 1985, p. 12. Reproduced by permission.

DETERMINING APPROPRIATE LEADER BEHAVIOUR STYLE*

Leader behaviour responds to the environmental diagnosis of self, the system, and the task plus applied leader behaviour theory. Diagnoses of the task will be discussed in Chapter 6. In this chapter, a bridge will join

---

* This section grew from the work of Hersey and Blanchard (1988).

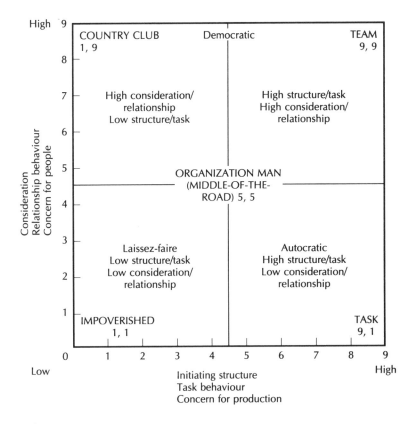

FIGURE 5.5 Theories of leadership: Ohio State model, Situational Leadership Theory, Managerial Grid®, and common leader behaviour styles. Adapted from Hersey & Blanchard, 1988.

the diagnosis of the system and the appropriate leader behaviour style. This bridge becomes the most important element in determining leader behaviour. Self-diagnosis, which was discussed in Chapter 3, is information for the leader concerning what needs to be done and/or thought about so that one can actually behave according to the theory-specified leader behaviour style in a given situation.

The leader behaviour that will be used in this section is the Ohio State model, shown in Figure 5.2. Chapter 4 contained a discussion of five theories that can be used to diagnose a system (see Table 4.6). These theories are combined in Figure 5.6.

The theories used to diagnose the system read in progression from right to left in Figure 5.6. In other words, the lowest level of development is on the right side and the highest level of development is on the left side. Also, leader behaviour numbers (LB1, LB2, LB3, and LB4) are placed in

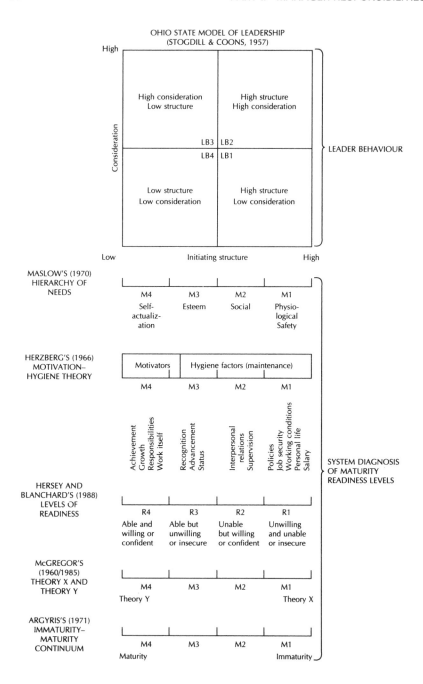

FIGURE 5.6 Theories for diagnosing a system and determining appropriate leader behaviour. Adapted from Hersey & Blanchard, 1988.

the four leader behaviour quadrants, moving counterclockwise from least to most mature.

In order to determine the appropriate leader behaviour style given a system's diagnosis, the bottom part of Figure 5.6 (system diagnosis) must be bridged to the top part of the figure (leader behaviour). Suppose that the task is to change from team nursing to primary care nursing as the model of nursing care delivery on one nursing unit. The leader uses Hersey and Blanchard's (1988) theory for diagnosing the maturity of the people in a system regarding their readiness to accomplish a goal. Suppose the readiness level is designated as R1. The group, therefore, is predominantly unwilling or insecure and unable to carry out the task. The numbers in the theories to diagnose the system and the numbers in the leadership model should be paired. Therefore, R1 level of readiness corresponds directly to LB1. In order to accomplish the task, therefore, the leader's best bet is to begin goal accomplishment by behaving according to LB1, high structure and low consideration. This leader behaviour style is the pivot on which alternate solutions and the ultimate recommended action are based. In the example given, task behaviour from the leader becomes paramount at this point in time. The leader must develop a strategy that gives people knowledge about primary care nursing and lets people know their responsibilities. In other words, the leader must take full responsibility for getting this task accomplished at this point in time.

The diagnosis and designation of a leader behaviour style gives the leader a place to start —a place that, according to research, has the highest probability for success. Once a start has been made, the changing maturity of the system should be reflected in the leader's behaviour, either moving forward one quadrant (growth) or backward one quadrant (regression). Recalling the example, if a leader started in LB1 and found that the group was becoming more receptive to primary care nursing, then the leader should gradually change from LB1 to LB2, high structure and high consideration. In LB2, group interaction is started, but the leader still maintains control of task accomplishment. If a leader is in LB2 and finds that the group is regressing in maturity, that is, becoming less willing to carry responsibility for the task, then a leader would have to move back to LB1. The stepwise move from LB1 to LB4 represents a gradual decrease in leader control concerning how the group accomplishes the goal and a gradual increase in follower control concerning the process of goal accomplishment. The opposite stepwise move, LB4 to LB1, represents increased leader control and decreased follower control.

Determination of the appropriate leader behaviour style is necessary before the leader develops solutions to a problem. Once in the leader behaviour model, move forward one quadrant or backward one quadrant in response to the growth or the regression of the system in relation to accomplishing the task. The speed with which leader behaviour movement occurs is variable, depending solely on the system. The goal of the leader is to move the system to requiring LB4, low structure and consideration. The right side of Figure 5.6 represents immaturity, and the left side represents maturity. When a system is mature, it can monitor itself and accomplish the task. The leader can then delegate to the system and be free to work toward getting another task accomplished. Delegation occurs only in LB4.

One simple example has been used to show how to bridge the system diagnosis with the leader behaviour that should be used as the pivot for solutions to a problem. The steps in the example were:

1. *Determine the system diagnosis* using one or more theories, depending on preference and ease in application.
2. *Pair the maturity/readiness number with the same leader behaviour number* to determine where leader behaviour should begin.
3. *Move one leader behaviour style forward or one leader behaviour style backward* depending on the growth or regression of the system in relation to task accomplishment. The leader's goal is ultimately to have the system require LB4.

Now that the basics for determining the appropriate leader behaviour style have been presented, examples from each theory or combination of theories will be discussed. A case study in Chapter 7 will amplify this discussion, and Urban City Hospital, an experiential exercise at the end of Part II, can be used for practice in applying the presented content.

It is most unlikely that a person or group can be diagnosed as mature using one theory and immature using another theory, given the same task. A leader makes a decision based on an individual's predominant need. If a follower is predominantly motivated to achieve (Maslow's theory), then it is most unlikely that he or she would be able but unwilling (Hersey and Blanchard's theory), primarily concerned with working conditions (Herzberg's theory), or passive and dependent (Argyris's theory). The variety of theories that can be used to diagnose offer different aspects or descriptions of the same process—the development of a person from immaturity to maturity. For this reason they can all be applied toward the same purpose. Each theory should offer information that can be helpful in building a specific strategy for goal accomplishment that *motivates* and *educates* people to accomplish a goal.

Maslow's Hierarchy of Needs

Suppose that a new nurse with the title "nurse manager" joins a community care unit. After six months, the nurse manager wishes to streamline the charting system, eradicating any routine nurses' notes. This need is based on feedback from the staff. The system is composed of the entire staff—ten RNs. After individually diagnosing each nurse on ability to accomplish the task, the modal level of maturity is at the esteem level on Maslow's (1970) hierarchy. Data suggest that the nurses are diligent, independent, motivated to achieve, and like to be noticed for quality and quantity of work done.

Esteem is M3; the corresponding leader behaviour style is high consideration and low structure, LB3. Strategies for accomplishing the task, therefore, should focus on getting the group working together on the problem. The leader, for example, could convene the group, broadly state the issue based on comments received from the group, and facilitate the group's work in further specifying the problem and developing solutions.

Maslow's theory is predominantly used to diagnose motivational needs and is best used in combination with another diagnostic theory in order to diagnose educational needs.

Herzberg's Motivation–Hygiene Theory

An acute-care hospital unit admits approximately three newly diagnosed clients with diabetes per week. No diabetic teaching programme has been formalized. The manager has been on the unit two years; the unit has RNs, SRNs, and orderlies on staff. The goal, therefore, is to develop a diabetic teaching programme. The system involves the RNs.

The manager assesses the system's ability to carry out the task and finds that members are often talking together about the idea, seem enthused about it, and have some knowledge about diabetic teaching; all want to be leaders in the process. Furthermore, they are pushing to plan the programme over dinners and after working hours. The system can be diagnosed as M2, because the focus is on interpersonal relations and supervision. The leader should start behaviour in LB2, high structure and high consideration, and be alert to the ability of the group to control how to accomplish the goal. If the leader believes that the group is able, then a gradual move into LB3 is appropriate, providing reinforcement for the group's work and some structure as needed. The manager could then function simply as a group member, letting the group establish its own informal leader and structure itself. The manager provides predominantly support and reinforcement in this quadrant.

Hersey and Blanchard's Levels of Readiness

Nursing care plans are not being done on clients and an audit from the King's Fund Audit Commission is six months away. Care plans are supposed to be written and updated by the team leaders on all shifts: the team leaders on the evening shift should make a nursing assessment and begin the process. The manager decides to start toward goal accomplishment with the three evening team leaders. The system is diagnosed as able but unwilling—R3. Rationale for this decision is that the team leaders have each worked on the unit a minimum of three years, they all have had formal education that taught the nursing process, and they have previously written excellent care plans.

High consideration and low structure, LB3, is the appropriate style to use for an R3 system diagnosis. Since the team leaders know what they are supposed to do, telling them in a high-structure style will probably only make them more defensive. It is necessary first to find out why they are unwilling to do the nursing care plans and then work from there. This involves two-way communication, which is high consideration. Once a manager knows why the team leaders are unwilling, solutions to these causes must be sought. Once the unwillingness is relieved, then the team leaders should be able and willing.

McGregor's Theory X and Theory Y

Suppose a director of inservice for nursing must set up an orientation programme for six newly registered nurses who have just graduated and will take their finals in eight weeks. They were hired as staff nurses. The director must plan the programme without having met the new nurses.

What would be safe to assume about the maturity level of the graduates using cues from McGregor's Theory X and Theory Y? It would be helpful for the director to think back to how he or she felt in the situation. This is likely to be a high stress state promoting unsafe feelings and a need for direction—definitely on the Theory X side at an M1 level. The director should therefore be high in structure and low in consideration—LB1. A detailed plan of activities should provide knowledge of the environment, practical experience with supervision, and clear expectations of the graduates. The director should be warm and caring but be the guide and leader in satisfying the graduates' needs for structure. At the same time, the director must be acutely alert for signs of growth from the new graduates; when evident a gradual move to LB2 is indicated.

Argyris's Immaturity–Maturity Continuum

The director of nursing services needs three nurses from the intensive care unit to revise the emergency resuscitation plan for the hospital. The nurse manager of the unit posts a notice on the desk asking each shift to nominate a full-time nurse who would be willing to serve.

The nurse manager's behaviour is low structure and low consideration—LB4. This choice was based on the following data about the nurses:

they (a) are all equal in ability, (b) have worked on the unit a minimum of three years, (c) are flexible and effectively meet the demands of a situation, (d) are all able to assume the role of charge nurse, and (e) are insightful. Given these data, the director can assume the nurses are at a mature point on Argyris's continuum—M4.

DISCUSSION OF APPLIED LEADER BEHAVIOUR THEORIES

The initial determination for the appropriate leader behaviour style is the leader's best bet at the start of goal accomplishment (Fiedler, 1987; Hammer & Turk, 1987; Vecchio, 1987; Zenger, 1985). It has the highest probability for motivating people to accomplish the task. How one operates within the style, given that it can be interpreted broadly, depends on the particular needs of the group that were identified during the diagnosis. These particulars are then used in the alternate solutions and recommended action. The umbrella leader behaviour style remains constant unless the system matures or regresses. Then movement is only one quadrant forward or backward—in systematic, gradual stepwise progression or regression.

A leader never jumps from LB1 to LB3, for example. Why? Because the leader behaviour model is designed from learning theory, which says that reinforcing behaviour increases the probability that the behaviour will continue. Because the task is the most important concern for the leader, it is primary in LB1. It is reinforced in LB2 but consideration for the individual employee/group becomes equal in importance. If the task is not getting accomplished, the manager must move back to LB1. Should LB1 be successful, reinforcement of the task behaviour would not occur if one jumped to LB3. Another example would be an employee to whom you have always delegated responsibilities (LB4). Noticing that quality in outcome is slipping, the manager should move to LB3 and use high consideration in order to discover why quality is slipping. Jumping back to any other style would be inappropriate at this time because the leader is aware that the employee knows what to do; high structure therefore would not be the leader's best bet unless LB3 failed to work and minimum quality standards were in jeopardy. Then the leader would need to become firmer and more structured, gradually moving back to LB2 and then to LB1.

The leader is advised that if any serious doubt exists concerning the system's readiness/maturity, then it is better to hold on to control until data are observed suggesting that followers are mature enough to carry effectively the responsibility that comes with control. A manager's move from LB2 to LB3, for example, is usually interpreted as a positive, rewarding change. Should a manager relinquish control too quickly and then have to take it back, such as a quick move from LB3 to LB2, this is often interpreted as punishment or leader dishonesty. Both interpretations are negative forces that may make goal accomplishment difficult because of the defensiveness that they engender in participants.

Another issue that is often raised concerns feelings that leader behaviour must be consistent. Leader behaviour responds to the context and system of resources; leader behaviour, therefore, changes as indicated from diagnoses. Experience has shown that employees respond negatively to changes in a leader's affect and tone but not to caring and respectful changes in how one carries out leader responsibilities. By using a situational approach, a manager essentially is giving employees what they need. Moodiness, however, is not what employees need—so self-diagnose before you act.

A leader behaviour application that is worthy of understanding is Ouchi's (1981a, 1981b) Theory Z. This is a term that represents management behaviour in successful Japanese organizations. Smith, Reinow, and Reid (1984) contrasted typical Theory Z Japanese management practices with those routinely used in the US. Japanese concepts involve permanent employment, few evaluations and promotions, nonspecialized career options, implicit managerial control, collective decision making (quality circles), work group responsibilities, and holistic concern for employees. Management practices in the US seem dissimilar. For example, the emphasis in the US is on specialization, accelerated evaluation and promotion, explicit organization control, individual accountability, and delegation of authority to individuals.

While much has been written applying Theory Z practices in the US, it is not considered to be the answer in all managerial problems, even though some adaptations may be beneficial (Adair & Nygard, 1982; Smith, Reinow, & Reid, 1984; Younger, 1983). Theory Z practices predominantly incorporate democratic approaches to leadership—leader behaviour styles 2 and 3— high relationships/consideration and high task/structure. Use of only these two styles assumes that followers are all at moderate levels of maturity/readiness and that followers should be kept at that level of maturity/readiness. The authors do not believe that those assumptions about followers hold in Western societies; however, they appear appropriate in Eastern cultures. Techniques that are used from Theory Z should therefore be carefully evaluated so that leader behaviour matches the needs of the majority of followers.

LEADER EFFECTIVENESS

A leader's behaviour or influence over an individual or group can be either successful or unsuccessful. If the desired goal is reached (approximately or exactly), then the specific leader behaviour used by the manager can be called successful. Conversely, if the desired goal is not reached within an acceptable range, then the leader behaviour can be called unsuccessful (Hersey & Blanchard, 1988). When leader behaviour fails to influence an individual or a group to achieve a specified goal, then the manager must evaluate what occurred using the steps of the management process and redesign the strategy for goal accomplishment.

When leader behaviour is successful, success can range from very ineffective to very effective depending on how followers feel about the leader's behaviour (Hersey & Blanchard, 1988). For example, if the leader used personal power to influence followers, thereby making goal accomplishment a personally rewarding experience for the followers, then the leader's behaviour is both successful (the goal was accomplished) and very effective (the followers feel terrific about their accomplishments).

On the other hand, followers can be coerced to accomplish by a manager who uses position power, close supervision, and the use of rewards and punishments. Even though the leader's behaviour was successful, the leader's behaviour is also very ineffective if the followers were unhappy and carrying negative feelings toward the leader. Generally, when leader behaviour is successful and effective, the followers are self-motivated to accomplish the goal even when the manager is not present. When leader behaviour is successful and ineffective, followers often relax the drive to accomplish when the manager is absent (Hersey & Blanchard, 1988).

ORGANIZATIONAL EFFECTIVENESS

The effectiveness of a leader's behaviour should be determined on the basis of its relationship to the growth of an organization during a specified period of time (Hersey & Blanchard, 1988). Likert (1967) identified three sets of variables: causal variables, intervening variables, and output variables. Hersey and Blanchard (1988) also looked at short-term and long-term goals. Organizational effectiveness should be a result of evaluating all four sets of variables in order to decrease the halo-horn effect, which was discussed in Chapter 3. Even though subjectivity is an element in any evaluation, looking at separate variables usually decreases the amount of subjectivity that will bias the incident. The following variables are used to evaluate the effectiveness of the organization over time.

Causal Variables

Causal variables have influence on the developments within an organization, including results or accomplishments (Hersey & Blanchard, 1988).

These variables are under management control; they can be changed or altered.

Causal variables refer to the following:

1. Appropriateness of leader behaviour to the system's level of maturity;
2. Accuracy of the system's diagnosis;
3. Appropriate involvement of the system in decision making;
4. Effectiveness of the organization's philosophy and objectives in guiding its constituents; and
5. Use of available technology in a particular organization.

Intervening Variables

Intervening variables refer to the resources (people) within an organization. Likert (1961) asserted that they represent the internal state of the organization. Intervening variables refer to employees' commitment, motivation, morale, and skills in leadership, communication, and conflict resolution (Hersey & Blanchard, 1988).

Output Variables

Output variables represent the achievements of the organization. Output variables are quantifiable and include production (output or services), costs, earnings, turnover, management-union relations, and so forth.

Long-Term Goals and Short-Term Goals

This aspect involves long-term and short-term planning. Long-term goals refer to the future development of the organization. A short-term perspective refers to immediate output (Hersey & Blanchard, 1988). An effective management team in an organization must balance both.

SUMMARY

Leadership has many definitions, all of which converge on several points. Leadership involves using communication processes to influence the activities of an individual or of a group toward the attainment of a goal in a unique situation. Democratic, autocratic, and laissez-faire are common labels for leader behaviour styles. Even though the democratic style is often connoted as a best style, each style is appropriate, depending on the unique situation.

Management theorists have designated two major components of leader behaviour: one refers to getting the task accomplished and the other is concerned with interpersonal behaviour. Theorists have different labels for these components. The Ohio State model of leadership has structure and consideration as its components. Structure refers to a leader's attempt to organize and define the roles and activities of group members. Consideration involves two-way communication—establishing trust, openness, respect, warmth, and effective interpersonal relationships between and among group members.

Several leadership models were presented, discussed, and compared. All of the models are appropriate to apply in nursing systems. The Ohio State model was applied in this chapter. The appropriate leader behaviour style for a given system is determined by diagnosing the system's level of maturity readiness and then pairing the maturity/readiness level with the parallel leader behaviour. This results in a place for the leader to start and represents the pivot upon which solutions for solving the problem are based. A leader then changes from one style to another, depending upon the growth or regression of the system. The ultimate goal of the leader should be to facilitate (1) getting the tasks accomplished and (2) moving the group members to the highest level of maturity and then delegating to them.

Leader behaviour can move on a range from successful or unsuccessful. If successful it can further range from very ineffective to very effective. The effectiveness of an organization over time should be evaluated on the stimuli (causal variables) that act upon an organism (intervening variables) to create responses (output) (Hersey & Blanchard, 1988). Long-term goals and short-term goals must also be considered.

REFERENCES

Adair, M., & Nygard, N. (1982) . Theory Z management: Can it work for nursing? *Nursing & Health Care, 4,* 489–491.

Allport, F. (1924). *Social psychology.* Boston: Houghton Mifflin.

Argyris, C. (1971). *Management and organizational development: The path from XA to YB.* New York: McGraw-Hill.

Bennis, W. (1959). Leadership theory and administrative behavior: The problems of authority. *Administrative Science Quarterly, 4,* 259–301.

Bingham, W. (1927). In H.C. Metcalf. *The psychological foundations of management.* New York: Shaw.

Bingham, W. (1973). In H.C. Metcalf. *The psychological foundations of management.* Easton, PA: Hive. (Original work published 1965)

Blake, R., & Mouton, J. (1964). *The Managerial Grid.* Houston, TX: Gulf Publishing.

Blake, R., & Mouton, J. (1978). *The new Managerial Grid.* Houston, TX: Gulf Publishing.

Blake, R., & Mouton, J. (1981). Management by Grid principles or situationalism: Which? *Group and Organization Studies, 6,* 439–455.

Blake, R., & Mouton, J. (1984). *The Managerial Grid III* (3rd ed.). Houston, TX: Gulf Publishing.

Blake, R., Mouton, J., & Tapper, M. (1981). *Grid approaches for managerial leadership in nursing.* St. Louis: Mosby.

Cattell, R. (1951). New concepts for measuring leadership in terms of group syntality. *Human Relations, 4,* 161–184.

Cooley, C. (1902). *Human nature and social order.* New York: Scribner.

Fiedler, F. (1967). *A theory of leadership effectiveness.* New York: McGraw-Hill.

Fiedler, F. (1987). When to lead, when to stand back. *Psychology Today, 21*(9), 26–27.

Fleishman, E. (1973). Twenty years of consideration and structure. In E. Fleishman, & J. G. Hunt (Eds.). *Current developments in the study of leadership.* Carbondale: Southern Illinois University Press.

Hammer, T., & Turk, J. (1987). Organizational determinants of leader behavior and authority. *Journal of Applied Psychology, 72*(4), 674–682.

Hersey, P., & Blanchard, K. (1988). *Management of organizational behavior: Utilizing human resources* (5th ed.). Englewood Cliffs, NJ: Prentice-Hall.

Herzberg, F. (1966). *Work and the nature of man.* Cleveland: World Publishing.

Homans, G. (1950). *The human group.* New York: Harcourt Brace Jovanovich.

Kerr, S., & Schriesheim, C. (1974). Consideration, initiating structure, and organizational criteria—an update of Korman's 1966 review. *Personnel Psychology, 27,* 555–568.

Kilbourne, C. (1935). The elements of leadership. *Journal of Coast Artillery, 78,* 437–439.

Knickerbocker, I. (1948). Leadership: A conception and some implications. *Journal of Social Issues, 4,* 23–40.

Koontz, H., & O'Donnell, C. (1986). *Essentials of management* (4th ed.). New York: McGraw-Hill.

Likert, R. (1961). *New patterns of management.* New York: McGraw-Hill.

Likert, R. (1967). *The human organization.* New York: McGraw-Hill.

McGregor, D. (1960). *The human side of enterprise.* New York: McGraw-Hill.

McGregor, D. (1985). *The human side of enterprise: 25th anniversary printing.* New York: McGraw-Hill. (Original work published 1960)

Maslow, A. (1970). *Motivation and personality* (2nd ed.). New York: Harper & Row.

Merton, R. (1969). The social nature of leadership. *American Journal of Nursing, 69,* 2614–2618.

Ouchi, W. (1981a). *Theory Z.* Reading, MA: Addison-Wesley.

Ouchi, W. (1981b). Organizational paradigms: A commentary on Japanese management and Theory Z organizations. *Organizational Dynamics, 9,* 36–43.

Shartle, C. (1951). Leader behavior in jobs. *Occupations, 30,* 164–166.

Sherif, M., & Sherif, C. (1956). *An outline of social psychology.* New York: Harper & Row.

Smith, H., Reinow, F., & Reid, R. (1984). Japanese management: Implications for nursing administration. *Journal of Nursing Administration, 14*(9), 33–39.

Stogdill, R. (1974). *Handbook of leadership.* New York: Free Press.

Stogdill, R., & Coons, A. (Eds.). (1957). *Leader behavior: Its description and measurement* (Research Monograph No. 88). Columbus: Bureau of Business Research, Ohio State University.

Tannenbaum, R., & Schmidt, W. (1958). How to choose a leadership pattern. *Harvard Business Review, 37,* 95–102.

Tannenbaum, R., Weschler, I., & Massarik, F. (1961). *Leadership and organization: A behavioral science approach.* New York: McGraw-Hill.

Urwick, L. (1953). *Leadership and morale.* Columbus: College of Commerce and Administration, Ohio State University.

Vecchio, R. (1987). Situational leadership theory: An examination of a prescriptive theory. *Journal of Applied Psychology, 72*(3), 444–451.

Younger, J. (1983). Theory Z management and health care organizations. *Nursing Economics, 1,* 40–45, 69.

Zenger, J. (1985). Leadership: Management's better half. *Training, 22*(12), 44–53.

CHAPTER 6

Diagnosing the Task

THE VROOM AND YETTON MANAGERIAL
  DECISION-MAKING MODEL
APPLICATION OF THE DECISION MODEL
DISCUSSION OF THE MODEL
SUMMARY

Part II of this book is devoted to identifying the appropriate leader behaviour for motivating people in a system to accomplish a goal. This process involves diagnosing the environment—self, system, and task—and applying leader behaviour theory.

Diagnosing self, presented in Chapter 3, is necessary in identifying the leader's personal point of view on the problem/goal and on the environment. Further, diagnosing one's personal leader behaviour style is helpful in order to approximate more closely behavioural intent with others' perceptions of behaviours. Diagnosing self is a consciousness-raising experience with an intent of reducing leader bias.

Chapter 4 contained a discussion of theories that can be used to diagnose a system. Once a diagnosis is made, leader behaviour theory is applied in order to determine the leader behaviour style that has the highest probability for motivating people to accomplish a task. This leader behaviour style is the umbrella or pivot upon which problem solutions are based.

Diagnosing the task is the last segment of leader responsibilities and completes the equation that forms the basis for this part of the book:

Manager behaviour = • diagnosis of organizational environment
                          —self

                                      ╱ motivational needs
                          —system ╱
                                      ╲ educational needs

                          —task

                       • plus applied leader behaviour theory

THE VROOM AND YETTON MANAGERIAL DECISION-MAKING MODEL

The conceptual framework for diagnosing the task is the Vroom and Yetton managerial decision-making model (Vroom, 1973; Vroom & Jago, 1974, 1978, 1988; Vroom & Yetton, 1973). This decision-making model is another theory destroying the myth that managers who use democratic styles are "good" and those who do not are "bad". The decision process used by the manager in a situation should depend on the nature of the unique situation. The model, therefore, provides a means to diagnose situations (tasks) in determining the most appropriate problem-solving technique for the manager to use in getting something accomplished. While diagnosing the nature of the task should be only one of three determinants of leader behaviour, the Vroom and Yetton decision-making model is a powerful one that reports validity for its purpose (Field, 1982; Vroom & Jago, 1978).

A general guide for diagnosing the task can be depicted by the following equation (La Monica & Finch, 1977):

$$\text{Effective decisions} =$$
$$\text{function of (quality + acceptance + time)}$$

Quality refers to whether there are a number of possible solutions to the problem and some alternatives could result in better outcomes than others—a qualitative judgment on the best solution must be made. *Acceptance* is concerned with whether staff members must accept the problem's solution in order for the problem to be eliminated—must the staff do anything? *Time* relates to how much time is available to work on the problem. The Vroom and Yetton managerial decision-making model integrates answers to these three variables and suggests a decision-making style that has the highest probability for effectiveness. These results will be combined with other diagnoses from previous chapters in determining leader behaviour.

Table 6.1 contains five different managerial decision styles. Read each and then study the case in Box 6.1 Select the decision-making style that you would use if you were the manager in the case. Write your response in the space provided after the case.

As you have probably noted, the five managerial decision styles can be considered as a continuum. AI and AII are autocratic styles, CI and CII are consultative styles, and GII is a group decision-making style. Delegation (DI) has been discussed by Vroom and Yetton (1973) and Vroom and Jago (1988) as one in a two-person superior/follower relationship; delegation is at the opposite end of the continuum from AI. These decision

TABLE 6.1 Management Decision Styles

Type	Description
AI	You solve the problem or make the decision yourself, using information available to you at that time.
AII	You obtain the necessary information from your subordinate(s), then decide on the solution to the problem yourself. You may or may not tell your subordinates what the problem is in getting the information from them. The role played by your subordinates in making the decision is clearly one of providing the necessary information to you, rather than generating or evaluating alternative solutions.
CI	You share the problem with relevant subordinates individually, getting their ideas and suggestions without bringing them together as a group. Then you make the decision that may or may not reflect your subordinates' influence.
CII	You share the problem with your subordinates as a group, collectively obtaining their ideas and suggestions. Then you make the decision that may or may not reflect your subordinates' influence.
GII	You share a problem with your subordinates as a group. Together you generate and evaluate alternatives and attempt to reach agreement (consensus) on a solution. Your role is much like that of chairman. You do not try to influence the group to adopt "your" solution, and you are willing to accept and implement any solution that has the support of the entire group.
DI	You delegate the problem to your subordinate(s), providing him [them] with any relevant information that you possess, but giving him [them] responsibility for solving the problem . . . you may or may not request him [the group] to tell you what solution . . . [has been] reached.

Source: AI-GII—Reprinted by permission of the publisher, from "A New Look at Managerial Decision Making", by Victor H. Vroom, *Organizational Dynamics*, Spring, 1973, © 1973. American Management Association, New York. All rights reserved.

DI—Vroom, V., Yetton, P., 1973. *Leadership and Decision Making*, p. 13.

styles can be paralleled with the Ohio State model of leadership, as shown in Figure 6.1. As a manager moves from AI to GII, the amount of time involved in solving the problem increases.

APPLICATION OF THE DECISION MODEL

Now that a decision-making style has been chosen for the case example, the Vroom and Yetton (1973) model should be applied in diagnosing the task. Vroom (1973) developed the decision model using a

BOX 6.1 Case Example

You are an assistant director of nursing in a large city hospital. The management has recently put into effect, at your request and consultation, the unit manager system on two floors. This was expected to relieve the nurses of administrative responsibility, increase their abilities to provide quality care to clients, ensure that health assessments and care plans could be accomplished for every client, and lower the nursing budget. Quality health care and nursing care plans reflected the suggestions made by the hospital accreditors. To the surprise of everyone, yourself included, little of the above has been realized. In fact, nurses are sitting in the conference room more, quality has maintained a status quo, and employees and patients are complaining more than ever.

You do not believe that there is anything wrong with the new system. You have had reports from other hospitals using it and they confirm this opinion. You have also had representatives from institutions using the system talk with your nursing personnel, and the representatives report that your nurses have full knowledge of the system and their altered responsibilities.

You suspect that a few people may be responsible for the situation, but this view is not widely shared among your two supervisors and four head nurses. The failure has been variously attributed to poor training of the unit managers, lack of financial incentives, and poor morale. Clearly, this is an issue about which there is considerable depth of feeling within individuals and potential disagreement among your subordinates.

This morning you received a phone call from the nursing director. She had just talked with the hospital administrator and was calling to express her deep concern. She indicated that the problem was yours to solve in any way you think best, but she would like to know within a week what steps you plan to take.

You share your director's concern and know that the personnel involved are equally concerned. The problem is to decide what steps to take to rectify the situation.

Decision style you would use: _____

Source: La Monica, E., & Finch, F. (1977). Managerial decision-making. *Journal of Nursing Administration 5*, 21. Reproduced by permission. This case was adapted into nursing from a business example. The original material is presented by Vroom, 1973, pp. 72–73.

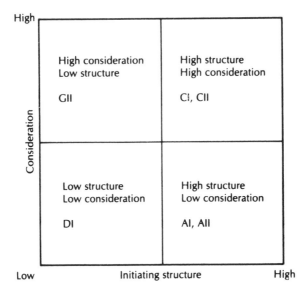

FIGURE 6.1 Vroom and Yetton's decision styles and the Ohio State model of leadership.

tree format; it is commonly referred to as the decision-making tree, shown in Figure 6.2.

Notice that there are seven questions across the top of Figure 6.2 Questions A, B, and C refer to the variable of quality and questions D through G refer to the variable of acceptance. Referring to a case, it is necessary to start at the left of the model, question A, and answer the question in a yes–no format. If the answer to question A is "no", then follow the "no" line to the next node and answer the question on top of the node. Follow this format until the tree ends with a decision-making style. It should be noted that each successive question in the quality and acceptance sets of variables asks more specific information concerning the variable—it is similar to programmed history taking when an answer of "history of familial diabetes", for example, results in more specific questions concerning this matter being asked.

The decision model is conceptually saying the following:

1. If acceptance of decision by followers is crucial, then get the group involved in solving the problem.
2. If quality is important, with expertise being a requirement, then find people who have the expertise and solve the problem.

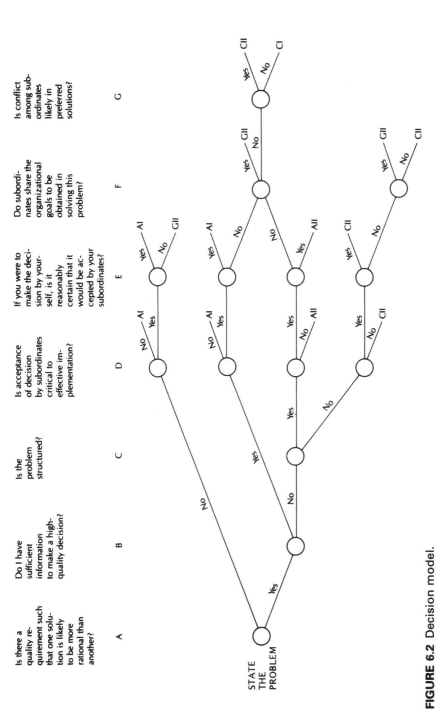

FIGURE 6.2 Decision model.

3. When both quality and acceptance are required, then bring the experts and the group together for problem solving.

The purpose of the tree, however, is to integrate these variables and to suggest a decision-making style that will take the shortest amount of time, considering the requirements of the task. Time increases as one moves down from AI to GII. Hence, if style CII is suggested at the end of the tree, quality and acceptance are important so one could not use styles AI, AII, or CI because the group would not be involved to the degree required in these styles. But one could use GII or DI if the leader thought that the group was mature enough to solve the problem using those styles *and* had the time available. The problem would be solved more quickly in style CII than in style GII. Simply, any decision-making style under the one indicated by the decision model is fine to use; more time would be needed to solve the problem. Decision-making styles above the one indicated by the decision model should not be used.

Let us walk through the case example using the decision model to see if Vroom agrees with your choice for the best style to use given the nature of the task. Start at the left and answer question A.

Question A: Quality—Yes
There is quality requirement in this case. A number of possible solutions to the problem exist, and one could be better than another; there are several ways to solve this problem, and one way could result in more effective outcomes than another.

Follow the "yes" line on the tree to the next node; question B must be answered.

Question B: Manager's information—No
The assistant director obviously has neither the information nor the expertise to make a high-quality decision and solve the problem.

Follow the "no" line to the next node and answer a further question on quality.

Question C: Structure—No
This question requires explanation. A structured problem is one in which the decision is based on quantitative (objective) data, and the location of those data is known. An unstructured problem has a subjective element; the decision is a qualitative assessment—a value judgment—and/or the location of the information is unknown. In the case example, information that is required for solving the problem is qualitative and its specific location is unknown.

Follow the "no" line to the next node and answer question D.

Question D: Acceptance—Yes
Another way of asking question D is: Do followers have to do anything in order for the problem to be solved? In this case, acceptance is

critical. In fact, one reason the system is failing may be that personnel were not involved in the initial planning.

Follow the "yes" line to question E.

Question E: Prior probability of acceptance—No
An autocratic decision in this case probably would not be tolerated.

Follow the "no" line to question F.

Question F: Goal congruence—Yes
Another way of asking this question is: If the problem is solved, will it benefit the people working in the environment? Obviously, the people will benefit in this case if the unit manager system works.

The resulting style that is suggested by the model is GII. Bring the two supervisors together with the four head nurses and proceed in solving the problem as a group.

Does the style you chose match Vroom's choice? If so, your intuition was on target. Now you can up your batting average continuously by using the theory. If no match existed, it would be advisable to follow Vroom's suggestion over your own. Vroom and Jago (1978) reported on an experimental study suggesting that managers who apply the decision model have significantly more effective outcomes—more technical quality and more follower acceptance—than managers who do not use the model.

DISCUSSION OF THE MODEL

The decision model just discussed is used to diagnose the task; this is just one part of the environmental diagnosis. Diagnosis of the system and self-diagnosis must be considered in determining leader behaviour.

Suppose that the system diagnosis in the case example resulted in followers being assessed at the M1 level of maturity, thereby requiring high structure and low consideration leader behaviour. The diagnosis of the task in the case suggested that group decision making is indicated—high consideration and low structure (see Figure 6.1) What should the manager do?

The best course for the leader is to bid for more time by presenting evidence to the superior that the nature of the task demands that the group become involved in solving this problem in order to have the best probability for an effective outcome. Further, the group is not mature enough to handle a group problem-solving activity. More time is needed to help the group mature to the level required for solving the problem. The manager's best bet, therefore, is to try to get the task tabled until the group is mature enough to handle it—get more time.

The manager should try, to the degree possible, to match the decision-making style required by the task with the leader behaviour suggested by the group maturity level—this is ideal. It is also a way to determine the problems/goals that should be the focus of group work at a given point in time. Tasks should be given to groups according to the group's ability to accomplish them effectively. Decision styles (AI through DI) can be used by the manager to help followers progressively mature in group problem solving. Decision styles are a ladder to maturity in this area.

If the superior of the manager says "the task must be done even though the group is not ready to handle it", even though a case against this has been made repeatedly and with strength, then the manager must act. Given that the situation is far from ideal, every effort must be taken to ensure the highest probability for success. The group must be involved even though the experts must maintain control of the group's process because quality and acceptance are both critical. The manager's best bet in this instance is to move into a leader behaviour style that falls between what the system requires and what the task requires—high structure and high consideration—CI or CII.

It must be noted that group decision making in the case example, indicated as best by the decision model, means that the manager presents the problem for the group members to solve. The problem is to determine how to make the unit manager system work effectively, producing the anticipated outcomes. The problem must be presented with clarity. Group members should not be given the opportunity to say that they do not want the system. The system exists, and now it must be made effective. This principle applies in all group decision-making processes.

Foresight in management is always better than hindsight. The manager should always try to prevent the situation just discussed by a complete and accurate diagnosis of essential elements in the environment. However, when prevention has not worked (and prevention does not always work), then the manager must do what is best in the given situation.

Self-diagnosis must also be matched because a manager who is most easily suited to the requirements of the system and task will have the smoothest journey through solving the problem. Should the leader's personal style not match, two alternatives are possible, given that the task must be accomplished by the system: (1) delegate leadership for solving the problem to an assistant whose personal leadership style matches the requirements or (2) provide the leader behaviour style that is required by the system and task by being conscious that one's behaviour must follow the style needed. In the second alternative, the manager must be diligent in thinking about the leader behaviour that must be provided for the system because one's personal inclination may be different from the desired behaviour.

SUMMARY

The task is the third aspect of the environment that must be diagnosed in order to determine leader behaviour. Vroom and Yetton's (1973) managerial decision-making model was discussed for this purpose. The variables of quality, acceptance, and time are considered important in specifying the task's requirements. A decision model (tree) can be used to integrate elements of quality and acceptance for a given situation and to suggest a decision style that requires the least amount of time and has the highest probability for effective outcome. One case was followed and discussed applying the decision model. The experiential exercises in this part of the book contain three additional cases for practice using the model. The manager should try to match the decision-making style required by the task with the leader behaviour suggested by the system's maturity level. The manager can use the model to decide on task priorities for a given group.

The next chapter contains a case application of the management process and problem-solving method.

REFERENCES

Field, R.H.G. (1982). A test of the Vroom–Yetton normative model of leadership. *Journal of Applied Psychology, 67*(5), 523–532.

La Monica, E., & Finch, F. (1977). Managerial decision-making. *Journal of Nursing Administration, 7*, 20-28.

Vroom, V. (1973). A new look at managerial decision-making. *Organizational Dynamics, 1*, 66–80.

Vroom, V., & Jago, A. (1974). Decision-making as a social process. *Decision Sciences, 5*, 743–769.

Vroom, V., & Jago, A. (1978). On the validity of the Vroom–Yetton model. *Journal of Applied Psychology, 63*, 151–162.

Vroom, V., & Jago, A. (1988). *The new leadership: Managing participation in organizations.* Englewood Cliffs, NJ: Prentice-Hall.

Vroom, V., & Yetton, P. (1973). *Leadership and decision-making.* Pittsburgh: University of Pittsburgh Press.

CHAPTER 7

Applying the Management Process and the Problem-Solving Method

This chapter provides an application of the theory that has been presented in Chapters 1 through 6. A case example is studied by following the steps of the problem-solving method, each of which has been discussed in separate chapters. As a review, this problem-solving method involves:

1. Problem identification
2. Problem definition and/or goal statement
3. Problem analysis
4. Alternative solutions
5. Recommended action
6. Implementation and evaluation

The management process—which is comprised of planning, organizing, motivating, and controlling—will then be interrelated in response to the manager's activities in the case example.

Box 7.1 contains a description of the case that forms the basis for this chapter. Assume the role of the leader/manager in this environment, reviewing the data presented in Box 7.1 in order to carry out the problem-solving method.

BOX 7.1 Case Example

You are the head nurse of a 54-bed orthopaedic unit in a 400-bed general hospital located in a northern city. You have held the position for five years and work the day shift. During the ski season, which lasts from December to April, the unit maintains a full capacity and often overflows with clients who are set up in the halls and in the solarium.

Clients are generally healthy, robust people who are forced into dependency by various incapacitating fractures, most frequently the broken tibia and/or fibula. Clients fall into two categories: those who require a short hospital stay (one to two days) and those who need a long stay (two to four weeks) due to the severity of the injuries.

The organization is old and traditional, sporting an excellent reputation for the quality of its services. There is a bureaucratic hierarchy of control in nursing, with power and authority belonging to the position rather than to the incumbent—there is a right way of doing things and a wrong way of doing things. The director of nursing generally makes the decisions regarding policy and passes the information down.

Team nursing is the model of nursing care delivery that is practised. Nurses have made team nursing into a packaged procedure, dividing the labours of the team, using flow charts, setting up informal routines for getting the work done, and compartmentalizing all team responsibilities. Nursing histories and care plans have been made up so that they can be applied to all clients; nurses simply check what applies to the particular client. Giving medications to all clients on the unit is the responsibility of one RN on each shift. Since the task is perceived as boring, it is rotated on a weekly schedule.

The quality of nursing care is considered good at the present time. Each team has 18 clients, and there is usually one RN, one licensed practical nurse or nurse's aide, and one orderly assigned to each team during the day shift. The staff has been fairly stable over the past year.

You meet with the staff every morning and afternoon for report and again for team conference when time permits. If there are problems, the team leaders come to you for assistance and vice versa. Otherwise you generally leave the team leaders alone. You try to make rounds every day but that is not always possible because managerial responsibilities have been increasing since the nursing organization was decentralized.

For the past several weeks, you have noticed increasing tardiness at morning report. Then, staff seemed to be more concerned with the individual functions of their position rather than with the *gestalt*. You believe that nursing care is not as individualized as it could be. Staff members are spending more and more time talking and complaining with each other in the conference room, reporting that their "work is finished". You check on this and they are right—the work they set out to do is done, and the clients seem happy.

Source: Selected aspects of this case were originally prepared by Anita R. Madea, Doctoral Candidate, Teachers College, Columbia University, Department of Nursing Education, 1981.

PROBLEM IDENTIFICATION

A problem is identified by the difference between what is actually happening in a situation (the actual) and what one would like to have occur (the optimal). The manager should first write down the problem areas. These are then narrowed down to one or two areas and defined succinctly, as shown in Table 7.1.

After thinking about these problem areas, it is necessary to focus on a particular problem. Several questions must be answered: (1) Are the problem areas related to one another? (2) Are any of the problem areas an effect of another problem? (3) Which problem is tractable and can be solved directly?

In looking at the three problem areas just delineated, it is possible that as nursing care is systematized, it is becoming repetitive, boring, and monotonous. Staff members may not have the opportunity to develop new skills and capacities, and work is getting done quickly. Innovation and creativity are suppressed as nursing care becomes procedure-bound.

The three problem areas are seen as related. Since nursing care is becoming a set routine, it gets done fast, leaving the staff with excess time. This may contribute to a lack of enthusiasm, accentuated by the paucity of

TABLE 7.1 Problem Identification

Actual	Problem	Optimal
1. Tardiness is increasing	Tardiness	1. No tardiness
2. Nursing care is becoming increasingly routine	Routine nursing care	2. Nursing care is becoming increasingly individualized
3. Nursing time spent with the client is decreasing	Decreased time spent with clients	3. Nursing time spent with the client is increasing

creativity, that is present in nursing care planning. The ward sister must now use the knowledge available and make a decision on the problem.

PROBLEM DEFINITION

The priority problem area of those stated in the previous portion of this chapter is that nursing care was becoming increasingly routine. The goal should be for nursing care to become more individualized. This problem area includes many aspects of nursing care. Since problem statements should be specific, what aspect of nursing care requires the first emphasis? Suppose the ward sister decides that the client should become involved in developing the care plan, using the established core care plans as baseline information and cues to nursing responsibilities in caring for clients with orthopaedic problems. The problem and goal might sound like the following:

> *Actual:* The client has no input into the nursing care plan, which is routine for all clients with orthopaedic problems.
>
> *Optimal:* The client and the team leader develop an individualized nursing care plan using the routine care plan as minimal expectations.
>
> *Problem:* Routine nursing care plans are not individualized; clients do not plan with the team leaders.
>
> *Goal:* To individualize nursing care plans by having the team leader and the client build on the routine care plan.

PROBLEM ANALYSIS

In problem analysis, the environment must be diagnosed in order to choose a leader behaviour style that has the highest probability for success in motivating the system to accomplish the task. It is the pivot upon which all solutions are based. In order to diagnose the environment, the system must first be specified.

In the case example, the ward sister decides to work with the three-day shift team leaders since they are mainly responsible for taking nursing histories and personalizing the routine care plan. The two regular staff nurses who cover the team leaders on days off are also considered part of the system. Nothing will be added to the normal material resources in solving the problem. In essence, the system consists of three team leaders and two staff nurses who act as team leaders when necessary. The environment can be diagnosed as follows.

Diagnosing Self

The manager sits back and considers why this problem has been specified—routine nursing care has always been considered boring and dull. As a client several years ago, the manager had found routine care dehumanizing and ritualistic—in other words noncaring, which is the antithesis of nursing practice.

Thinking more, the manager realizes that the staff has generally been left alone concerning their task responsibilities; support was offered often and the presence of a manager was constant. This style of leadership seemed easy and was most enjoyable and rewarding.

Diagnosing the System

The manager decides to use the following two theories to diagnose the system: (1) Maslow's hierarchy of needs to diagnose motivational needs and (2) Hersey and Blanchard's (1988) levels of readiness to diagnose educational needs. Staff members are diagnosed individually regarding their ability and willingness to fulfil the goal and/or to solve the problem. Remember that Hersey and Blanchard's theory requires a "yes" or "no" response—if not totally "yes", then the answer is "no".

> Team leader 1 is a bright, energetic nurse with four years' experience on this unit who has learned the position's responsibilities quickly but lacks ability to solve problems scientifically. The person has procedures for everything.
> *Diagnosis:*   M2—Social
>   R2—Unable but willing or confident
>
> Team leader 2 is a Bachelor of Nursing (BN) graduate who has been on the unit in this position for seven years. Responsibility for establishing a routine history form rested predominantly with this team leader, who always enjoys starting new things once a cue has been given. Planning nursing care with the client, however, has never been part of nursing practice. This nurse spends the most time sharing information about clients with associates.
> *Diagnosis:*   M2—Social
>   R2—Unable but willing or confident
>
> Team leader 3 is an RN and adores team nursing. The nurse is flexible and goes along with all new ideas, giving much of self to accomplishing new projects especially if she is working with friends. This nurse has had little experience since graduation.
> *Diagnosis:*   M2—Social
>   R2—Unable but willing or confident
>
> Staff nurse 1 has a wide knowledge base but seems bitter. The nurse always carries out and individualizes responsibilities with pride and

makes thoughtful comments in reports about clients, yet often resists group efforts toward change.

Diagnosis: M3—Self-Esteem
              R3—Able but unwilling or insecure

Staff nurse 2 is a new nursing graduate. This nurse's chief complaint on the unit is insufficient time to sit and talk with clients. This nurse is used to having the time to collaborate with the client in developing the care plan, being a graduate of a school of nursing that used Orem's (1985) theory of nursing as a conceptual framework. However, this nurse always seems frustrated and she rarely feels satisfied with the work completed.

Diagnosis: M1—Safety
              R2—Unable but willing or confident

The manager must identify the modal level of maturity/readiness. The majority of people in the system are at R2 and M2—unable but willing or confident and motivated at the social level. The leader behaviour style that is indicated for an M2/R2 level of maturity/readiness is leader behaviour style two (LB2), high structure and high consideration. This style becomes the pivot upon which alternative actions and the recommended action are based. The level of maturity of the system suggests that the leader must give direction to the group concerning the task—what is to be done—and also involve them in problem-solving activities. The leader should meet with the group on a regular basis, suggesting solutions to issues as they arise and offering directions after receiving the group's advice. When talking with the two staff nurses individually, the manager can behave according to the leader behaviour style that is indicated by their individual levels of maturity. But, when communicating with the group, LB2 is indicated as the best beginning leader behaviour style on the journey to goal accomplishment.

Diagnosing the Task

The last diagnosis to be made by the leader is of the nature of the task. Using the Vroom and Yetton managerial decision model (Vroom, 1973; Vroom & Jago, 1974, 1978, 1988; Vroom & Yetton, 1973), the questions shown in Figure 6.2 must be answered, starting with question A.

Question A: Quality—Yes. Clearly, there are a number of possible solutions, and one could be more effective than another.

Follow the "yes" line to the next node and respond to question B.

Question B: Manager's information—No. The manager would certainly have ideas on how this can best be accomplished. Given that there are a variety of client problems and that the system has been directly involved in planning care, the staff would obviously have information and expertise that is not possessed by the leader.

Follow the "no" line and answer question C.

Question C: Structure—No. The manager has to make a subjective decision on how this problem will be solved. The decision will not be based on objective (quantitative) data. Further, the exact location of the data that will be used to solve the problem is unknown.

Follow the "no" line to question D.

Question D: Acceptance—Yes. The team leaders must accept the decision in order for the goal to be accomplished.

Proceed to question E.

Question E: Prior probability of acceptance—No. This is a sticky question in this case. There are neither data to suggest that the manager's decision would be followed nor that the manager's decision would be rejected. The "no" response is based on the team leaders' deep involvement in developing and implementing the current procedure. Moreover, when in doubt on this question, always favour group discussion; this covers the possibility of group rejection, and the only thing lost is a little time.

Follow the "no" line to question F.

Question F: Goal congruence—Yes. The staff will certainly gain from the experience of collaborating with clients and from the feeling of helping another in this personalized way. The resulting style that is suggested by the model is GII. Bring the system together and solve the problem as a group. As shown in Figure 6.1, GII is LB3, high consideration and low structure.

Synthesizing the Diagnosis

As the manager, you diagnose yourself as committed to solving the problem because of personal and managerial reasons. You enjoy LB3, and that seems to be the one in which you function most often with the team leaders.

Upon diagnosing the system, you find that the modal level of maturity readiness is M2/R2 (socially motivated and unable but willing or confident), requiring LB2, high structure and high consideration. This is moving one quadrant back from your preferred style of LB3. The nature of the task requires LB3, group decision making with high consideration and low structure. The group should be involved in how the problem will be solved.

The manager must first follow the leader behaviour style suggested by the system's maturity—LB2. It must be recognized that the problem cannot be totally solved until the system understands the "whys" and "hows" of collaborating with clients in developing nursing care plans.

Once this is accomplished, then the group will be both able and willing; the manager can then go into LB3, which is required by the task. Even though an able and willing group requires LB4, remember that once in the leadership model, you move one quadrant forward for a progressing group or one quadrant backward for a regressing group. This provides reinforcement for learning (change). The manager must also be aware that conscious effort must be made to give the initial high task behaviour to the group—given the preferences of this manager, such a style may be neither involuntary nor most pleasing for the manager even if necessary. In introducing the problem to the staff, the manager should share the cues that led to the problem definitions, including one's own feelings. This is included in high relationship behaviour. Also, a social flavour to the meetings should be staged.

ALTERNATIVE ACTIONS

The alternative actions should be ways of solving the problem that use the indicated leader behaviour style—high structure and high consideration. Expected positive and negative results should be delineated for each alternative action (see Table 7.2).

TABLE 7.2 Alternative Actions and Results

Action	Possible Results
1. Set up an informal potluck dinner at the leader's house, inviting the system members. Introduce the problem after dinner. Explain everything that has led up to the problem as you see it—tardiness, lack of creativity, and so forth. Positively reinforce the excellent care plans that are being done and suggest that collaboratively planned individualized care seems like the next step in growth. Explain your perception of the problem solution and stress that this is just one way to solve the problem. What you would like is to spend time discussing concerns and getting and sharing information about	Staff nurse 2 offers to develop a protocol and try it with several clients. The nurse will report on the strengths and weaknesses of the protocol and revise it with all of the team leaders before going any further. − This result may dampen group involvement in learning about the problem. + It may be a good idea later on. − All of the system does not come to the informal dinner. + The group decides to meet once a week in order to get more information about what they are going to do, prior to designing or implementing anything.

(continued)

TABLE 7.2 (*continued*)

Action	Possible Results
the problem; the team leaders would develop a plan for designing the new care plan protocol and implementing it. Prior to leaving, a series of information sessions is planned. In this action, the manager is being high task in delineating the problem and its rationale. Knowledge is the first priority, and then the manager states that group problem solving is expected. The manager provides reinforcement in a group discussion. This all characterizes starting at LB2, high structure and high consideration, with a planned shift to LB3, high consideration and low structure.	+ The three regular team leaders express insecurity in their ability to do this; they request help from someone who has done this before. − Staff nurse 1 expounds that it will not work because clients expect to be told what to do. + The group openly discusses the problem, asking questions of the manager and of each other.
2. Announce a meeting for team leaders during the conference time slot on the regular shift. Then introduce the goal and follow the same agenda as in the first alternative. Provide coffee and snacks.	− Those nurses not scheduled on that day will not attend. + All positive possible results stated in the first alternative. − The negative result from the first alternative concerning staff nurse 1.
3. Invite the unit supervisor to the first meeting that has been set up during a team conference time slot. The problem and goal is introduced in the same way as alternative actions one and two. In addition the supervisor emphasizes that the goal is favourable with administration.	+ The staff members may be encouraged by support from higher administration. − The staff members may be resentful that an authority figure not in the direct system was aware of the problem/goal before they were.

Note. +   Possible positive outcome
       −   Possible negative outcome

RECOMMENDED ACTION

The manager decides that alternative action two is the most favourable because the team leaders are not accustomed to meeting together socially. Further, they never meet outside of the work environment, even for work-related issues. The meeting would be scheduled, if possible, on a day that all members of the system were working. If not possible, the greatest number in the system would be on duty. The person(s) not on would be asked whether it would be possible to come in for this meeting. Compensation time would be offered. The manager should attempt to neutralize negative outcomes of this alternative action.

Following delineation of the recommended action, it must be implemented and then evaluated.

IMPLEMENTATION AND EVALUATION

To implement simply means "to do" or "to put into action". It follows that after one has specified a recommended action, it must be implemented. Prior to implementation, evaluation emerges as a responsibility and continues to be important until after the action is completed.

Evaluation is most effective when it includes all three types. These are discussed by Newman (1975) as types of control, a broader concept that includes evaluation.

1. *Steering controls.* In this form of evaluation, results are predicted prior to implementation. If things are not going along as desired, corrective action is taken during implementation.

   Referring back to the example, if at the team conference the nurses were not responding in general accordance with the expected positive results, the manager might change the action strategy immediately.

2. *Yes–no controls.* This is a check point where action does not proceed to another step until quality and effectiveness with the previous step are confirmed.

   Again going to the case example, all members should generally be satisfied with the first meeting's outcomes and be clear and agreed on the agenda for the next meeting prior to adjourning.

3. *Post-action controls.* This form of evaluation is after-the-fact—action has been completed; the problem is solved. Now accomplishments and what is being done regarding care plan development are compared with the leader's original intent.

THE MANAGEMENT PROCESS

Chapter 1 contained a discussion of the four components of the management process—planning, organizing, motivating, and controlling. These relationships are discussed regarding the case example.

In order to plan for all of these areas, the areas requiring attention had to be organized logically. What was to be done first and why? Further, the system was organized to contain only the people who were primary in solving the problem.

The determination of a leader behaviour style that responded to the modal level of maturity of the system was a planned intervention that intended to motivate the system to accomplish by giving the nurses what they needed. The manager had to (1) plan for behaviours that filled the indicated leader behaviour style requirements and (2) organize alternative actions and a recommended action to respond to the group's needs.

In each of the three components of the management process, the manager is also comparing accomplishments with intent. Are all necessary nurses included in the system? Should anyone be added? Is my diagnosis accurate—do I need more data? Did my recommended action provide a structured taking-off place for the system? Did it kindle interest in the problem? Will high structure be required for the second session? Was the entire group involved?

SUMMARY

This chapter used a case study to apply all of the material in Chapters 1 through 6. Theory was applied in the problem-solving method. The chapter concluded with a discussion of the interrelatedness of the management process given the described case example. The experiential exercises at the conclusion of Part II contain guidelines for applying the problem-solving method to a case from the learner's real world.

REFERENCES

Hersey, P., & Blanchard, K. (1988). *Management of organizational behavior: Utilizing human resources* (5th ed.). Englewood Cliffs, NJ: Prentice-Hall.

Newman, W. (1975). *Constructive control.* Englewood Cliffs, NJ: Prentice-Hall.

Orem, D. (1985). *Nursing: Concepts of practice* (3rd ed.). New York: McGraw-Hill.

Vroom, V. (1973). A new look at managerial decision-making. *Organizational Dynamics, 1,* 66–80.

Vroom, V., & Jago, A. (1974). Decision-making as a social process. *Decision Sciences, 5,* 743–769.

Vroom, V., & Jago, A. (1978). On the validity of the Vroom–Yetton model. *Journal of Applied Psychology, 63*, 151–162.

Vroom, V., & Jago, A. (1988). *The new leadership: Managing participation in organizations.* Englewood Cliffs, NJ: Prentice-Hall.

Vroom, V., & Yetton, P. (1973). *Leadership and decision-making.* Pittsburgh: University of Pittsburgh Press.

Managerial Ethics
*Elizabeth M. Maloney, Ed.D.**

In May 1922, 68 years ago, The American Academy of Political and Social Science devoted an entire issue to the ethics of the professions and business. It is clear that concern with ethics is far from new. However, it is the content of that concern that has changed so much over the years in

*Elizabeth M. Maloney, EdD, RN, is Chair of the Department of Nursing Education and an Associate Professor of Nursing Education at Teachers College, Columbia University, New York. She is a former member of the New York State Nurses Association Council on Ethical Practice and she currently teaches ethics for health care professionals. Dr Maloney has written and spoken extensively in the area of ethical nursing practice and in psychiatric nursing.

the health field. The individual struggle with justice—right and wrong—remains essentially the same. Meanwhile, in the last two decades particularly, there has been mounting concern with the ethical management of society's organizations. This concern ranges from national government to structures closer at hand, particularly the health care system. Specifically this chapter is concerned with management in the spectrum of organizations devoted to health and illness.

BACKGROUND TO ETHICAL CONCERNS

There is little doubt that the old "service to humanity" credo contained most of the elements of the Christian–Judeo belief system that undergirds ethics in the Western world. Almost without exception, early literature in this area was a blend of commenting on professional organizations and their structure, admission standards, and legal aspects of licensing. There were, of course, no discussions of ethical dilemmas in a high technology illness system as one knows of them today.

It is highly probable that early content was emphasized precisely because there existed a natural limit to what health workers could do (or were expected by the public to be able to do). Indeed, the early 1900s was an era when it was freely acknowledged at some identifiable point what was good nursing care. There was, in short, a limit to the possibilities. At the edge of the limit was death, when it could no longer be held at bay. It is important to recognize that this was the generally held opinion or consensus; a matter of public acknowledgment. Today there is a vast array of available technology and there is high expectation of more to come. The increased debates in the public realm are best measured by the flood of literature in the press, both popular and professional. Ethics is in fact one of the persistent themes of our time.

Emmanuel (1987, p. 16) indicated that people now live "in a liberal polity" where a multiplicity of views are entertained as to what constitutes the meaning and value of life. Directly associated with these terms is another: the "quality" of life. Hypothetically, part of the discussions around and about the patient's right to die have to do with this latter concept. However, to simply discuss "quality" of life is to say little. Anyone capable of rational thought has a different definition of the quality of life. Basically, as in all ethical decisions, the final outcome of care is dependent on reconciliation of multiple personal value systems. These systems are in turn based on religious and family experiences and the specific context in which the "quality" must be defined. Briefly it all depends on whose ox is being gored, as the saying goes—whose life; whose family; and under what circumstances? And what are the restrictions legally?

It is important to note here again that cultural concerns have a great deal more to do with attitudes about right and wrong than any of us realize. Assuming that professional literature reflects the immediate concerns of a profession, it can clearly be seen that these concerns ebb and flow over time. For example, Anderson (1949) reviewed articles on ethics in the *American Journal of Nursing* in 10-year intervals starting with 1900 and ending in 1948. Briefly, a curve peaking in the years 1930 to 1940 showed 30 articles; the number of articles descended to zero from 1941 to 1945, indicating a national concern with other matters, most likely the years at war. Certainly, speculation could be pursued also with the unprecedented concern with ethical matters manifested in the 1970s and 1980s. This concern, grounded in the use of ever-more sophisticated, expensive technology and its use, has culminated in the employment of philosophers in medical centres and in the rise of ethical committees in well over half of US hospitals. It has also resulted in the development of a group of nurses commonly called nurse-ethicists. It is of interest that many (but not all) came from a psychiatric nursing background. Working with philosophers and studying at centres dealing with ethical concerns, these experts have produced a solid body of literature aimed directly at problems found in nursing practice. It is these same problems that the nurse manager confronts each day. The solution to these ethical dilemmas is almost never clear-cut and oftentimes remains open-ended. Still, from the currently available theoretical material, there are strong markers for the resolution of some of these dilemmas. It is reasonable to emphasize that the more pressing ethical dilemmas are, in the end, so urgent that they are concretized into law, thus providing relief from ambiguity for all concerned personnel. For example, there is the New York State law, effective in 1988, which requires that health care facilities have a written policy on "do not resuscitate" (or DNR) orders (Brawer & Miller, 1987).

As well as the foregoing legal direction, professional codes are helpful in counteracting institutional pressures. Recognition of the part played by these pressures has increased in the literature of managerial ethics. Utilizing the argument that the "most obvious link between nursing and the great moral ideas is health", Packard and Ferrara (1988, p. 60) objected to the conventionally held idea that nurses' moral freedom is constrained by institutional and other pressures so great as to restrict their ethical freedom. Citing the need for a code of ethics for corporate employees, Rue and Byars (1986) noted that "a code of ethics also reduces the organizational pressures to compromise personal ethics for the sake of organizational goals" (p. 2). It would seem then that there are almost universal pressures—political, organizational, and others—that militate against moving toward the right and just solution to ethical dilemmas. Managers everywhere share common problems.

ETHICS AND MORALITY DEFINED

Rue and Byars (1986) defined ethics as "standards or principles of conduct used to govern the behavior of an individual or group of individuals" (p. 2). Ethics are generally concerned with questions of right and wrong or with moral duties. Hosmer (1987) pointed out that the term ethics is used in the plural since most people have a system of beliefs rather than one single value by which to live.

What then is morality? Hosmer (1987) stated that morality is a set of standards by which people judge one another. He noted also that one usually speaks of "moral standards of behavior and systems of belief" (p. 92). One could say then that morals are the way that people expect other people to behave, according to established group norms.

Aroskar (1987a, 1987b) added that ethics, as an area of philosophy, refers to moral conduct; not what is *actually* done, but what ought to be done. She further cited some of the realities that act as barriers to doing what should be done. Some of these constraints are constant in the daily lives of nurse managers: cost-containment factors, limitations and short-ages of personnel, internal and external politics, and others. Germane to the work of the health care manager is Aroskar's comment that medical ethics is concerned with moral decision making both in day-to-day affairs and in the larger world of policy making. Modern-day nursing practice and management is rife with situations where value-laden conflicts arise. As Benjamin (1988) and others have pointed out, it has not been widely recognized that nurses are involved in pivotal and complex ethical situations and that willingly or not, they are involved in and often make ethical decisions. These decisions are made within an intricate system of formal and informal relationships where conflicting value systems are often found. These problems are compounded by an organization whose goals at any given time may be in conflict with those of individuals or groups within it. It is managerial leadership that often must set the scene for the ethical decisions that the total group must make.

Peculiar to health care professionals is the fact that the majority are employees of health organizations. As employees, they are bound to accede to lawful demands of the employing institutions. Compounding this is the presence of the doctor, who most frequently is not hospital-employed but who uses hospital facilities primarily for nursing care and multiple other technological personnel and/or resources. The fact is that there are many examples where health professionals have been caught between their own personal values and legal demands to obey the lawful orders of doctors or superiors. Even more important are situations where demands may be lawful, but they conflict with other moral values and emphasize the legal–moral conflict that will continue to occupy students of moral dilemmas. For example, it may be lawful to have an order to discontinue aggressive treatment, but in the day-to-day care of the patient, it might be that the advocate's role would imply a different stance. The legalities are not always clear as to what constitutes interference in the patient–doctor role, as amply demonstrated in the now famous Tuma case (Veatch & Fry, 1987). There are a number of writers in the field who have considered the major world views from which primary ethical systems arise (Kant, 1909; Rawls, 1971; Ross, 1939). Their work serves as a starting point for the formulation of a coherent set of principles or guidelines for decision making in the ethical realm.

PRINCIPLES OF ETHICS—GUIDELINES

Principles arise from the ethical systems that have developed from a lifelong exposure to fundamental beliefs about how a human being behaves in a given situation. Obviously, these go back to a group of beliefs in one of the two major ethical systems. Add to that a particular cultural system of beliefs and some normative directions for what to do come into being. It would seem that the concept of "normative" comes into consideration immediately in ethical dilemmas. The principles are as follows: autonomy, beneficence, nonmaleficence, veracity, justice, and confidentiality. A brief discussion of each principle follows.

Autonomy

Basically, this is the freedom to decide what persons will or will not do with their lives, their bodies, and their selves, all of course within the limits of what is possible and what does not infringe upon the rights of others. It does mean that one accords others the same freedom and independence of action as accorded self and that one respects the dignity of others. Autonomy means never looking upon another as a means to some end unless that person is in entire agreement with the clearly understood end. For example, in the health field informed consent emerges from this concept. If, as in some past instances, patients have become part of a research study without consenting and without being informed, then this is a clear violation of an ethical principle. Freedom to act upon information given is an integral part of informed consent. If by one means or another the element of coercion enters the situation, then free choice cannot be exercised. Sometimes professionals are not entirely aware that their position intimidates their lay audience, the patient, and that patients will go along because they think they have received what amounts to a definitive statement about their condition.

Beneficence

This is a situation where one is not only minimally responsible for doing no harm; rather, in various service professions, one is bound also to do good. Hospitals, doctors, and nurses exist "to do no harm" but also to institute activity that will be beneficial to all of the clients encountered. Since patients enter the health care system for the solution of a health problem, to do nothing about their problems is acting counter to the principle of beneficence. Of course, in the instances where doing nothing is of therapeutic value, there is an exception to this principle.

Nonmaleficence

This principle requires the professional to prevent harm whenever possible and to never use a particular treatment or medication to harm patients. Lifton (1986) in *The Nazi Doctors* described in detail how a whole group cooperated in the malevolent use of formerly benevolent treatment and research efforts. The process by which this took place is worthy of study, particularly the concepts of climate or milieu or the importance of the context in which malevolent actions take root. The idea of the "slippery slope" is important here and can partially be described as that having accepted the possibility of what once was unthinkable, the rapid descent into unethical activity becomes commonplace. The unacceptable becomes acceptable. If unit staff decides that it is too time-consuming to take all of the vital signs of recovering patients, then this nonactivity at some point becomes institutionalized or commonplace; the next step may be to enter ficticious figures.

Veracity

In the health care field, truth-telling has long been debated in the literature. In recent years, opinion has come down hard on the patient's right to know the truth. Certainly the professional's obligation to present the full array of information to patients is unquestioned, with however some notable exceptions. There are instances where bald truth-telling may destroy the last vestige of hope available to the patient. There are still people who communicate in every manner possible that they do not wish to hear bad news. One could argue that by failing to make certain professional statements, one is in essence lying. Bok (1978) explored the concept of lying in effective detail, including the giving of placebos as lying. Included in her work also is the consideration of references given by management that might, among other things, fail to include serious behavioural deficits on the part of a departing employee. To say nothing then can be to lie.

This has always been a troubled area. In more paternalistic times, the problem did not arise as frequently. The patient was told what he or she was supposed to know. The content of what the patient was offered was based on values and perceptions of the health worker offering the information. Certainly no one would argue today that in most instances autonomy is involved; patients have a right to information about themselves. There are still people who argue that the individual with a terminal health problem simply does not want to know, on the grounds that such information would do more harm than good. Thus the teleological approach is tempting—to produce good feeling without too much thought about the moral value of the patients' right to know, along with the moral duty to make the information available. (In reality, however, there are many combinations possible.) Here also can be summoned Kant's (1909) concept that everyone has the duty to tell the truth, thus answering the question "are lies ever justified?" in the negative.

The bare bones of a common practice dilemma are that situations will arise wherein health care professionals must make value judgments about whether lying might be the best thing to do for a patient (beneficence). Thus two principles are involved; to do good and to tell the truth. Sissela Bok (1978) said that liars in such circumstances comfort themselves with the thought of their benevolence but that, in the long run, the liar loses some measure of credibility and damages the system that supports the lie. Characteristic of the dilemma is conflict among principles and the need to formulate some personal guidelines as to how one solves the problem, based on, among other things, some alternatives relevant to a moral solution of the dilemma.

Justice

Germane to the health field is the expectation that people with like problems will be treated equally or alike. It is central to the principle of justice that fairness and rights be considered always. Perhaps in no other area is the question so pressing as in how scarce resources will be distributed in the health care field. Faced with cost-containment and ever-rising expectations about the efficacy of modern health technology, the dilemma persists concerning who is to receive the scarce organ or the expensive or novel treatment. Should people, for example, be moved to the head of the transplant list for any reason at all?

Justice also demands that differences be handled differently if a patient is so unequal in some respect to all of the others for whom a policy has been applied. When then should exceptions be made? If so, on what grounds? Are professionals willing to deny health care to such exceptions because of the rules?

Confidentiality

The contract often unspoken between health care professional and client/patient exists in part because the patient (in this instance) makes the assumption that whatever is divulged will be held in confidence. So sure of this are most people that they do not even think about the matter. In short, all of us make assumptions about our private matters that may be just that—assumptions. Excluding all of the inroads on privacy that have arisen in late years, largely due to computers, situations in the health field certainly exist where the patient's right to keep information private infringes on the rights of others. Nowhere is this more glaring than in the question of Acquired Immune Deficiency Syndrome (AIDS) and the right-to-know of those closest to the patient.

The control of information about ourselves is, whether people are aware of it or not, subject to gradation—that is, people quantify who will receive what part of our store of information about ourselves and others. The most common way to do this is by degree of closeness. Spouses may know what the outer world does not; but in order to solve various problems, selected others must also know. Every professional group then becomes privy to information that their patients or clients do not wish to have known widely. Confidentiality becomes a duty and the patient or client has a right not to have specified information released. Health care managers are privy to information about employees that may be confidential. To whom and under what circumstances is such information released?

MANAGEMENT AND THE DEVELOPMENT OF A MORAL CLIMATE

Turning to Aroskar (1987a, 1987b) for a definition of moral and ethical leadership, the following perception is found: leaders describe moral leadership as taking responsibility for one's commitments—taking responsibility for one's choices. Drawing on prominent ethicists, Aroskar also noted other characteristics that emerged, such as leadership being a particular kind of social–ethical practice evoked by health issues that require caring. Other adjectives invoked are responsibility, involvement, fairness, concern for others—all of these words describing moral leadership. Ethical dilemmas, it goes without saying, do not arise every day but must be part of a carefully defined situation. Bok (1988) and others have, for example, pointed out the fate of "whistleblowers" in our society. It should be an act of last resort; all other reasonable avenues having been exhausted. Whistleblowers are, in the long run, not treated well in our society.

Although it is seldom discussed overtly, the work environment on a particular plane of behaviour makes implicit assumptions. These assumptions are based on cues taken from those already in place on a nursing unit. These cues can be as concrete as a warning from a fellow worker—"never cut a corner where x is here"—to an aura of openness about mistakes; there may be a generalized assumption that "right" and "justice and regard for others" will prevail in that particular environment. Admittedly the "right" attitude or the "just" response are influenced by different value systems. Often responses to ethical dilemmas have to be developed through interdisciplinary debate based on known principles of ethics.

Managers are at a pivotal place in an organizational structure and are expected to accomplish organizational goals as smoothly as possible. Clearly this brings them into conflict at times with staff and patient goals. Indeed, part of the nurse manager's dilemma arises from serving multiple masters. Specifically, the constituencies to be served are: (1) the patient or client for whom the health organization exists; (2) the nursing staff and related others *for* whom management is responsible; and (3) the agency administration *to* whom the nurse in a managerial position is responsible. By way of illustration, a simple situation is described and found in Part II experiential exercises; it is one that is perhaps destined to become more common as the current nursing shortage persists. A series of questions is posed in Exercise 5, Ethics—A Managerial Dilemma, and the opportunity to utilize the answers based on ethical principles is open to the learner.

Framework for Managerial Activity—General Considerations

It would be useful at this point to identify some of the most commonly experienced or perceived ethical problems by health care staff. With the end in view of establishing an ethics committee, which would provide assistance to professional staff, a survey was conducted by Edwards and Haddad (1988). The purposes of the study were to assess the educational needs and primary ethical problems that were perceived by health care staff. It is the identification of the staff members' ethical concerns that may provide guidance to the nurse manager in dealing with ethical dilemmas. The findings were reduced to two factors:

1. The justification of life-support and resuscitative efforts in futile or gravely burdensome cases; and
2. Professional competency issues, such as truth-telling, withholding information, and questioning the competency of the medical staff and nursing colleagues.

In general, all of the available literature in the field bears out the foregoing findings, albeit expressed in somewhat different language. It says little for (either medicine or nursing) that the most common reason cited by these subjects for compromising their ethical values was a doctor's or a superior's request. It does, however, add verisimilitude to the picture of the nurse as the person "caught in the middle" in terms of not only ethical dilemmas but many other situations as well. On the other hand, it is important to point out that many corporations have developed codes of ethics for their personnel, since hierarchical pressure (those perceived to be in authority) and a work climate where corners are cut are by no means unique to the health field.

Health Care Cost-Containment

The control of health care costs eventually translates itself into allocation of scarce resources. The technology that allows for life, where there once would have been death, is extremely expensive. Who then will be designated to receive it—everyone who establishes need? Or, will it be selected individuals based on stated criteria? Who will set the criteria? How long will these criteria be used and who decides when they will be terminated? These are but a few of the significant questions that health care managers will be obliged to consider in concert with other professionals from the health disciplines. The second problem that emerges in the managerial realm is the pressure to employ less qualified personnel to deal with an increasingly complex care situation. There are two sources for this pressure, the first being a shortage of qualified personnel and the second, the cost of qualified personnel.

Scarce Research and Personnel

Part of the manager's ethical dilemma is generally related to staffing and to the quality of patient care. The increasing impetus to provide cost-effective care may take the form of pressure to employ and use less qualified personnel in situations where greater knowledge and skill are required. The concept that Fry (1985) used to describe this dilemma is based on the idea that nursing and management in nursing are assumed social roles. Not only does one act as an individual or in one's private capacity, but one also bears the moral responsibility for actions carried out in the name of a particular profession. Fry called this the "morality of role acceptance" (pp. 135–136). Fry illustrated this dilemma graphically in describing a nursing home director faced with quality of care concerns (legislation allowing unlicensed personnel to administer medications) and measures to assure cost-effectiveness. Although there were other issues involved, Fry stated that this was a classic example of a common dilemma in health care: "between what is right according to universal moral norms and what is right according to outcomes or consequences" (pp. 135–136). It is right that medications be dispensed, but the situation becomes problematic if lack of expertise leads to undesirable ends. Related to ethical principles, the following principle might be invoked; clearly nonmaleficence is appropriate, that is, do no harm.

As resources become ever-more scarce, what is "due" to whom and what are the criteria to determine this? A classic focal point in ethics is the lifeboat dilemma. Briefly, in order to survive as a group, someone must go overboard. On what basis is this decided? Is it age, evidence of a productive life, or possibilities for future contributions to mankind? Who will receive the organ transplant? What are the criteria and who develops them? Are the answers based on a first-come-first-served basis, or do other factors pre-empt the waiting list? And how do health care staff react to the decision? The amount of national resources allocated to the NHS care is finite and probably will always operate in competition with other well-defined national concerns. Since the situation will undoubtedly become more urgent, then the impact will be felt in hospitals and will often become priority staff-management problems. The tendency to solve economic problems by bringing in less skilled workers is evident in the health field in the US and the pattern could be copied in the UK.

Staff Concern with "Do Not Resuscitate" Orders

This area appears to be a focal point for a great many ethical concerns, primarily because decisions one way or the other have such profound implications for everyone concerned. These implications are both moral and legal. Further, they are of extreme importance to nursing since many experts in ethics point out that it is nurses who are caught in the middle. If there are, as has happened in the past, ambiguous unwritten directives, it is nurses who have called the code or not; nurses have dealt with directions for "no codes" and "slow codes", at least before the era of public debate and subsequent clarification of the situation. This clarification has been achieved by a steadily expanding series of legal decisions in the US such as the Quinlan and Fox cases (Jameton, 1984). These were cases where substitute judgments were invoked because of incapacity; but what of the patient who decides that it is time to terminate treatment— or to refuse a specific operation, such as limb amputation? For health care managers, Tamborlane's (1987) comment concerning the agency and administrative role when a patient makes a personal decision to terminate treatment is to the point: "Agency personnel's moral or ethical beliefs should not be allowed to infringe upon a competent individual's rights to discontinue treatment when he or she wishes to let the disease take its natural course" (pp. 30–31). These are the kinds of decisions that management-instituted ethics committees regularly discuss.

Competence

Managers spend considerable time wrestling with the problem of personnel who for one reason or another may be providing care that does not come up to standard. Recognition of problem personnel generally "comes up" from the unit in the form of an oral or written report. The nature of the incompetence can range from repeated mistakes to lying, and those reported behaviours may have their origin in several sources. One of the most common is substance abuse. Such impairment is expensive in human and monetary terms and gives rise to ethical dilemmas among those who are most closely associated with the individual concerned. The danger to patients is clearly identified to be greater than, for example, the substitution of medication, which is such a frequent outcome of an employee's addiction. This is only one area for concern.

Formerly, attitudes toward substance abuse in the workplace were moralistic and often resulted in harsh disciplinary measures. People were reluctant to report colleagues and probably still are. At least two studies demonstrated that there remains an apparent disinclination to cooperate with managers in the identification of substance abuses. For example, as late as 1985, *Nursing Life* reported that 53% of the respondents to their survey stated that they would not help management and appeared to perceive such identification as management's responsibility. There are two strong factors working for management in the solution of dilemmas thus presented to colleagues of the abuser. One is the legal necessity to report incompetence and the other is the much more therapeutic approach to such problems that is demonstrated through organization-wide assistance programmes. In asking why ethical dilemmas should arise in situations such as the foregoing, a good question is raised. Between the obligation to report and the now very common practice of directing identified abusers into special programmes for assistance, why would anyone consider this a dilemma? First, there is the common or shared humanity—what will happen to this person if they lose their job or licence? Second, most people have a perceived loyalty to colleagues. As Winslow (1988) noted, most people are unwilling to expose publically the shortcomings of a colleague. Based on the childhood tradition of not telling on a peer or being tagged as a tattletale, there is an element of felt injustice for the other if one does take steps to expose the abuse.

MANAGERIAL OPTIONS

In attempting to provide leadership in situations where ethical dilemmas are identified, there are several things that managers are able to do. Some of these things are concrete, such as establishment of ethics committees. Other steps include assurance that everyone for whom management is responsible is aware of guidelines related to confidentiality of sensitive patient material. All personnel need to have complete information about how one begins dealing with incompetence in colleagues and the like. Managers can address the underlying ethical principles through specifically oriented continuing education programmes. Perhaps one of the most effective means of maintaining a reasonably open and moral climate is to hold a genuine belief in staff capacity to identify and solve ethical problems. As Aroskar (1987a, 1987b) pointed out, both staff and patients are persons who are worthy of respect. More to the point, she noted that there may be coercive forces or elements such as threats and peer pressure if one refuses dubious medical orders. "Such actions or an environment that condones such actions may jeopardize an individual nurse's personal and professional integrity in any practice setting and require change" (Aroskar, 1987a, p. 26).

Although health care managers are sometimes involved as patient advocates, it is more likely that there will be situations where advocacy of an embattled staff nurse may be the issue. Noting the complexity of the health care professional's role *vis-à-vis* the ever-expanding technology of patient care, many ethicists writing about medical ethics have taken note of the great responsibility that many carry which must be based on an equally great degree of necessary skill and knowledge. The same ethicists have noted the lack of power to make decisions—the frequent and classic case of the man or woman in the middle. What are some of the operative ways that the manager can deal with situations involving the foregoing factors?

Establishment of an Ethics Committee

The hospital ethics committee is now commonplace in institutional life. In the US, over 50 to 60% of the hospitals now have such committees; some of the larger medical centres employ philosophers who have extensive backgrounds in ethics and the solution of ethical dilemmas. In larger practice settings these committees often deal with matters that do not filter down to daily life on the unit. To provide for nursing staff, Edwards and Haddad (1988) described the establishment of an ethics committee specifically for nursing staff. One activity included the separation of ethical problems from management problems. Essentially, tackling ethical problems involves the elements and steps in problem solving, thus allowing for a reasoned and principled solution.

Another similar effort is described by Jaeger (1988). Although confined to one unit staff, many of the elements were the same. First, staff frustration with ethical concerns in which there seemed to be no clear cut means of dealing with these questions was identified. Essentially, the health care manager described an identification of a staff problem (ethical concerns and no apparent means of dealing with these problems), the mobilization of the staff through unit meetings, the encouragement of staff members' identification of the problem(s) as they saw it, and provision of an environment where staff felt free to verbalize ethical concerns. This was followed by an educational phase. Literature was provided and discussions ensued, thereby tying the abstract literature to the setting. Although the first problem to be clearly defined was the code status of patients, after several months it became apparent that there were many other dilemmas involved. It was at this point that the need for ethical health conferences became evident. Therefore, guidelines were set up and the goal of the conferences was to provide a continuing pattern of open communication and mutual support among patients, family, and the health care team. Finally, a structure for data collection was established. The report of both of these efforts emphasized that the support and commitment of the top-level health care managers is tantamount to survival of such efforts. Thus, as can be seen from a brief summary of two committee efforts, such activity provides one of the most useful means for management to solve ethical dilemmas. Out of such infrastructure comes identification of education needs in the ethical area. Essentially, the classic steps of problem solving emerge from the foregoing examples.

WHAT OF THE FUTURE?

Jameton (1984), a philosopher who has studied ethics in nursing, wrote that "nursing is the morally central health care profession. Philosophers of nursing, not medicine, should determine the image of health care and its future direction" (pp. 196–197).

Recently two efforts to provide a moral foundation for nursing and another to ground the "nursing ethic in a convenantal relationship" may offer a glimpse of where a specifically nursing ethic may be going. In one direction Yarling and McElmurry (1986) called for the reform of the hospital and the social structure it embodies as being essential to autonomy for nursing practitioners, and thus to a moral basis for nursing. Bishop and Scudder (1987) objected on the grounds that nursing autonomy is secondary to the nurse's primary concern, that of patient welfare.

Winslow (1988) argued that there is a need to be aware of and to change metaphors about nursing, noting that such metaphors interact with nursing ethics (stated rules or principles), which in turn interact with the more explicit features of nursing ethics. The metaphors touch on roles in that, for example, the traditional loyal, servant–mother roles are being slowly replaced by contractual advocacy roles. Concomitant alterations in expectations will eventually create a focus on different realities in the nurse–patient–institutional context. It is to be noted that these are only a few of the many roles played in an ever-changing health care scene.

SUMMARY

Ethical dilemmas in the health care field, hospital, community, and home can be expected to intensify in the future. As new technology is perfected and as resource allocation becomes a more acute problem, health care management will predictably draw more and more on ethical committees as devices for support and as development vehicles for at least working consensus among staff when ethical dilemmas present themselves. Some of the dilemmas will be at least partially resolved (after prolonged public debate) by legal means. Certainly euthanasia is much on the public mind and is closely allied to its more concrete form labelled "do not resuscitate". As Edwards and Haddad (1988) noted, a basic knowledge of ethical theories and related principles is a necessity both for the practising nurse and the nurse manager. It is a necessity to deal with the moral–ethical issues that arise in the work day. Certainly, every barometer reads that there will be more, not less, technology; therefore there will be probably more, not less, concern with moral and ethical problems in the future.

REFERENCES

American Academy of Political and Social Sciences. (1922). The ethics of professions and business. *The Annals, C1.*

Anderson, B. (1949, July). Discussion of ethics in the curriculum. Lecture at Teachers College, Columbia University, New York, NY.

Aroskar, M. (1987a). Commentary. *Hastings Center Report, 17*(2), 26.

Aroskar, M. (1987b, September). *Ethics in the leadership equation.* Distinguished Lecture at Columbia University Health Sciences Campus, New York, NY.

Benjamin, M. (1988). Nursing ethics: An emerging integrity. *Hastings Center Report, 18*(2), 38–39.

Bishop, A., & Scudder, J. (1987). Nursing ethics in an age of controversy. *Advances in Nursing Science, 9*(3), 34–37.

Bok, S. (1978). Lying: Moral choice in public and private life. New York: Pantheon.

Bok, S. (1988). Whistleblowing and professional responsibilities. In J. Callahan (Ed.). *Ethical issues in professional life.* New York: Oxford Press.

Brawer, I., & Miller, T. (1987). New York to provide comprehensive guidelines for do not resuscitate orders. *Journal of the New York State Nurses Association, 18*(5), 3.

Edwards, B., & Haddad. A. (1988). Establishing a nursing bioethics committee. *Journal of Nursing Administration, 18*(3), 30–33.

Emmanuel, E. (1987). A communal vision of care for incompetent patients. *Hastings Center Report, 17*(5), 15–20.

Fry, S. (1985). Political activities and the professional role. In S. Talbot & D. Mason (Eds.). *Political action*. Menlo Park, CA: Addison-Wesley.

Hosmer, L. (1987). *The ethics of management*. Homewood, IL: Irwin.

Jaeger, T. (1988). A head nurse's approach to multidisciplinary ethical conferences. *Nursing Management, 10*(1), 61–62.

Jameton, A. (1984). *Nursing Practice: The ethical issues*. Englewood Cliffs, NJ: Prentice-Hall.

Kant, I. (1909). *Critique of practical reason*. London: Longmans.

Lifton, R. (1986). *The Nazi doctors*. New York: Basic Books.

Nursing Life. (1985). What our readers said about entrapping a colleague. *Nursing Life, 3*(5), 54–55.

Packard, J., & Ferrara, M. (1988). In search of the moral foundation of nursing. *Advances in Nursing Science, 10*(4), 60–71.

Rawls, J. (1971). *Theory of justice*. Cambridge, MA: Belknap.

Ross, W. (1939). *The right and the good*. Oxford: Oxford University Press.

Rue, L., & Byars, L. (1986). *Management: Theory and application* (4th ed.). Homewood, IL: Irwin.

Tamborlane, T. (1987). A patient's right to refuse or discontinue treatment. *Caring, 4*, 30–31.

Veatch, T., & Fry, S. (1987). *Case studies in nursing ethics*. Philadelphia: Lippincott.

Winslow, G. (1988). From loyalty to advocacy: A new metaphor for nursing. In J. Callahan (Ed.). *Ethical issues in professional life*. New York: Oxford Press.

Yarling, R., & McElmurry, B. (1986). The moral foundation of nursing. *Advances in Nursing Science, 8*(2), 63–73.

Part II

Manager Responsibilities: Experiential Exercises

EXERCISE 1 Diagnosing Personal Leader Behaviour Style*

Purposes

1. To diagnose one's personal leader behaviour style.

2. To identify one's expectations of leader behaviour.

3. To explore the implications of one's personal leadership style.

4. To explore the similarity or disparity between one's personal style and one's expectations of leader behaviour.

Facility

Classroom.

Materials

Worksheet A: Leader Behaviour (Self) Questionnaire.

Worksheet B: Scoring Key for "Initiating Structure".

Worksheet C: Scoring Key for "Consideration".

Worksheet D: Locating Scores on the Ohio State Leadership Studies Model.

Pencil or pen.

Time Required

Forty-five minutes to one hour.

Group Size

Unlimited.

Design

1. Instruct members to respond individually to the items in Worksheet A, following the directions on the instrument.

2. After completing Step 1, go to Worksheets B and C and follow the directions for scoring.

(*continued*)

*Adapted by permission from La Monica, Elaine L., *The Nursing Process: A Humanistic Approach*, pp. 376–384. Copyright © 1979 by Addison-Wesley Publishing Company, Inc., Menlo Park, CA.

EXERCISE 1   (continued)

3. Go to Worksheet D and interpret scores on the model.

4. Discuss findings. Compare self with expectations.

Variations

Worksheet A can be given to an associate, a supervisor, and/or a follower. Their task is to rate you on how they feel you behave. Instruments can then be scored and compared with perceptions of self. Since behaviour is as perceived by others, ratings scales filled out on your behaviour lend support to your perceptions of self. A discussion of differences in perceptions among raters can be an excellent consciousness-raising activity. The mean score of different raters (including self) is the best indicator of leader behaviour style.

EXERCISE 1
WORKSHEET A: Leader Behaviour (Self) Questionnaire

This questionnaire is to determine your leadership style. Following is a list of items that may be used to describe your behaviour as you think you act. This is not a test of ability. It simply asks you to describe how you believe you act as a leader of a group.

DIRECTIONS:

a. Read each item carefully.

b. Think about how frequently you engage in the behaviour described by the item.

c. Decide whether you *always, often, occasionally, seldom*, or *never* act as described by the item.

d. Draw a circle around one of the five letters following the item to show the answer you have selected: A = always, B = often, C = occasionally, D = seldom, E = never.

When acting as a leader, I:

1. Do personal favours for group members.	A	B	C	D	E
2. Make my attitudes clear to the group.	A	B	C	D	E
3. Do little things to make it pleasant to be a member of the group.	A	B	C	D	E
4. Try out my new ideas with the group.	A	B	C	D	E
5. Act as the real leader of the group.	A	B	C	D	E
6. Am easy to understand.	A	B	C	D	E
7. Rule with an iron hand.	A	B	C	D	E
8. Find time to listen to group members.	A	B	C	D	E
9. Criticize poor work.	A	B	C	D	E
10. Give advance notice of changes.	A	B	C	D	E
11. Speak in a manner not to be questioned.	A	B	C	D	E
12. Keep to myself.	A	B	C	D	E
13. Look out for the personal welfare of individual group members.	A	B	C	D	E
14. Assign group members to particular tasks.	A	B	C	D	E
15. Am the spokesperson of the group.	A	B	C	D	E
16. Schedule the work to be done.	A	B	C	D	E

(*continued*)

EXERCISE 1
WORKSHEET A   *(continued)*

17. Maintain definite standards of performance.	A B C D E
18. Refuse to explain my actions.	A B C D E
19. Keep the group informed.	A B C D E
20. Act without consulting the group.	A B C D E
21. Back up the members in their actions.	A B C D E
22. Emphasize the meeting of deadlines.	A B C D E
23. Treat all group members as my equals.	A B C D E
24. Encourage the use of uniform procedures.	A B C D E
25. Get what I ask for from my superiors.	A B C D E
26. Am willing to make changes.	A B C D E
27. Make sure that my part in the organization is understood by group members.	A B C D E
28. Am friendly and approachable.	A B C D E
29. Ask that group members follow standard rules and regulations.	A B C D E
30. Fail to take necessary action.	A B C D E
31. Make group members feel at ease when talking with them.	A B C D E
32. Let group members know what is expected of them.	A B C D E
33. Speak as the representative of the group.	A B C D E
34. Put suggestions made by the group into operation.	A B C D E
35. See to it that group members are working up to capacity.	A B C D E
36. Let other people take away my leadership in the group.	A B C D E
37. Get my superiors to act for the welfare of the group members.	A B C D E
38. Get group approval in important matters before going ahead.	A B C D E
39. See to it that the work of group members is coordinated.	A B C D E
40. Keep the group working together as a team.	A B C D E

Source: Worksheets A, B, and C copyright Ohio State University. Developed by staff members of the Ohio State Leadership Studies, Center for Business and Economic Research, Division of Research, College of Administrative Science, Ohio State University, Columbus, Reproduced by permission.

EXERCISE 1
WORKSHEET B: Scoring Key for "Initiating Structure"

SCORING INSTRUCTIONS: On the Leader Behaviour (Self) Questionnaire, draw a circle around the questionnaire item numbers noted below (2, 4, 7, 9, etc.). On the left side of the questionnaire, beside each such item, write the score you get for each item. The appropriate score is determined by noting, as indicated below, the points for the response you made on the questionnaire. For example, if your response to question 2 was "seldom" you would put a "1" by question number 2 on your questionnaire. Do this for each of the 15 questions below. Add these 15 scores together. The total is your score for initiating structure. Transcribe the score in the space provided on Worksheet D.

Item No.	A Always	B Often	C Occasionally	D Seldom	E Never
2	4	3	2	1	0
4	4	3	2	1	0
7	4	3	2	1	0
9	4	3	2	1	0
11	4	3	2	1	0
14	4	3	2	1	0
16	4	3	2	1	0
17	4	3	2	1	0
22	4	3	2	1	0
24	4	3	2	1	0
27	4	3	2	1	0
29	4	3	2	1	0
32	4	3	2	1	0
35	4	3	2	1	0
39	4	3	2	1	0

(continued)

EXERCISE 1 (continued)
WORKSHEET C: Scoring Key for "Consideration"

SCORING INSTRUCTIONS: On the Leader Behaviour (Self) Questionnaire, circle the questionnaire item numbers noted below (1, 3, 6, 8, etc.). On the left side of the questionnaire, beside each circled item, write the score you get for each item. The appropriate score is determined by noting, as indicated below, the points for the response you made on the questionnaire. For example, if your response to question 1 was "often" you would put a "3" by question number 1 on your questionnaire. Do this for each of the 15 questions below. Add the 15 scores. The total is your score for consideration. Transcribe this score in the space provided on Worksheet D. (Note that there are 10 questions "left over", which are not scored. These are in the questionnaire in order to maintain conditions comparable to when the questionnaire was standardized.)

Item No.	A Always	B Often	C Occasionally	D Seldom	E Never
1	4	3	2	1	0
3	4	3	2	1	0
6	4	3	2	1	0
8	4	3	2	1	0
12	0	1	2	3	4
13	4	3	2	1	0
18	0	1	2	3	4
20	0	1	2	3	4
21	4	3	2	1	0
23	4	3	2	1	0
26	4	3	2	1	0
28	4	3	2	1	0
31	4	3	2	1	0
34	4	3	2	1	0
38	4	3	2	1	0

EXERCISE 1
WORKSHEET D: Locating Scores on the Ohio State Leadership Studies Model

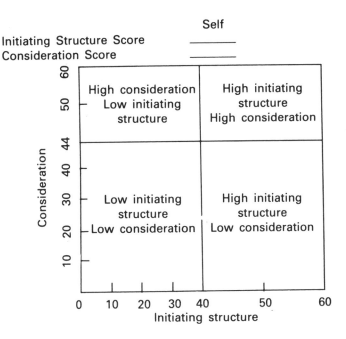

Self

Initiating Structure Score   _____
Consideration Score   _____

DIRECTIONS: After scoring the instrument, Worksheets B and C, indicate where your initiating structure scores place on that continuum, followed by your consideration scores. Draw the horizontal and vertical line from each axis until both meet. The box in which lines meet indicates your leadership style. Scores above 40 on the initiating structure dimension indicate you are above the mean. If you scored above 44 on the consideration dimension, you would also be above the mean.

The purpose of using this instrument is to begin the process of gaining awareness of your leader behaviour. The Leader Behaviour (Self) Questionnaire is a rough indicator. If your scores conform to your experience in dealing with others and their perception of you, then the instrument provides an excellent basis for further self-study.

Source: Copyright Ohio State University. Developed by staff members of the Ohio State Leadership Studies, Center for Business and Economic Research, Division of Research, College of Administrative Science, Ohio State University, Columbus. Reproduced by permission.

EXERCISE 2   Diagnosing the System

Purposes	1. To gain experience in specifying the priority problem in a case.
	2. To practise identifying particular leader behaviour styles.
	3. To determine leader effectiveness.
	4. To develop a problem solution.
Facility	Large room to accommodate learners working around tables of six to eight.
Materials	Worksheet A: Case—Urban City Hospital.
	Worksheet B: Diagnostic Skills Worksheet.
	Pencils or pens.
	Blackboard and chalk.
	Experts' Diagnosis and Rationale.
Time Required	Two and one-half hours.
Group Size	Unlimited groups of six to eight.
Design	1. Each individual working independently and viewing self as an outside consultant is to:
	A. specify the priority problem goal in Urban City Hospital;
	B. identify the dominant leader behaviour styles used by George Jones and May Conte;
	C. determine the organizational effectiveness of Urban City Hospital under the management of George Jones and May Conte;
	D. develop a problem solution; and

Source: Adapted by permission from La Monica, Elaine L., *The Nursing Process: A Humanistic Approach*, pp. 385–394. Copyright © 1979 by Addison-Wesley Publishing Company, Inc., Menlo Park, CA.

E. write down detailed rationale for A–D. The rationale will serve as a basis for discussion in reaching group consensus (Step 2). Record individual determinations on the Diagnostic Skills Worksheet (30 minutes).

2. Following the individual diagnosis, each work group of six to eight should then reach consensus as to the problem goal, solution, leader behaviour styles of the characters, and their organizational effectiveness. The group should attempt to reach unanimous consensus. A group recorder must be chosen to record the group decisions (45 minutes to one hour).

3. Form into a total group and have each recorder share the work group's decisions and discuss rationale. Record decisions on a blackboard using the following suggested format:

PROBLEM/GOAL	LEADERSHIP STYLE		EFFECTIVENESS		SOLUTION
	Jones	Conte	Jones	Conte	
Group 1					
Group 2					
Group 3					

4. Refer to the discussion section and share the interpretations from the experts' diagnosis and rationale.

5. Discuss the experience.

(continued)

EXERCISE 2 *(continued)*

Variations

1. The individual diagnosis can be given as a homework assignment.

2. The exercise can be used only to identify leader behaviour styles and leader effectiveness, deleting the aspects of specifying a problem and developing a solution. This is recommended if the exercise is used after studying Chapters 4 and 5 and prior to completing Chapters 6 and 7.

Discussion Based on Experts' Diagnosis and Rationale: *

Problem/Goal

The problem is that the time clock policy is being applied inconsistently. There may be other potential problems in the case, but managers should identify the simplest, most tractable present problem and attack it. The time clock problem has the potential for erupting in such a way that people may be labelled dishonest or commanded to attend to a policy under threat; such would undoubtedly decrease productivity.

Leadership Styles

Leader behaviour is as perceived by others. George Jones exhibited low structure and low consideration behaviour—he was not constantly telling followers what needed to be done, how to do it, when to do it, and so forth. Neither was he observed involving staff members in two-way communication or in establishing interpersonal rapport.

Given the data provided, May Conte was considered to be high consideration and low structure because she was observed relating with the group, giving support and reinforcement, and establishing a team. One did not observe Conte defining facets of task

*The experts are K. Blanchard and P. Hersey. Oral presentation, School of Education, University of Massachusetts, 1974.

accomplishment. Even though the case did not portray Conte as high task, it could be assumed safely that such a manager also directed the task. It can be said, therefore, that Conte's basic style was high consideration and low structure, while her supporting style was high structure and high consideration.

Effectiveness   Organizational effectiveness under the management of May Conte and George Jones should be evaluated on the four variables discussed in Chapter 5. It is easy to create a halo or horn effect and judge a manager's overall effectiveness on the basis of one or two traits that are important to the evaluator. If the manager has the trait, then the manager is good in everything, and vice versa. This effect is tempered significantly by rating a manager on each variable, summing the ratings and dividing by the number of variables to get an average effectiveness rating.

Since the scale of −4 to +4 is arbitrary, it is simplest to say that Jones and Conte were +4 unless a negative point in the area is noted. Remember that manager effectiveness should be judged on the basis of the majority of who or what is being evaluated. There will always be the unreachable or the spurious.

Both managers were considered excellent. Jones, however, was slightly more effective than Conte. The case is designed to bring out the halo-horn effect because most groups see Conte as the more effective manager. Conte is certainly more likeable because one gets a feel for her personality and one knows more about her. Also, it is easy to say that Jones should not be credited with success because he does not do anything. Such a conclusion relates only to the evaluator's past experience with a low structure and low consideration manager who behaved that way because she or he did not

(*continued*)

EXERCISE 2 *(continued)*

care. LB4, however, is a legitimate strategy, and one must believe that Jones is behaving this way because that is what his followers require. To think otherwise would be aiming to perpetuate a previous negative experience. What would have happened to Conte's group if Jones had started to tell Conte what to do and sought invitation to the group's social events? This author sees beginning disaster.

Solution

The solution is to get rid of the time clock or to appoint a committee to make recommendations on this problem. Policies are placed because of a need by the majority of the group. Once passed, policies tend to live forever, even though this should not occur. Policies need to be re-evaluated to see if they best serve the majority of people in the organization. Is the policy what is needed given their level of maturity? A time clock is a high-task intervention and obviously is not required given the majority at Urban City Hospital. The hospital is running beautifully, and the work is getting done. There will always be a couple of freedom abusers as will there be obsessive workers. *Policies, however, must reflect the needs of the majority.*

Experts' Diagnosis of Organizational Effectiveness

Variable	Jones	Conte	Discussion
1. Causal Variables • Leadership strategies • Management's decisions • Organizational philosophy, policies, and objectives.	+ 2		Two points were deducted because Jones had a policy in the hospital that was abused. His management style was appropriate given the level of maturity of his immediate followers.
		+ 2	Two points were deducted because Conte did not attend to the time clock policy. While a policy is in effect, it

Experts' Diagnosis of Organizational Effectiveness

Variable	Jones	Conte	Discussion
			should be supported. If the policy seems inappropriate, do something to change it—it should not be ignored. Conte's management style was appropriate given the follower's level of maturity.
2. Intervening Variables • Employees' personal commitment to objectives and growth • Motivation and morale	+ 4	+ 4	The majority of people being led by Jones and Conte were happy, committed, and growing within the organization.
3. Output variables • Production • Costs • Earnings • Turnover	+ 4	+ 4	From the perspective of both managers, output was excellent. The hospital was not in the red, clients were satisfied, quality of care was very good, and people would rather work there than any place else. Conte's group also always got their work done.
4. Long-term and short-term goals	+ 4		Immediate output of the hospital was excellent, and there is no reason not to believe that this would continue. Jones's followers functioned effectively when he was in LB4—low structure and low consideration.
		+ 3	Output of Conte's group was excellent, and this would most likely continue. Conte's group was not able to function effectively without steady input from her, however, which is evident since Conte was appropriately

(continued)

EXERCISE 2   *(continued)*

Experts' Diagnosis of Organizational Effectiveness

Variable	Jones	Conte	Discussion
			in LB2 or LB3—high structure and consider- ation or high consider- ation and low structure.
Totals:	14	13	
	+ 4 = 3.50	+ 4 = 3.25	

Generally speaking, Urban City Hospital was an effectively running organization and both Conte and Jones were excellent leaders. There is every reason to believe that this time clock issue would be handled effectively and that both managers would continue to improve.

EXERCISE 2
WORKSHEET A: CASE—Urban City Hospital*

Janis Monroe, Unit General Manager (UGM) of Urban City Hospital, was concerned by reports of absenteeism among some of the staff. From reliable sources, she had learned that some of the staff were punching the time cards of fellow workers who were arriving late or leaving early. Monroe had only recently been appointed to head Urban City Hospital. She judged from conversations with the previous director and other administrators that people were, in general, pleased with the overall performance of the hospital.

Urban City Hospital has a reputation for quality medical care with a particularly good reputation in the areas of coronary care, intensive care, and emergency care. Located in the centre of Urban City, the hospital draws many lower socioeconomic families from that area but also services many clients from the suburban areas. The staff, with various educational backgrounds and training, were generally from the small state in which Urban City is located. In fact, a number of nurses are graduates of the hospital's nursing programme.

---

*Source: The author of this case is unknown. This author received it at the School of Education, University of Massachusetts, 1974.

It is thought that clients usually enter Urban Hospital for one of the following reasons:

■ High quality of care

■ Somewhat lower costs than other nearby facilities

■ Variety of medical care available.

George Jones, a long-time employee in the hospital, was administrator of Urban City Hospital. He generally left the staff alone, spending most of his time scheduling personnel, procuring funds and supplies, overseeing budget matters, and tending to related issues. Jones had an assistant, Rudy Lucas. When he needed to communicate with people in a particular area, George would just call them together or talk to an individual in the area and ask him to "pass the word". The latter was his usual approach.

Work situations at the hospital were quite varied. Some laboratories were cramped and less than adequate by some standards for the job required, whereas others more than met minimum criteria. Work efficiency did not seem to be related to these circumstances.

It should be noted that as far as hospitals are concerned, Urban City Hospital was one of the finest in the area. Clients generally liked their care and spoke highly of the facility.

The pay scale for the staff was low compared with other similar facilities. The average starting salary for a nurse was about £150 per week, and the age of the building made working conditions generally more difficult than might be desirable.

Judy Mulry, a first-year administrative assistant to the director, provided the data for this case. After she had been working at the hospital for a month or so, Mulry noted that certain members of the staff tended to seek each other out during free time and after hours. She then observed that these informal associations were enduring, built upon common activities and shared ideas about what was and what was not legitimate behaviour in the hospital. Her estimate of these associations is diagrammed in Exhibit 1. The hospital responsibility for each person is given.

The Conte group, so named because May Conte was its most respected member and the one who seemed to take responsibility for maintaining good relations within the group, was the largest. The group invariably tried to eat lunch together and operated as a team, regardless of the differences in individual assignments. Off the job,

(*continued*)

EXERCISE 2
WORKSHEET A   (continued)

Conte's group members often joined parties or got together for weekend trips. Conte's summer camp was a frequent rendezvous.

Conte's group was also the most cohesive one in the hospital in terms of its organized punch-in, punch-out systems. The time clock system for the staff had been started three years before by the Board of Trustees, which had been taken over by a conservative element. There might be times, however, when an individual staff member would have completed any specific responsibilities from one-half to three-quarters of an hour prior to the scheduled time to leave. If there were errands or other things to do in that extra free time, another member of the group would punch out for the one who left early. The "right" to leave early was informally balanced among the members of the group. In addition, the group members would punch a staff member "in" if he or she were unavoidably late.

Conte explained the logic behind the system to Mulry.

"You know we don't get paid as well here as in other hospitals," she said. "What makes this the best hospital to work in is that we are not continually bothered by administrators. When things are under control, as they are now, and the clients are satisfied, the top brass seems to be happy. It seems silly to have to stay to punch out on those few occasions when a little extra free time would be of help to you. Of course, some people abuse this sort of thing. . . like Marsha . . . but the members of our group get the job done and it all averages out."

"When there is extra work, naturally I stay as late as necessary. So do a lot of others. I believe that if I stay until the work is done and everything is in order, that's all the administration expects of us. They leave us alone and expect the job to get done. . . and we do."

When Mulry asked Conte if she would not rather work at a newer hospital at a higher salary, she just laughed and said, "Never".

The members of Conte's group were explicit about what constituted a good job. Customarily, they cited Marsha Jones, who happened to be the administrator's sister, as a woman who continually let others down. Mulry received an informal orientation from Marsha during her first few days at the hospital. As Marsha put it: "I've worked at this hospital for years, and I expect to stay here a good many more. You're just starting out, and you don't know the lay of the land yet. Working in a hospital is tough enough without breaking your neck. You can wear yourself out fast if you're not smart. Look at Manfred, the director of plant operations. There's a guy who's just

McBride
  Executive
  housekeeper

Harris
  Assistant
  housekeeper

Mulry
  Administrative
  assistant

Smith
  Accountant

Lucas
  Assistant
  administrator

G. Jones
  Administrator

Blanche
  Food service
  manager

Kane
  Dietician

Roberto
  Assistant
  laboratory
  manager

Conte
  Laboratory
  manager

Pellegrini
  Pharmacist

Luciano
  Inservice
  education

Venko
  Pharmacist

Impolitto
  Physical
  therapist

Nappa
  X-ray
  technologist

Roberts
  Controller
      Leighton
      Credit
      manager

Parant
  Business office
  manager

Manfred
  Director, plant
  operations

Patti
  Supervisor,
  admitting

Proctor
  Operating room
  supervisor

Roman
  Supervisor, records

Pope
  Assistant
  supervisor,
  RN

Johnson
  Supervisor,
  RN

Jones
  Supervisor,
  RN

Spaulding
  Discharge planner,
  RN

EXHIBIT 1: Urban City Hospital Staff, Informal Groupings

(continued)

EXERCISE 2
WORKSHEET A   (*continued*)

going to burn himself out, and for what? He makes it tough on everybody and on himself, too."

Mulry reported further on her observations of the group activities: "May and her group couldn't understand Marsha. While Marsha arrived late a good deal of the time, May was usually early. If a series of emergency situations had created a backlog of work, almost everyone but Marsha would spend extra time to help catch up. May and members of her group would always stay later. While most of the staff seemed to find a rather full life in their work, Marsha never got really involved. No wonder they couldn't understand each other."

"There was quite a different feeling about Bob Manfred, the director of plant operations. Not only did he work his full shift, but he often scheduled meetings with maintenance and other plant personnel on other shifts to consider better ways of getting their jobs done. He was also taking courses in the evening to complete the requirements for a degree. He often worked many Saturdays and Sundays. . . and all for 'peanuts'. He hardly got paid a cent extra. Because of the tremendous variance in responsibilities, it was hard to make comparisons, but I'm sure I wouldn't be far wrong in saying that Bob worked twice as hard as Marsha and 50% more than almost anyone else in the hospital. No one but Marsha and a few old-timers criticized him for his efforts. May and her group seemed to feel a distant affection for Bob, but the only contact they or anyone else had with him consisted of brief greetings."

"To the members of May's group, the most severe penalty that could be inflicted was exclusion. This they did to both Manfred and Marsha. Manfred, however, was tolerated; Marsha was not. Evidently, Marsha felt her exclusion keenly, though she answered it with derision and aggression. Marsha kept up a steady stream of stories concerning her attempt to gain acceptance outside working hours. She wrote popular music, which was always rejected by publishers. She attempted to join several social and literary clubs, mostly without success. Her favourite pastime was attending concerts. She told me that 'music lovers' were friendly, and she enjoyed meeting new people whenever she went to a concert. But she was particularly quick to explain that she preferred to keep her distance from the other people on the staff at the hospital."

"May's group emphasized more than just effort in judging a person's work. Among them had grown a confidence that they could develop and improve on the efficiency of any responsibility.

May herself symbolized this. Before her, May's father had been an effective laboratory manager and helped May a great deal. When problems arose, the director and other staff would frequently consult with May, and she would give counsel willingly. She had a special feeling for her job. For example, when a young lab technician couldn't seem to get off the ground, May was the only one who successfully stepped in and probably saved a promising young technician. To a lesser degree, the other members of the group were also imaginative about solving problems that arose in their own areas."

"Marsha, for her part, talked incessantly about her accomplishments. As far as I could tell during the year I worked in the hospital, there was little evidence to support these stories. In fact, many of the other staff members laughed at her. What's more, I never saw anyone seek Marsha's help."

"Willingness to be of help was a trait the staff associated with Conte and was prized. The most valued help of all was of a personal kind, though the jobs were also important."

"The members of Conte's group were constantly lending and borrowing money, cars, and equipment among themselves and, less frequently, with other members of the hospital staff."

"Marsha refused to help others in any way. She never tried to aid those around her who were in the midst of a rush of work, though this was customary throughout most of the hospital. I can distinctly recall the picture of the day supervisor trying to handle an emergency situation at about 3 P.M. one day while Marsha continued a casual telephone conversation. She acted as if she didn't even notice the supervisor. She, of course, expected me to act this same way, and it was this attitude in her I found virtually intolerable."

"More than this, Marsha took little responsibility for breaking in new nurses, leaving this entirely to the assistant supervisor. There had been four new nurses on her shift in the space of a year. Each had asked for a transfer to another shift, publicly citing personal reasons associated with the 7–3 shift but privately blaming Marsha. May was the one who taught me the ropes when I first joined the staff."

"The staff who congregated around Pat Johnson were primarily nursing supervisors, but as a group tended to behave similarly to the Conte group, though they did not quite approach the creativity or the amount of helping activities that May's group did. They were, however, all considered 'good' in their jobs. Sometimes the Johnson group sought outside social contact with the Conte group. Even though they worked in different areas, both groups seemed to

(continued)

EXERCISE 2
WORKSHEET A   *(continued)*

respect each other; and several times a year, the two groups went out on the town together."

"The remainder of the people in the hospital stayed pretty much to themselves or associated in pairs or triplets. None of these people were as inventive, as helpful, or as productive as Conte's or Johnson's groups, but most of them gave verbal support to the same values as those groups held."

"The distinction between the two organized groups and the rest of the hospital was clearest in the punching-out routine. McBride and Harris, Blanche and Kane, and Roberts, Parant, and Leighton arranged within their small groups for any early punch-outs. George Jones was frequently out of the building during any punch-outs, and he didn't seem to pay attention to such things like the time clock anyway. His assistant, Lucas, although always in the hospital, wasn't seen by many people. He seemed to 'hide' in his office. Jones and Patti had no early punch-out organization to rely upon. Marsha was reported to have established an arrangement with Patti whereby the latter would punch Marsha out for a fee. Such a practice was unthinkable from the point of view of Conte's group. Marsha constantly complained about the dishonesty of other members of the staff in the hospital."

"Just before I left Urban City to take another position, I casually met Ms Monroe (the UGM) on the street. She asked me how I had enjoyed my experience at Urban City Hospital. During the conversation, I learned that she knew of the punch-out system. What's more, she told me she was wondering if she ought to 'blow the lid off the whole mess'."

EXERCISE 2   *(continued)*
WORKSHEET B: Diagnostic Skills Worksheet

Problem (Individual Diagnosis) _____

_____

_____

Problem (Group Diagnosis) _____

_____

_____

LEADER BEHAVIOUR STYLE—Indicate dominant style with a checkmark for each character.

LEADERSHIP STYLE	INDIVIDUAL DIAGNOSIS		GROUP DIAGNOSIS	
	George Jones	May Conte	George Jones	May Conte
High structure and low consideration				
High structure and high consideration				
High consideration and low structure				
Low structure and low consideration				

EFFECTIVENESS DIMENSION—Indicate by a checkmark your determination of the degree of effectiveness or ineffectiveness for each character in the case.

	Ineffective							Effective
	−4	−3	−2	−1	+1	+2	+3	+4
INDIVIDUAL DIAGNOSIS:								
George Jones								
May Conte								
GROUP DIAGNOSIS:								
George Jones								
May Conte								

Solution (Individual) _____

_____

_____

Solution (Group) _____

_____

_____

EXERCISE 3   Diagnosing the Task

Purpose
To practise applying the Vroom and Yetton managerial decision-making model.

Facility
Large room to accommodate learners working in groups of six to eight.

Materials
Table 6.1: Management Decision Styles.

Worksheet A: Cases 1, 2, and 3.

Figure 6.2: Decision Model.

Blackboard and chalk.

Time Required
One and one-half hours.

Group Size
Unlimited groups of six to eight.

Design
1. Individuals working alone are to read each case on Worksheet A and choose the decision style they (as individuals) would use if they were the manager in each situation. Record responses and rationale for decisions in the spaces provided after each case (15 minutes).

2. After completing Step 1, individuals in each work group of six to eight should then discuss their choices for decision styles with each other, citing reasons for each selection. A recorder for each group should write down the group consensus by majority vote (30 to 45 minutes).

3. Following discussion in small groups, form into a total group and have the recorders share the group's decisions and rationale. Record decisions on a blackboard using the following suggested format:

	Case 1	Case 2	Case 3
Group 1			
Group 2			
Group 3			

4. In the total group, use the decision model to determine the diagnosis of each task. Refer to the discussion section and hold an open discussion case by case for each of the three examples. Compare decision styles arrived at by consensus (displayed on the blackboard) with those determined by application of the decision model.

Discussion

Case #1:

A. Quality	Yes
B. Manager's information	Yes
C. Acceptance	No
Minimum-time decision style	AI

There is a quality requirement, and since the ward sister has been in that position for ten years, it is reasonably certain that he or she would possess the information to make a high-quality decision. The nurses are only concerned that supplies be available; therefore they have to accept nothing. Once supplies are ordered and stocked, the problem is alleviated; people must live with the results. Since AI can be used given the task, all styles could be used depending on how much time is available. A ward sister who wanted to develop problem-solving skills in followers could use this task to accomplish it.

(*continued*)

EXERCISE 3   *(continued)*

Case #2:

A. Quality	No
B. Acceptance	Yes
C. Prior probability of acceptance	No
Minimum-time decision style	GII

There is no quality requirement since who attends the conference does not affect staffing. The decision must be accepted by the staff, and it is doubtful whether a supervisor's judgement would be accepted. The wise supervisor, therefore, would not use any style above GII and might even delegate the task (DI) by letting the nurses make a decision among themselves.

Case #3:

A. Quality	Yes
B. Manager's information	No
C. Structure	No
D. Acceptance	Yes
E. Prior probability of acceptance	Yes
Minimum-time decision style	CII

There is definitely a quality requirement; one location may be better than another. The manager needs to have the staff assess the district in order to make a wise choice. The problem is not structured because there is a subjective element in making the decision—"what feels right"—and the executive director does not know exactly what information is needed to make the decision. The case says that the staff are willing to accede to the director's judgement. CII is the decision style that would require the least amount of time but GII might be used, especially if the manager wishes the group to mature so that there is less of a need for manager reliance.

Variations

1. Teaching designs for inservice education and for ongoing units can be found in the original article: La Monica, E., & Finch, F. (1977). Managerial decision-making. *Journal of Nursing Administration, 7,* 20–28.

2. Further cases that have been adapted from business examples are in the following: Taylor, A. (1978). Decision making in nursing: An analytical approach. *Journal of Nursing Administration, 8,* 22–30.

3. Cases can be developed by individuals as a homework assignment and then discussed in small groups.

EXERCISE 3
WORKSHEET A: Case 1

You are the ward sister of a 50-bed orthopaedic unit that is the first group to move to a new wing in one week. You must estimate the supplies and medications necessary to stock on the new floor so that nursing care can be maintained smoothly and without interruption.

Since you have been ward sister for ten years on this unit, you have the knowledge and experience necessary to evaluate approximately what you will need. It is important that nothing be forgotten since surgery will be uninterrupted, and fresh postoperative patients will be arriving from surgery as well as preoperative patients needing preparation. Absent supplies may result in delayed surgery, confusion, frustrated personnel, and poor nursing care. It is your practice to meet regularly with your managerial subordinates to discuss the problems of running the floor. These meetings have resulted in the creation and development of a very effective team.

Decision style you would use: _____

Rationale: _____

_____

_____

Case 2

You are the nursing coordinator of 12 RNs in an intensive care unit. Their formal education, responsibilities, and experience are very similar, providing for an extremely close-knit group who share responsibilities. Yesterday, your director of nurses informed you that she would supply funds for four of your nurses to attend the Royal College of Nursing's Annual Conference at Brighton.

It is your perception that all of your nurses would very much like to attend, and from the standpoint of staffing there is no particular reason why any one should attend over any other. The problem is somewhat complicated by the fact that all of the nurses are active officers and members of the local organization.

Decision style you would use: _____
Rationale: _____
_____
_____

Case 3

You are the executive director of a small but growing Visiting Nurse's Association. The rural location and consumer needs are factors that contribute to the emphasis on expanded roles in nursing practice at all levels.

When you took the position five years ago, the nursing care was poor, and finances were slim. Under your leadership, much progress has been made. You obtained state and federal monies and personally educated your nursing resources. This progress has been achieved while the economy has moved into a mild recession, and, as a result, your prestige among your colleagues and staff is very high. Your success, which you are inclined to attribute principally to good luck and to a few timely decisions on your part, has, in your judgement, one unfortunate by-product. It has caused your staff to look to you for leadership and guidance in decision making beyond what you consider necessary. You have no doubts about their capabilities, but wish they were not quite so willing to accede to your judgment.

You have recently acquired a grant to permit opening a satellite branch. Your problem is to decide on the best location. You believe that there is no formula in this selection process; it will be made by assessment of community needs, lack of available resources, and "what feels right". You have asked your staff to assess their districts since their knowledge about the community in which they practice should be extremely useful in making a wise choice.

Their support is essential because the success of the satellite will be highly dependent on their willingness to initially staff and then educate and assist new nurses during its early days. Currently, your staff is small enough for everyone to feel and function as a team; you want this to continue.

The success of the satellite will benefit everybody. Directly they will benefit from the expansion, and indirectly they will reap the

(continued)

EXERCISE 3
WORKSHEET A: *(continued)*

personal and professional advantages of being involved in the building and expansion of nursing services.

Decision style you would use: _____

Rationale: _____

_____

_____

_____

Source: La Monica, E., & Finch, F. (1977). Managerial decision-making. *Journal of Nursing Administration, 7*, 21–22. Reproduced by permission.

The first two nursing situations were adapted from business examples. The original material is represented in Vroom, V. H. (1973). A new look at managerial decision making. *Organization Dynamics, 1*, 72–73. The third adaptation is originally found in Vroom, V. H., & Jago, A. G. (1974). Decision making as a social process. *Decision Sciences, 5*, 750.

EXERCISE 4 Term Project—Independent Case Analysis

Purposes

1. To carry out the steps of the problem-solving method.

2. To apply theory and research findings in analysing a health care or management situation.

3. To report the results formally.

Facility

A clinical setting where learners work with a group of people (professional and nonprofessional) in the delivery of health care.

Materials

Worksheet A: Evaluation of Written Assignment. Paper and a typewriter.

Time Required

Variable, but generally a term project.

Group Size

Not applicable.

Design

1. Each learner is to develop a personal case experience as a leader, a follower, or a consultant/advisor, and analyse what is happening (or has happened) in the situation.

2. The problem-solving method should be applied using individually selected theories to diagnose the system and choose the appropriate leader behaviour style.

3. The paper is a formal project. It must be typed double-spaced, using an approved style and format. References must be included and the paper's maximum length should be 30 pages.

4. Worksheet A: Evaluation of Written Assignment will be the basis on which the paper will be graded. This worksheet can be used as an outline for the paper.

Variation

Grade determinations can be adjusted according to teacher preference.

(*continued*)

EXERCISE 4
WORKSHEET A: Evaluation of Written Assignment

I.   Synthesis of Theoretic Framework Used in Analysis (10 points)

II. Problem Identification and Definition (20 points)

III. Problem Analysis (30 points)

IV. Alternative Actions with Anticipated Results for Each (20 points)

V.   Recommended Action and Rationale (10 points)

VI. Style and Format (10 points)

EXERCISE 4
Worksheet A *(continued)*

GRADING SCALE:

A+	100	B+	90–92	C+	80–82
A	97–99	B	87–89	C	77–79
A–	93–96	B–	83–86	C–	73–76
				F	72 and below

EXERCISE 5   Ethics—A Managerial Dilemma

Purpose   To gain experience in discussing and problem solving managerial dilemmas that have ethical implications.

Facility   Large room to accommodate participants seated in groups of six.

Materials   Worksheet A: A Managerial Dilemma.

                     Paper and pencil or pen.

Time Required   One hour.

Group Size   Unlimited groups of six.

Design   1. Participants should consider themselves as nurse managers. Using the managerial dilemma described in Worksheet A, ask participants to individually respond to the following questions:
                     A. What is the problem? Is there an ethical problem?
                     B. Who is involved?
                     C. What is the context?
                     D. Is anything interfering or possibly interfering with an individual's rights to freedom while away from the employing organization? Is privacy invaded or potentially invaded?
                     E. Are patients' rights involved? Are staff members' rights involved?
                     F. What alternatives exist?

                     2. In groups of six, participants should share and discuss their responses. Different perceptions between/among learners should receive particular attention.

Source: The content for this exercise was prepared by Elizabeth M. Maloney, author of Chapter 8 on Managerial Ethics. The exercise was put into the format used in this book by Elaine L. La Monica.

3. Small groups should report on their thoughts to the large group of the whole.

Variations
1. Step 1 may be done as a homework assignment.

2. Individuals or small groups can develop other managerial dilemmas and use the same process for discussion and problem solving. The dilemmas may be done as part of a homework assignment.

3. The entire exercise can be a written homework assignment that is carried out by individual learners or dyads.

EXERCISE 5
WORKSHEET A: A Managerial Dilemma

Due to the shortage of RNs, your agency employs nurses three days a week, in 12-hour shifts. Susan Jones, one of these employed nurses, begins to make small but important errors at work. She oversleeps and is often late enough that co-workers have begun to complain. Susan also seems irritable and tired.

It comes to your attention indirectly that this individual, Susan Jones, is working the same three-day pattern at another hospital. You feel strongly that it is only a matter of time before serious mistakes in patient care will occur. There are no regulations prohibiting such employment practices.

Part III

MANAGEMENT SKILLS

The purpose of Part III of this book is to discuss the skills managers need to carry out the steps of the management process—planning, organizing, motivating, and controlling—described in Part I.

Chapter topics are related specifically to management and leadership and are not meant to be all-inclusive. A conceptual framework is provided for each area, and discussion focuses on basic skills that can be augmented and amplified by the manager through experience and continued education. The basic management skills are discussed in separate chapters even though all of the topics are interrelated. Areas that are covered in this part of the book are: communication, change, power, teaching, interviewing, assertiveness, group dynamics, conflict resolution, time management, and performance evaluation. Experiential exercises for topics conclude Part III.

Communication

Communication is the most important skill in management and leadership. As a matter of fact, it is probably the most important concept in life. Communication occurs in every step of the management process; **everything** that a manager does involves communication—with followers, with superiors, and with associates. Kepler (1980) accepted communication as the most critical task that leaders must master; this position has been widely supported in research investigations (Anderson, 1984; Pincus, 1986; Tjosvold, 1984).

Chapter 9 begins with a definition of communication followed by a theoretic perspective on the communication process and the purposes of communication. Types of communications are then presented; how leaders communicate concludes the chapter.

DEFINITION OF COMMUNICATION

Communication would not be necessary if human beings existed in a vacuum, autonomously going through life in an impermeable cell; if they were born, lived, and died in isolation from others; or if individuals reached only within the self to fulfil needs. Humans are social beings who are dependent, independent, and interdependent on others in the environment. The only vehicle for reaching out to closely related others in the environment is communication through languages—both verbal

173

(French, Italian, German, and so forth) and nonverbal (body language and gestures understood by particular cultures) (La Monica, 1985).

Shannon and Weaver (1949) defined communication as all that occurs between two or more minds. Since behaviour is what other people perceive, all behaviour is communication, and all communication produces behaviour. Davis and Newstrom (1985) defined communication as "the transfer of information and understanding from one person to another person" (p. 424). It is the bridge between people. Johnson (1986) saw the concept as a means for one person to relay a message to another, expecting a response.

Communication, therefore, always involves a sender and a receiver. Even though Gibran (1951) said that one can verbally speak with self, communication in organizations always includes at least two people and both roles of sender and receiver. Davis and Newstrom (1985) aptly pointed out that a manager sending a written message to a follower has communicated the message only when the follower receives, reads, and understands the message.

THE COMMUNICATION PROCESS

The communication process involves five basic steps, portrayed in Figure 9.1 (Berlo, 1960; Chartier, 1981; Davis & Newstrom, 1985; Hein, 1980; Hewitt, 1981; Johnson, 1986; Long & Prophit, 1981; Miller, 1966; Pluckhan, 1978).

The sender has an idea and a wish to communicate that idea to another person. Davis and Newstrom (1985) cogently asserted that senders must think before sending a message; this step is critical. Once a sender has the idea clearly in mind, then the appropriate language(s) for communicating the idea must be selected. It is necessary to consider nonverbal body language as well as verbal language. Remember that management and leadership involve conscious, identifiable strategies for all behaviours. Choose language that has the highest probability for sending the message accurately and for being received accurately.

After a message has been encoded, it is transmitted by the sender over selected nonverbal and/or verbal channels. The receiver, who must be tuned into the sender's channels, receives the message and decodes it back from language to an idea. The receiver acts in response to the decoded message. The message may be stored or ignored; the receiver may communicate another idea back to the sender, or the receiver may simply perform a task in response to the message.

Whatever the receiver does in response to the sender's message is called feedback, which is a message sent back to the sender. The receiver then becomes the sender and the communication process begins again. Such circularity continues until communication ceases.

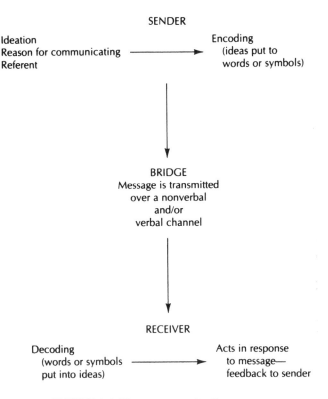

FIGURE 9.1 The communication process.

Evaluating feedback is a way for the sender to validate that the message has been perceived according to intent. The goal of any communication, of course, is congruence between the sender's intended message and the receiver's perceived message. Validation is essential because people communicate and perceive in response to individual attitudes, knowledge, and experience (Berlo, 1960). Perception is selective. Hence, what is transmitted on "the bridge" (Figure 9.1) may not be perceived as such. If necessary, further messages may be used to clarify original intent.

PURPOSES OF COMMUNICATION

The overall purpose for managing and leading is to motivate systems to accomplish goals. Communication to and with others is "the bridge" by which the manager and the human resources in a system relate. A manager must be able to communicate effectively in order to truly fulfil the role. Furthermore, it is the manager's responsibility to build and to maintain the bridge even though other human resources participate in its design and structure; the manager is the leader. Davis and Newstrom (1985) identified the following equation when discussing the purposes of communication:

The skill to work + the will to work = teamwork

It is evident from von Bertalanffy's (1968, 1975) general system theory that teamwork has a high probability for resulting in high quality, decreased costs, and high employee morale. Communication is the bridge on which teamwork rests.

The equation in the previous paragraph can be related to Hersey and Blanchard's (1988) theory on job maturity and psychological maturity. In the theory, the manager wishes to have human resources in a goal-directed system both willing and able. Then the system will accomplish the task because the people are intrinsically motivated and have the required knowledge and experience. Hersey and Blanchard's label *ability* seems parallel with Davis's (1985) term *skill*. Human resources who are not able must be provided with the information necessary to make them skilful. The attitude of willingness, which fosters teamwork, motivation, and job satisfaction, is communicated also.

Hewitt (1981) delineated more specific purposes for which communication processes are used. It is pointed out that the following purposes are rarely, if ever, used in isolation of one another.

1. To learn or to teach something;
2. To influence someone's behaviour;
3. To express feelings;
4. To explain one's own behaviour or to clarify another's behaviour;
5. To relate with others;
6. To untangle a problem;
7. To accomplish a goal;
8. To reduce tension or to resolve conflict; and
9. To stimulate interest in self or in others.

TYPES OF COMMUNICATION

There are two basic types of communication: verbal and nonverbal. Each type can be further broken into one-way or two-way communication. Figure 9.2 illustrates these points.

Everything that is written or spoken is included in verbal communication. Verbal interactions, between/among superiors and followers,

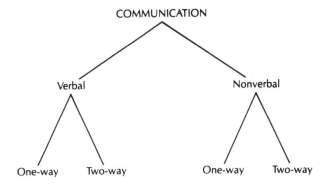

FIGURE 9.2 Types of communication.

associates and associates, nurses and patients, nurses and other members of the health care team, and so forth, form the bases for verbal communication. Written memoranda, bulletin board notices and meeting announcements, newspaper items, written requests, written assignments, and other similar items are also verbal communications.

Nonverbal communication is body language—it is unspoken and unwritten but nevertheless powerfully communicated through the body's behaviour. People nonverbally communicate through gestures, posture, eye contact, facial expressions, space variations, voice volume and tone, and so forth. Both the content and the intensity of interactions between or among individuals is greatly influenced by nonverbal communication. Differences between what a speaker is feeling and saying are often nonverbally communicated to the listener. Even though nonverbal communication amplifies, contradicts, and/or augments what is being communicated verbally, nonverbal communication, like silence, can stand alone.

James (1932) attempted to organize available information into a method for analysing behaviour. It was suggested that leaning the body forward communicated a positive attitude toward the addressee whereas leaning the body backward communicated a negative attitude. There are many early research findings in this area: Fast (1970), Hall (1966), Mehrabian (1968, 1969), and Scheflin (1964), to name a few. Walters (1977) concisely specified research findings in various nonverbal attending skills with effective and ineffective uses of each—Table 9.1.

One-way communication means that the message is sent from the sender to the receiver; it involves no feedback from the receiver back to the sender. Two-way communication uses feedback. Johnson (1986) continued this basic definition by saying that one-way communication occurs when the sender cannot perceive how the receiver is decoding

TABLE 9.1 Attending Skills

Ineffective Use	Nonverbal Modes of Communication	Effective Use
Doing any of these things will probably close off or slow down the conversation.		These behaviours encourage talk because they show acceptance and respect for the other person.
Distant; very close	Space	Approximate arms-length
Spread among activities	Attention	Given fully to talker
Away	Movement	Toward
Slouching; rigid; seated leaning away	Posture	Relaxed but attentive; seated leaning slightly toward
Absent; defiant; jittery	Eye contact	Regular
You continue with what you are doing before responding; in a hurry	Time	Respond at first opportunity; share time with them
Used to keep distance between the persons	Feet and legs (in sitting)	Unobtrusive
Used as a barrier	Furniture	Used to draw persons together
Sloppy; garish; provocative	Dress; grooming	Tasteful
Does not match feelings; scowl; blank look	Facial expression	Matches your own or other's feelings; smile
Compete for attention with your words	Gestures	Highlight your words; unobtrusive; smooth
Obvious, distracting	Mannerisms	None, or unobtrusive
Very loud or very soft	Voice: volume	Clearly audible
Impatient or staccato; very slow or hesitant	Voice: rate	Average, or a bit slower
Apathetic; sleepy; jumpy; pushy	Energy level	Alert; stays alert throughout a long conversation

Source: From "The Amity Book: Exercises in Friendship and Helping Skills," by R. Walters. In G. Gazda, F. Asbury, F. Balzer, W. Childers, & R. Walters (Eds.) (1977), *Human Relations Development: A Manual for Educators*. Copyright © 1977 by R. Walters. Boston: Allyn & Bacon. Reprinted by permission of the author.

the message. Two-way communication takes place when the sender receives feedback or validation. Referring back to the components of leader behaviour discussed in Chapter 5, structure involves one-way communication, and consideration involves two-way communication. Both types of communication are used for verbal and nonverbal inter-actions in leadership and management. Some examples of each are provided.

1. Sender gives verbal message and does not provide an avenue or time for feedback (one-way). *Example*: Manager announces a luncheon staff meeting by posting notices on bulletin boards.

2. Sender gives verbal message and provides an avenue for feedback but receiver does not comply with the request (one-way). *Example:* In-service educator sends out a memo-randum requesting staff nurses to specify one of three areas that they would prefer to be the topic of the next staff devel-opment meeting. A space is provided on the memorandum to respond. No responses, however, are received.

3. Sender gives verbal messages and waits for a response; receiver replies (two-way). *Example:*

Director to supervisor: "You have been using Primary Nursing on your unit for six months. Have you had any reactions from the clients?"

Supervisor to director: "Not specifically to Primary Nursing, but our recent survey of patient satisfaction shows that our clients are generally more satisfied now than they were when surveyed last year at this time."

The literature is replete with discussions of types of communications. Basics have been discussed in this chapter. The next section looks at how managers communicate.

HOW MANAGERS COMMUNICATE

Managers communicate in the following ways: telling, selling, partici-pating, delegating, listening, and giving and receiving feedback. Figure 9.3 portrays the relationship between how managers communicate and the Ohio State leadership model that was discussed in Chapter 5. The leadership model represents how leaders behave toward followers; leaders behave by communicating to (one-way communication) and with (two-way communication) followers.

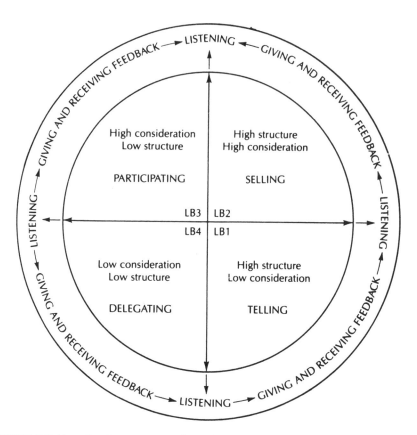

FIGURE 9.3 How leaders communicate in the Ohio State leader behaviour model.

Telling, Selling, Participating and Delegating

Hersey and Blanchard (1988) used situational leadership theory to specify and explain the active verbs for each leader behaviour style:

High Structure and Low Consideration (LB1) is referred to as "telling" because this style is characterized by one-way communication in which the manager defines the roles of followers by telling them what, how, when, and where to do the identified tasks. The manager guides and structures.

High Structure and High Consideration (LB2) is referred to as "selling" because most of the direction is provided by the manager, even though dialogue and clarification is encouraged. Through two-way communication and socio-emotional support, the manager tries to get the follower(s) psychologically to buy into decisions that have to be made. This is often called persuasion (Kipnis & Schmidt, 1985).

High Consideration and Low Structure (LB3) is called "participating" because the manager and follower(s) jointly share in decision making through two-way communication, discussion, group process, and problem solving. The manager reinforces, encourages, and calms.

Low Consideration and Low Structure (LB4) is labelled "delegating" because the style involves letting follower(s) develop and implement their own goal-accomplishing strategies. General supervision is minimal since the follower(s) are high in ability, willingness, and security.

Listening and giving/receiving feedback are represented in Figure 9.3 as a circle that runs around all of the leader behaviour styles. A manager behaves by communicating to and with followers in the leader behaviour style that has the highest probability for motivating them to accomplish the task. The manager should then listen to the feedback that is verbally and nonverbally provided by followers in response to the message given by the leader through one of the leader behaviour styles. Then the manager decodes the feedback and sends another message to the followers. This process occurs until communication ceases; hence, no further message is required at that time.

Listening

Listening involves the ability to tune into people, the environment, and the meanings of messages that are spoken and unspoken (La Monica, 1985). Davis and Newstrom (1985) asserted that one hears with one's ears but listening occurs in the mind. Listening is the ability to perceive the exact message that the sender intended, to the degree that is humanly possible. When messages are perceived accurately, better decisions result because the information inputs are sounder. Time is also saved when people listen because more—qualitatively and quantitatively—is learned in a given period of time. Davis and Newstrom further pointed out that good listening skills represent good manners and are forms of behaviour modelling that may enable others to listen more effectively in return. Table 9.2 provides guides for effective listening.

Giving and Receiving Feedback

Wang and Hawkins (1980) suggested that effective communication requires feedback. The purposes of feedback are to increase shared understanding about behaviour, feelings, and motivations; to facilitate

TABLE 9.2 Ten Guides for Effective Listening

1. *Stop talking!*
   You cannot listen if you are talking.
   Polonius *(Hamlet):* "Give every man thine ear, but few thy voice."
2. *Put the talker at ease.*
   Help the person feel free to talk.
   This is often called a permissive environment.
3. *Show the talker that you want to listen.*
   Look and act interested. Do not read your mail while someone talks.
   Listen to understand rather than to oppose.
4. *Remove distractions.*
   Don't doodle, tap, or shuffle papers.
   Will it be quieter if you shut the door?
5. *Empathize with the talker.*
   Try to help yourself see the other person's point of view.
6. *Be patient.*
   Allow plenty of time. Do not interrupt the talker.
   Don't start for the door or walk away.
7. *Hold your temper.*
   An angry person takes the wrong meaning from words.
8. *Go easy on argument and criticism.*
   This puts people on the defensive, and they may "clam up" or become angry.
   Do not argue: Even if you win, you lose.
9. *Ask questions.*
   This encourages the talker and shows that you are listening. It helps to develop points further.
10. *Stop talking!*
    This is first and last, because all other guides depend on it. You cannot do an effective listening job while you are talking.
    - Nature gave people two ears but only one tongue, which is a gentle hint that they should listen more than they talk.
    - Listening requires two ears, one for meaning and one for feeling.
    - Decision makers who do not listen have less information for making sound decisions.

Source: Davis, K., & Newstrom, J. (1985). *Human Behavior at Work: Organizational Behavior.* New York: McGraw-Hill, p. 438. Reproduced by permission.

development of a trusting and open relationship among people; and to give information concerning the effects of individual behaviour on others (La Monica, 1985). Feedback is also "the process of adjusting future actions based upon information about past performance" (Haynes, Massie, & Wallace, 1975, p. 260). It refers to the return of generated behaviour (Luft, 1984). Feedback can be verbal and/or nonverbal.

Feedback can be given and received in a variety of formal and informal ways. Time can be set aside at the conclusion of meetings for the group to discuss how it functioned. The exercises at the conclusion of this section of the book provide some paper and pencil instruments for encouraging this form of feedback. People can ask for feedback in formal or informal interactions. Performance appraisals at six-month intervals involve feedback; a simple comment like "you have really worked hard today" is also feedback. A casual, understanding nod (nonverbally) is feedback, too. Feedback, therefore, occurs whenever the receiver of a message sends a message back to the sender regarding the message received. In a casual sense, feedback is given constantly. In a more designed sense, however, feedback should be elicited and given by managers so that information on which decisions are based is as accurate as possible.

Napier and Gershenfeld (1985) believed that feedback involves upward communication, thereby making it a high-risk activity for followers. Giving and receiving feedback can do more damage than good by increasing risk and defensiveness if certain criteria are not followed. Managers can dampen this risk factor, minimizing defences and maximizing acceptance. This is accomplished if feedback is useful; giving and receiving feedback is a skill. The National Training Laboratory (NTL) Institute for Applied Behavioral Science suggested characteristics of useful feedback (*Laboratories in Human Relations Training*, 1971, pp. 27–28):*

1. *It is descriptive rather than evaluative.* By describing one's own reaction, it leaves the individual free to use it or not to use it as he sees fit. By avoiding evaluative language, it reduces the need for the individual to react defensively.

2. *It is specific rather than general.* To be told that one is "dominating" will probably not be as useful as to be told that "just now when we were deciding the issue you did not listen to what others said, and I felt forced to accept your arguments or face attack from you."

3. *It takes into account the needs of both the receiver and giver of the feedback.* Feedback can be destructive when it serves only our own needs and fails to consider the needs of the person on the receiving end.

4. *It is directed toward behavior which the receiver can do something about.* Frustration is only increased when a person is reminded of some shortcoming over which he has no control.

---

*Source: Adapted with permission from NTL Institute, "Feedback: The Art of Giving and Receiving Help," by Cyril R. Mill, pp. 18–19, *Reading Book for Laboratories in Human Relations Training*, edited by Cyril R. Mill and Lawrence C. Porter, copyright 1972.

5. *It is solicited, rather than imposed.* Feedback is most useful when the receiver . . . has formulated the kind of question which those observing can . . . answer.

6. *It is well-timed.* In general, feedback is most useful at the earliest opportunity after the given behavior (depending of course on the person's readiness to hear it, support available from others, etc.).

7. *It is checked to ensure clear communication.* One way of doing this is to have the receiver try to rephrase the feedback he has received to see if it corresponds to what the sender had in mind.

SUMMARY

Communication is the most important skill in management and leadership; everything that a manager does involves relating to others. It is defined as a process of passing information (messages) between or among people. Therefore, it involves a sender, a message, and a receiver who may give feedback to the sender on the message that was received. Since the purpose of managing is to motivate systems to accomplish goals, communication is necessary to give the system the skill to work and to facilitate the system's will to work as a team in goal accomplishment.

Two types of communication exist: verbal and nonverbal. In each type, communication can be one-way or two-way. Verbal communication involves the written or spoken word. Nonverbal communication involves body language. One-way communication means that a message is sent from a sender to a receiver, and it involves no feedback. Two-way communication also involves a sent message, but it includes feedback. Managers communicate by telling, selling, participating, delegating, listening, and giving and receiving feedback.

REFERENCES

Anderson, E. (1984). Communication patterns: A tool for memorable leadership training. *Training, 21*(1), 55–57.

Berlo, D. (1960). *The process of communication.* New York: Holt, Rinehart, & Winston.

Chartier, M. (1981). Clarity of expression in interpersonal communication. *Journal of Nursing Administration, 11,* 42–46.

Davis, K., & Newstrom, J. (1985). *Human behavior at work: Organizational behavior* (7th ed.). New York: McGraw-Hill.

Fast, J. (1970). *Body language.* New York: M. Evans.

Gibran, K. (1951). *The prophet.* New York: Knopf.

Hall, E. (1966). *Hidden dimension.* Garden City, NY: Doubleday.

Haynes, W., Massie, J., & Wallace, M. (1975). *Management: Analysis, concepts, and cases.* Englewood Cliffs, NJ: Prentice-Hall.

Hein, E. (1980). *Communication in nursing practice.* Boston: Little, Brown.

Hersey, P., & Blanchard, K. (1988). *Management of organizational behavior: Utilizing human resources* (5th ed.). Englewood Cliffs, NJ: Prentice-Hall.

Hewitt, F. (1981). Introduction to communication. *Nursing Times, 77,* center pages.

James, W. (1932). Study of the expression of bodily posture. *Journal of General Psychology, 7,* 405–437.

Johnson, D. (1986). *Reaching out: Interpersonal effectiveness and self-actualization* (3rd ed.). Englewood Cliffs, NJ: Prentice-Hall.

Kepler, T. (1980). Mastering the people skills. *Journal of Nursing Administration, 10,* 15–20.

Kipnis, D., & Schmidt, S. (1985). The language of persuasion. *Psychology Today, 19*(4), 40–44+.

Laboratories in human relationship training: Book of readings. (1971). Washington, DC: National Training Laboratory Institute for Applied Behavioral Science.

La Monica, E. (1985). *The humanistic nursing process.* Boston: Jones and Bartlett.

Long, L., & Prophit, P. (1981). *Understanding—responding: A communication manual for nurses.* Belmont, CA: Wadsworth.

Luft, J. (1984) *Group processes: An introduction to group dynamics* (3rd ed.). Mountain View, CA: Mayfield Publishers.

Mehrabian, A. (1968). Influence of attitude from the posture, orientation, and distance of a communication. *Journal of Consulting and Clinical Psychology, 32,* 296–308.

Mehrabian, A. (1969). Significance of posture and positions in the communication of attitude and status relationships. *Psychological Bulletin, 71,* 359–372.

Miller, G. (1966). *Speech communication: A behavioral approach.* Indianapolis: Bobbs-Merrill.

Napier, R., & Gershenfeld, M. (1985). *Groups: Theory and experience* (3rd ed.). Boston: Houghton-Mifflin.

Pincus, J.D. (1986). Communication: Key contributor to effectiveness—The research. *Journal of Nursing Administration, 16*(9), 19–28.

Pluckhan, M. (1978). *Human communication: The matrix of nursing.* New York: McGraw-Hill.

Scheflin, A. (1964). The significance of posture in communication systems. *Psychiatry, 27,* 316–331.

Shannon, C., & Weaver, W. (1949). *The mathematical theory of communication.* Urbana: University of Illinois Press.

Tjosvold, D. (1984). Effects of leader warmth and directiveness on subordinate performance on a subsequent task. *Journal of Applied Psychology, 69*(3), 422–427.

von Bertalanffy, L. (1968). *General system theory.* New York: Braziller.

von Bertalanffy, L. (1975). *Perspectives on general system theory: Scientific-philosophical studies.* New York: Braziller.

Walters, R. (1977). The amity book: Exercises in friendship and helping skills. In G. Gazda, F. Asbury, F. Balzer, W. Childers, & R. Walters. *Human relations development: A manual for educators* (2nd ed.). Boston: Allyn & Bacon.

Wang, R., & Hawkins, J. (1980). Interpersonal feedback for nursing supervisors. *Supervisor Nurse, 11,* 26–28.

Change

Everyone exerts influence on another—changes another—implicitly and explicitly, covertly and overtly. This fact is especially important in management and leadership. At an informal level, each time a person interacts with another by sending a message, the receiver's response to the sender is shaped by the message received. In a sense, the receiver has formed a response to fit a message sent by another. The sender, therefore, has influenced the receiver. To influence another means that a person elicits something from another or engenders something in another. This is change, and recalling from previous chapters, change is learning, and learning is change. Humans do not interact in a vacuum; people are part of a system that exerts constant influence over individual behaviour. This is a sociological perspective, of course, and contemporary management practice embraces this approach.

At a more formal level, managers are constantly attempting to change a system—to move the system from where it is in a given area (the actual) to where the manager wishes it to be in a particular area (the optimal). The processes for accomplishing this change were discussed in Parts I and II of this book. At this point, a major assumption (a given) of this book is that managers change people and people change managers. Changing a system is not simply one aspect of a manager's responsibilities—if one is managing and leading, one is changing people.

In the pursuit of knowledge and in order to understand more thoroughly leader behaviour and, therefore, be able to exert greater productive control over oneself and others, the following theories and concepts on change are presented and discussed in this chapter: force field analysis (field theory), levels of change, the change process, strategies of change, resistance to change, and combatting this resistance.

FORCE FIELD ANALYSIS

Lewin's (1951) force field analysis is a useful theory for understanding what is happening when a manager wishes to move a system from actual to optimal in a particular area. A problem was defined in Chapter 1 as the difference between actual and optimal (see Figure 1.3). This "difference" can be further explained using force field analysis. An example might help in explaining this concept. The problem definition is:

Actual: Staff on Ward 5 are continuously late to the day shift.

Optimal: Staff arrive on time for the day shift so that report can be given and the night staff released.

Problem: Lateness on the morning shift.

Goal: To have day staff arrive on time.

A manager wants to move actual to optimal, thereby eradicating the problem and accomplishing the goal. Figure 10.1 portrays this movement. Imagine the line symbolizing actual as a state that is suspended between forces that are working toward moving actual to optimal (driving forces) and forces that are working against the move from actual to optimal (restraining forces). Weights can be added to these forces to portray the relative importance of each force. Figure 10.2 contains such a force field.

If an equal amount of restraining and driving forces were operative in the field, there could be no movement in the actual line, which would be

FIGURE 10.1 Movement for goal accomplishment.

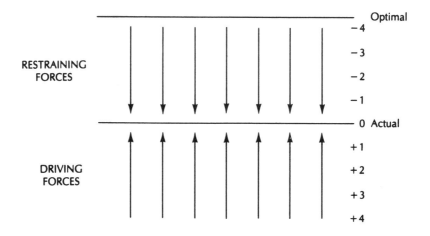

FIGURE 10.2 Force field.

in a state of equilibrium. If driving forces outweigh restraining forces, then actual would shift toward optimal. A manager can accomplish change, therefore, by either increasing and/or amplifying the driving forces or eradicating and/or suppressing the restraining forces. In either case, the actual line would move toward the optimal line. This type of discriminating analysis can provide the manager with items of concentration for the solution phase of problem solving.

Going back to the example, a force field analysis of the problem might look like that shown in Figure 10.3. The manager must assign a weight to each force—it is a relative figure that reflects one's best judgement on the importance of the identified forces. In the example provided, the driving

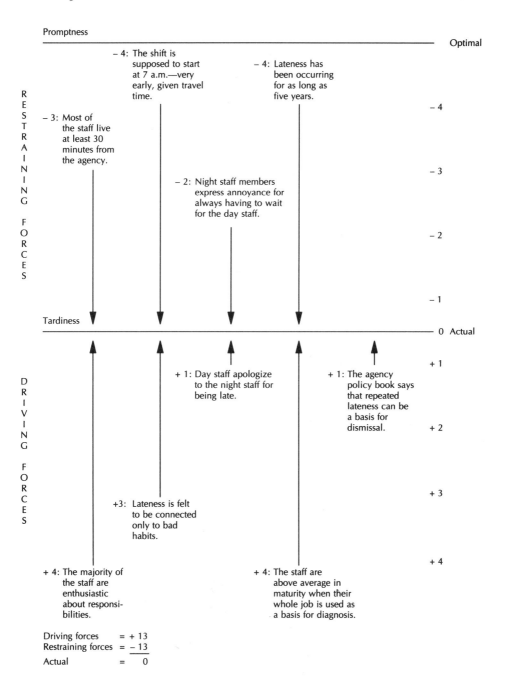

Promptness — Optimal

RESTRAINING FORCES

− 4: The shift is
supposed to start
at 7 a.m.—very
early, given travel
time.

− 4: Lateness has
been occurring
for as long as
five years.

− 4

− 3: Most of
the staff live
at least 30
minutes from
the agency.

− 3

− 2: Night staff members
express annoyance for
always having to wait
for the day staff.

− 2

− 1

Tardiness — 0 Actual

+ 1

DRIVING FORCES

+ 1: Day staff apologize
to the night staff for
being late.

+ 1: The agency
policy book says
that repeated
lateness can be
a basis for
dismissal.

+ 2

+ 3

+3: Lateness is felt
to be connected
only to bad
habits.

+ 4

+ 4: The majority of
the staff are
enthusiastic
about responsi-
bilities.

+ 4: The staff are
above average in
maturity when their
whole job is used as
a basis for diagnosis.

Driving forces   = + 13
Restraining forces = − 13
Actual   =   0

FIGURE 10.3 Driving and restraining forces in a case example.

forces equal the restraining forces. The manager can focus on either set of forces or both sets of forces to engender change. It is the belief of the authors, however, that the positive should always be amplified. When this is done, the negative looks less formidable. Force field analysis is a way to document this belief quantitatively.

A problem must still be analysed to diagnose self, the system, and the task and arrive at a leader behaviour style that has the highest probability for accomplishing the goal. The manager can then choose forces that become the content in developing the solutions. The forces relate to what is focused on in the strategy; how a manager focuses is the leader behaviour style. Any leader behaviour style can be applied to any force; *what* and *how* coexist as separate entities. Any single force or a combination of forces, even driving and restraining ones, can be the content of a problem solution. A manager is advised, however, to focus on the forces with the highest weights since they have the greatest impact on producing change.

LEVELS OF CHANGE

Once a problem has been analysed including a delineation of the force field, understanding the levels of change and change cycles can be useful. Hersey and Blanchard (1988) cited and discussed four levels of change: knowledge, attitudes, individual behaviour, and group behaviour.

Changes in knowledge tend to be easiest to make since they can result from reading a book or listening to a respected lecturer. Attitude structures are emotionally charged in a positive and/or negative way. They are, therefore, more difficult to change than knowledge. Moving to greater difficulty, individual behaviour comes next. A manager may know about and understand primary care nursing, for example, like it, and still not behaviourally apply it for a variety of reasons, like feeling uncomfortable with the behaviours. Group behaviour is the hardest to change because of the numbers of people. Trying to change customs, mores, and traditions is also difficult (Hersey & Blanchard, 1988). Figure 10.4 shows the four change levels.

Two change cycles are identified from the four levels of change: participative change and directive or coercive change (Hersey & Blanchard, 1988).

Participative Change

A participative change cycle occurs when change proceeds from knowledge to group behaviour, as shown in Figure 10.5. Followers are first provided with knowledge, with the intent that they will develop positive attitudes on a subject. Since research suggests that people behave on the

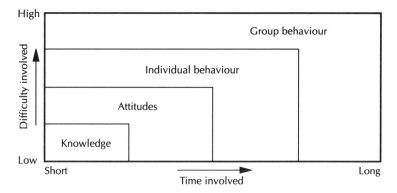

FIGURE 10.4 Change levels.
Source: This figure was adapted from one used by Paul Hersey and Kenneth H. Blanchard, *Management of Organizational Behavior: Utilizing Human Resources*, 5th ed., p. 4, © 1988. Reprinted by permission of Prentice-Hall, Inc., Englewood Cliffs, NJ.

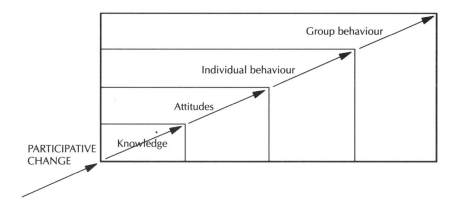

FIGURE 10.5 Participative change cycle.
Source: This figure was adapted from one used by Paul Hersey and Kenneth H. Blanchard, *Management of Organizational Behavior: Utilizing Human Resources*, 5th ed., p. 340. © 1988. Reprinted by permission of Prentice-Hall, Inc., Englewood Cliffs, NJ.

basis of their attitudes, a manager's desire is that this hold true. Once individuals behave in a certain way, these people become teachers and therefore influence others to behave accordingly—group behaviour then tends to change also. Participative change cycles can be used by managers with personal and/or positive power. Change is somewhat slow and evolutionary, but it tends to last because followers generally believe in what they are doing—the change is intrinsically imposed rather than extrinsically demanded (Hersey & Blanchard, 1988).

Directive (Coercive) Change

Figure 10.6 shows that directive change occurs in the opposite direction from participative change. Using position power, higher management gives directions about the mode of behaviour for the system of concern; actually an entire organization may be the focus. The dicta are set into place and followers are expected to attend to and abide by them. The hope of managers is that once followers see the plan in operation, they will develop positive attitudes about it and then gain further knowledge. This type of change is volatile; it tends to disappear when managers are not present to enforce it (Hersey & Blanchard, 1988). Position power is essential in this cycle.

Implications for Change Cycles

There is informal agreement among managers that participative change is the best. There are, however, specific instances when a leader must use a directive style. These instances relate to the implications for different leader behaviour styles (Haffer, 1986).

A directive style is necessary when an organization is in crisis and when people must behave in a certain way immediately in order for the organization to continue viably. The participative cycle is usually appropriate for followers who are average to above average in maturity, whereas those followers who are below average to average in maturity may need and prefer a directive cycle.

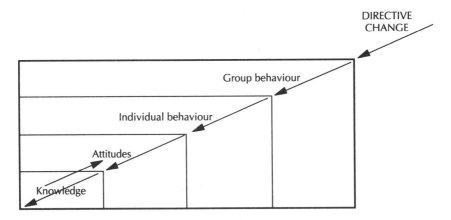

FIGURE 10.6 Directive (coercive) change cycle.

Source: This figure was adapted from one used by Paul Hersey and Kenneth H. Blanchard, *Management of Organizational Behavior: Utilizing Human Resources*, 5th ed., p. 341, © 1988. Reprinted by permission of Prentice-Hall, Inc., Englewood Cliffs, NJ.

These two change cycles can be used by a manager regardless of the maturity of the system. A participative cycle, for example, can be used with followers who require high structure and low consideration leader behaviour. The solution or strategy for accomplishing a goal simply starts with knowledge—the manager can require followers to attend lectures, to read, and so forth. A directive cycle can be used with mature followers even though such an intervention is risky. The benefits of this intervention must outweigh the probable consequences. If a manager used a participative change cycle with followers who required high consideration and low structure leader behaviour, the group might sit together and plan how they would like to gain the knowledge—maybe they could suggest guest speakers and so forth.

THE CHANGE PROCESS

The change process, as defined and discussed by Lewin (1947), Schein (1968), and Kelman (1958), lent further understanding to the experience of changing. It also can guide the manager in developing problem solutions that have a high probability for being effective because they are based on what is known about human behaviour. Lewin identified three phases in the change process: unfreezing, changing, and refreezing.

Unfreezing

Unfreezing involves breaking down the normal way people do things—interrupting patterns, customs, and routines—so that a person is ready to accept new alternatives (Hersey & Blanchard, 1988). Forces that act on and within an individual are "melted down" or "thawed". This phase involves externally motivating someone to take the journey toward goal accomplishment. (If necessary, refer back to Chapter 2 for a discussion on motivation.)

Changing

Once people are motivated to change, they are primed to accept new patterns of behaviour. Taking on these new behaviours involves changing attitudes. Kelman (1958) suggested three ways this happens: compliance, identification, and internalization.

Compliance occurs when change is forced by someone with position power who manipulates rewards and punishments. Identification means that role models for the new behaviour are available and individuals learn by identifying with them and trying to be like them. Internalization occurs when individuals are left to change on their own power. The need and desire to change is present, and people must learn the new patterns of behaviour by employing intrinsic resources. Self-learning and self-discovery fall into this last category.

Refreezing

Refreezing occurs when new behaviours become part of one's personality. The behaviour occurs because one has knowledge, positive attitudes, and experience with these new behaviours. Refreezing has occurred in followers when a leader has accomplished long-term goals whereby followers function effectively in a task when the leader is in LB4—low structure and low consideration. New behaviours should be positively reinforced by leaders to ensure that refreezing occurs within followers (Ferster & Skinner, 1957).

STRATEGIES OF CHANGE

Problems of change can be approached by individuals and groups in a variety of ways, and each strategy by each manager is unique—one's strategy did not, cannot, and will not exist again in an exact form. Strategies are usually a melding of a variety of methods, modes, and substrategies that are employed by the leader. Themes in change strategies, however, are evident. Olmosk (1972) identified and discussed the following seven pure strategies of change: fellowship, political, economic, academic, engineering, military, and confrontation. Some of these may sound familiar. In reality, a manager's strategy combines two or more of these pure strategies; however, one may stand out over the others.

Fellowship Strategy

Everyone is treated equally and emphasis is placed on team building in a group, getting to know group members, and building social bonds among members. This strategy is ideal for followers who have high social and esteem needs. Hence, it is ideal when LB3 is required by a system—high consideration and low structure. Getting people together at an informal dinner party to discuss new directions for a unit is an example of this strategy.

Political Strategy

A political strategy means identifying the formal and informal power structures. Once these structures are identified, efforts are made to influence those in power. The assumption of this strategy is that something will get accomplished if the influential people in a system wish it to be carried out. Directors who want to change from having nurses write separate notes to having them record on the progress notes might identify the key people in hospital policy-making and discuss with them individually prior to bringing the recommendation to a formal gathering.

Economic Strategy

Money talks! Emphasis is on acquiring or controlling material goods. With material resources, anything and anybody can be influenced—that is, bought and sold. Inclusion in a group is often based on possession or control of marketable resources. Fundraisers often employ this strategy.

Academic Strategy

In academia, knowledge or the pursuit of knowledge is the primary influencer. The belief is that people are logical, rational, and objective; that decisions will be based on what research suggests is the best path to follow. Emotions are not usually acknowledged in an academic strategy, even though it is known that people can never be entirely objective on anything. A bias that can range from narrow to wide always exists. In suggesting ways that result in more effective outcomes of patient care, a manager might cite research studies that support the identified goal for a unit.

Engineering Strategy

This method for facilitating change in people tends to ignore the subjects by attending to the surrounding environment. It is, therefore, a sociological approach with the belief that if the surroundings change, the people in those surroundings will also change. Health care planners use this strategy when designing patient units so that beds are in close proximity to the nurse's station. The logic is that if nurses are close to patients, they will spend more time "at the bedside", and the quality of care will increase.

Military Strategy

Physical force and real threats are the names of this game. "Ruling with an iron hand" and "running a tight ship" describe the climate in this environment. Position power is used in the form of threats and punishment if the leader's wishes are not obeyed. This is a high-structure strategy. The iron hand may be disguised in a warm, sweet velvet glove; all concerned, however, are fully aware that the iron fist exists and will be used if necessary. An example in this area is hardly needed. Be cognizant, however, that physical force may be used in hospitals by health care personnel on patients. Posey restraints are one such example. A manager must assess the need for such a strategy—it should be the last possible approach.

Confrontation Strategy

This approach induces non-violent and non-physical conflict within people. By doing this, a manager forces people to hear and see what is happening in a situation. The intent is that once people are aware of what is occurring, change will follow. People are often polarized into groups or cults as a result of this strategy. When groups feel that they will not or cannot be heard in any other way, this strategy is often employed. A union strike is one example.

RESISTANCE TO CHANGE

The literature on change is riddled with articles on the manager's responsibility for changing the health care system and on the role of the "change agent" (Beyers, 1984; Claus & Bailey, 1979; Lancaster, 1980; Levenstein, 1979; New & Couillard, 1981; Smith, 1970; Spradley, 1980; Stevens, 1977, 1985). Just the term *change agent* can arouse defensiveness in the subjects of change and can threaten the agent. No one really wants to change, because people like the comfort of behaviours that have worked in the past. Who wants to trade in their security blankets, and who wants to be "the one" to say that old security blankets must be burned in favour of new ones?

To say that people will change or that someone is a change agent engenders resistance. Davis and Newstrom (1985) explained this resistance as one of two types: resistance based on rational opposition to change and resistance based on emotional and selfish desires. In the former type of resistance, followers may believe and provide evidence substantiating their belief that the costs of the change exceed the benefits. The term · *costs* is used literally and figuratively. In the latter type of resistance, followers ignore the benefits of the outcomes of change because of their own personal needs and fears.

COMBATING RESISTANCE TO CHANGE

One of the best ways to combat resistance to change is by believing that change is a natural process that occurs continuously in everyone's life at every minute. The label of change is the insidious wart; the process of changing is simply cell regeneration—it happens without cognitive awareness, and no one really feels it. Managers should do their job, lead people, and forget labels. Change will happen.

Moving away from a philosophical but most important approach that should underlie the more concrete ways to combat resistance, various authors offer suggestions. Stevens (1975) suggested providing answers to the following questions that are commonly felt by those being changed: Will the change cause my position to be different? Will my status, power, job content, freedom, and so forth be affected? Will my financial status be improved? Schweiger (1980) stated that the manager should make the tangible benefits of change clear. Furthermore, the change should reflect the followers' existing values and ideas. Davis and Newstrom (1985) and Stogdill (1974) both believed that follower participation is the best way to gain support for change. This principle is also evident in the theory for diagnosing the task that was discussed in Chapter 6 (Vroom, 1973; Vroom & Jago, 1974, 1988; Vroom & Yetton, 1973). If followers must accept a decision, that is, if followers must do something in order to solve the problem, then they must be involved in problem solving.

SUMMARY

Change occurs constantly. Change is learning, and learning is change. Managers are constantly trying to move a system from one point to another—to solve a problem. Managers, therefore, are constantly developing strategies to change people and to solve problems. This is leadership.

The force field analysis theory is used to explain the forces that operate within the discrepancy between where a system is on an issue (the actual) and where a manager wishes it to be on that same issue (the optimal). Driving and restraining forces are identified, and change can occur by amplifying the driving forces, and/or suppressing the restraining forces.

The four levels of change are knowledge, attitudes, individual behaviour, and group behaviour. A participative change cycle moves from knowledge to group behaviour, and a directive cycle moves in the opposite direction. The change process involves unfreezing old patterns of behaviour, introducing a change, and refreezing the new mode of behaviour.

Strategies for change in a given situation are all unique and usually involve several approaches, with one or two dominant approaches. Seven pure strategies were identified and discussed: fellowship, political, economic, academic, engineering, military, and confrontation. Resistance to change can be expected. Philosophical and concrete approaches to combatting this resistance were offered in conclusion of this chapter.

REFERENCES

Beyers, M. (1984). Getting on top of organizational change: Part 1. Process and development. *Journal of Nursing Administration, 14,* 32–39.

Claus, K., & Bailey, J. (1979). Facilitating change: A problem-solving decision-making tool. *Nursing Leadership, 2,* 30–39.

Davis, K., & Newstrom, J. (1985) *Human behavior at work: Organizational behavior* (7th ed.). New York: McGraw-Hill.

Ferster, C., & Skinner, B. (1957). *Schedules of reinforcement.* New York: Appleton-Century-Crofts.

Haffer, A. (1986). Facilitating change: Choosing the appropriate strategy. *Journal of Nursing Administration, 16*(4), 18–22.

Hersey, P., & Blanchard, K. (1988). *Management of organizational behavior: Utilizing human resources* (5th ed.). Englewood Cliffs, NJ: Prentice-Hall.

Kelman, H. (1958). Compliance, identification and internalization: Three processes of attitude change. *Conflict Resolution, 2,* 51–60.

Lancaster, J. (1980). An ecological orientation toward change: Considerations for leadership in nursing. *Nursing Leadership, 3,* 12–15.

Levenstein, A. (1979). Effective change requires a change agent. *Journal of Nursing Administration, 9,* 12–15.

Lewin, K. (1947). Frontiers in group dynamics: Concept, method, and reality in social science; social equilibria and social change. *Human Relations, 1,* 5–41.

Lewin, K. (1951). In D. Cartwright (Ed). *Field theory in social science.* New York: Harper and Row.

New, J., & Couillard, N. (1981). Guidelines for introducing change. *Journal of Nursing Administration, 11,* 17–21.

Olmosk, K. (1972). Seven pure strategies of change. In J. Pfeiffer, & J. Jones (Eds.). *The 1972 annual handbook for group facilitators.* La Jolla, CA: University Associates.

Schein, E. (1968). Management development as a process of influence. In D. Hampton (Ed.). *Behavioral concepts in management.* Belmont, CA: Dickinson Publishing.

Schweiger, J. (1980). *The nursing as manager.* New York: Wiley.

Smith, D. (1970). Change: How shall we respond to it? *Nursing Forum, 9,* 391–399.

Spradley, B. (1980). Managing change creatively, *Journal of Nursing Administration, 10,* 32–37.

Stevens, B. (1975). *The nurse as executive.* Wakefield, MA: Contemporary Publishing.

Stevens, B. (1977). Management of continuity and change in nursing. *Journal of Nursing Administration, 7,* 26–31.

Stevens, B. (1985). *The nurse as executive* (3rd ed.). Rockville, MD: Aspen.

Stogdill, R. (1974). *Handbook of leadership.* New York: Free Press.

Vroom, V. (1973). A new look at managerial decision-making. *Organizational Dynamics, 1,* 66–80.

Vroom, V., & Jago, A. (1974). Decision-making as a social process. *Decision Sciences, 5,* 743–769.

Vroom, V., & Jago, A. (1988). *The new leadership: Managing participation in organizations.* Englewood Cliffs, NJ: Prentice-Hall.

Vroom, V., & Yetton, P. (1973). *Leadership and decision-making,* Pittsburgh: University of Pittsburgh Press.

Power

Managers and leaders must have knowledge about the phenomenon of power and be astutely able and willing to put its forces to work effectively in accomplishing specified goals. A manager without such ability and willingness is relatively impotent. The purpose of this chapter is to discuss power by first looking at various definitions of the concept. The types and sources of power followed by uses of power are then presented.

POWER DEFINED

Power is simply the exercise of control or influence over another person or over a group. Given the spirit of inquiry, however, researchers have been diligent in specifying more discriminating theories of social power.

Early theorists define power as intentional force or control (Adler, 1938, 1964; Ansbacher & Ansbacher, 1956, 1964; Bierstedt, 1950; Russell, 1938; Wrong, 1968). Others believe that power is inferred from observing the effects of interactions on those engaged. Simon (1957) called this an asymmetrical influence relation. Still another school of thought describes power as a social exchange (Adams & Romney, 1959; Blau, 1964; Gouldner, 1960; Harsanyi, 1962a, 1962b; Homans, 1958; Thibaut & Kelley, 1959). Contemporary theorists conceptualized power as one's potential for influencing another person (Hersey & Blanchard, 1988; Rogers, 1973; Nyberg, 1983).

TYPES OF POWER

Etzioni (1961) delineated two types of power: *position power* and *personal power*. He viewed power as one's ability to induce or influence behaviour of another person.

Position Power

Position power is derived from within an organization. A manager who can influence a group to accomplish a goal because of one's position in an organization is said to use position power (Etzioni, 1961). Hersey and Blanchard (1988) asserted that position power flows down in an organization—superiors delegate authority and responsibility to followers, who repeat the process again. In a sense, one's position power may be related to the amount of authority and responsibility that is given to and/or taken from one's superior. Simply having a position of management, therefore, does not always mean that one has position power.

An essential aspect of position power is the concept of authority. Bennis (1959) saw authority as "the process by which an agent induces a subordinate to behave in a desired manner" (p. 295). In a sense, authority is thereby granted to a leader—it is a legitimate right (Moloney, 1979) that may or may not be given by superiors in an organization. Authority is also granted by right of office—parent, manager, bishop—and by right of knowledge—lawyer, doctor, nurse (Francis, 1982). Power is the intrinsic ability to influence or control others; authority is a possession of granted or delegated power; leader behaviour or any behaviour is required in order to use or operationalize power. Power can only be communicated through behaviour.

Personal Power

According to Etzioni (1961), personal power is derived from followers. It flows upward to a manager and is the extent to which followers respect and are committed to their leader (Hersey & Blanchard, 1988). Personal power is informal power and position power is formal power. Informal power is seen as a day-to-day phenomenon since it can be earned from followers and also can be taken away (Hersey & Blanchard, 1988). Informal leaders in groups are examples of people who have been given and/or have taken personal power.

Reference has been made in the preceding paragraphs to power being given and/or taken. Each person has control over his or her own power—not complete control because of the social interacting system, but control nevertheless. Superiors give position power by delegating authority and responsibility to a manager; a manager earns the trust of superiors by behaving in a confident, able, willing, and trustful manner. Followers give personal power to a manager—they allow themselves to be led. A manager earns personal power by treating people with respect, by being fair, and by having and using the knowledge and experience necessary to lead others in accomplishing goals.

Power is a tension between or among people. To say that one is given power puts power in the control of the giver, not the receiver. To say that power is taken implies that the giver has none. Power can and usually does exist implicitly in all parts of a system. Behavioural evidence of its existence, however, is observable in different people at different times in various contexts. All people cannot exert control at the same time—not without a massive, dysfunctional power struggle.

Etzioni (1961) and Machiavelli (1950) believed that it is best to have both position power and personal power—to be both feared and loved at the same time. What happens if such a combination is not feasible? Hersey and Blanchard (1988) said that if one cannot have both position and personal power, then personal power alone is better than position power alone. This author tends to agree with this assertion—a manager soon becomes impotent if followers collectively choose not to follow. Machiavelli (1950) believed that a relationship based on fear of retaliation (position power) tends to endure longer than one based on love because the latter relationship can be terminated quickly with no sanction or price. Terminating the former relationship may carry a price. Even though contemporary managers do not follow Machiavellian guidelines as principles for their behaviour, Machiavelli made statements that all managers should understand.

SOURCES OF POWER

Power is derived from a variety of sources. These sources are also called power bases (Hersey & Blanchard, 1988; Stogdill, 1974). Each source is discussed separately, even though a manager may possess and use several sources at any given time.

> *Coercive Power*—This power source is based on fear. Compliance is induced because failure to comply will result in punishment or penalties (French & Raven, 1959).
>
> *Connection Power*—A manager with connection power has bonds with influential and important people within and outside of an organization. By complying with the manager, followers believe that favour will be gained with the important people connected with their leader (Hersey, Blanchard, & Natemeyer, 1979).

Reward Power—This is grounded on the belief of followers that the manager can provide rewards for them. Compliance with the manager's strategies results in gains such as increased pay, recognition, and so forth (French & Raven, 1959).

Legitimate Power—Based on a manager's position, followers believe that the manager has the right to influence them; their compliance follows. The higher one's position, the more legitimate power one possesses (French & Raven, 1959).

Referent Power—This source is based on the manager's personality trait; it is a part of one's personal power. A manager who is admired, liked, and identified with can induce compliance from followers (French & Raven, 1959).

Information Power—Information power is based on possession of or access to information. This can influence people because of the belief that compliance will result in sharing of information—followers often have the need to be "in on things" (Raven & Kruglanski, 1975).

Expert Power—Competence—knowledge, expertise, and skill—comprise expert power. Followers are influenced because their manager is seen as possessing the ability to facilitate accomplishment of their work assignments (French & Raven, 1959).

Even though these power sources are discussed distinctly, they are related to one another. Coercive power and reward power are two ends of the same continuum; a manager can give rewards to those who comply and can punish those who fail to comply. Such authority may be granted by the nature of a position, that is, legitimate power. Referent power and expert power are contained within a person and therefore can be labelled as personal power. Connection power can involve position or can refer to those connected to the manager regardless of the position held. Connection power, therefore, can be both position power and personal power. Information power also can be both personal and position power because a manager can have access to information given the nature of one's position or because of personal reasons. Table 11.1 provides a list of the sources and types of power.

USES OF POWER

Management literature is replete with suggestions that power should be an essential aspect of managers' personalities (Courtade, 1978; Heineken, 1985; Janik, 1984; Masson, 1979; Peterson, 1979; Shiflett & McFarland, 1978). Managers must therefore know about and exercise power.

TABLE 11.1 Sources and Types of Power

Sources of Power	Types of Power
Coercive	Position
Connection	Position and/or personal
Reward	Position
Legitimate	Position
Referent	Personal
Information	Position and/or personal
Expert	Personal

In addition to the sources from which power is gained, the manager can employ power strategies to accomplish goals.

1. *Rules and regulations* can be used to thwart attempted change by followers that is not in line with specified goals (Claus & Bailey, 1977; Scheff, 1961).

2. *Direct confrontation* in facts and figures is a manoeuvre that can be used to push toward a desired end (Peterson, 1979).

3. *Attractive personal attributes* can be amplified when selling a position since research has suggested that the more personable and attractive an individual is, the more influence that person has over others (Claus & Bailey, 1977).

4. *Coalitions* or group alliances, formed so that varied resources are pooled and a united front exists, can be used to overcome opposition (Claus & Bailey, 1977; Peterson, 1979).

5. *Social space* is a phenomenon Korda (1975) studied. The position and arrangement of desks and chairs can be a strategy to gain power. Sitting spaciously behind a desk while positioning a visitor or follower in a cramped area decreases the visitor's psychological comfort. Being situated in the "middle of things" also results in power because of access to information.

6. *Assertiveness* is a method of communication that powerful people know about and use in daily interactions. It is vitally important in management and is discussed in a subsequent chapter.

7. *Reciprocal open consultation*, in which managers and followers are open to be influenced by another. Equality and reciprocity are essential features of this strategy (Mulder, Koppelaar, de Jong & Verhage, 1986).

SUMMARY

Power is the ability to exercise control or influence over another person or a group. Two types of power exist: (1) position power, which is formally derived, and (2) personal power, which is informally derived. Authority is part of position power.

Seven sources of power are noted in the literature: coercive power, connection power, reward power, legitimate power, referent power, information power, and expert power. Various strategies for using power were discussed. These include confronting directly, falling back on existing rules and regulations, amplifying attractive personal attributes, forming coalitions, and using space powerfully.

REFERENCES

Adams, J., & Romney, A. (1959). A functional analysis of authority. *Psychological Review, 66*, 234–251.

Adler, A. (1938). *Social interest*. London: Faber & Faber.

Alder, A. (1964). *Social interest: A challenge to mankind* (J. Linton & R. Vaughn, Trans.). New York: Capricorn Books.

Ansbacher, H., & Ansbacher, R. (Eds.). (1956). *The individual psychology of Alfred Adler*. New York: Basic Books.

Ansbacher, H., & Ansbacher, R. (Eds.), (1964). *Superiority and social interest: A collection of later writings*. Evanston, IL: Northwest University Press.

Bennis, W. (1959). Leadership theory and administrative behavior: The problem of authority. *Administrative Science Quarterly, 4*, 259–301.

Bierstedt, R. (1950). An analysis of social power. *American Sociological Review, 15*, 730–736.

Blau, P. (1964). *Exchange and power in social life*. New York: Wiley.

Claus, K., & Bailey, J. (1977). *Power and influence in health care*. St. Louis: Mosby.

Courtade, S. (1978). The role of the head nurse: Power and practice. *Supervisor Nurse, 9*, 16–23.

Etzioni, A. (1961). *A comparative analysis of complex organizations*. New York: Free Press.

Francis, E. (1982). Using your power. *Health Services Manager, 15*(5), 7–9.

French, J., & Raven, B. (1959). The bases of social power. In D. Cartwright (Ed.), *Studies in social power*. Ann Arbor: Institute for Social Research, University of Michigan.

Gouldner, A. (1960). The norm of reciprocity: A preliminary statement. *American Sociological Review, 25*, 161–178.

Harsanyi, J. (1962a). Measurement of social power, opportunity costs, and the theory of two-person bargaining games. *Behavioral Science, 7*, 67–80.

Harsanyi J. (1962b). Measurement of social power in *n*-person reciprocal power situations. *Behavioral Science, 7*, 81–91.

Heineken, J. (1985). Power: Conflicting views. *Journal of Nursing Administration, 15*(11), 36–39.

Hersey, P., & Blanchard, K. (1988). *Management of organizational behavior: Utilizing human resources* (5th ed.). Englewood Cliffs, NJ: Prentice-Hall.

Hersey, P., & Blanchard, K., & Natemeyer, W. (1979). *Situational leadership, perception, and the impact of power.* La Jolla, CA: Learning Resources Corporation.

Homans, G. (1958). Social behavior as exchange. *American Journal of Sociology, 63,* 597–606.

Janik, A. (1984). Power base of nursing in bargaining relationships. *Image: The Journal of Nursing Scholarship, 16*(3), 93–96.

Korda, M. (1975). *Power: How to get it, how to use it.* New York: Random House.

Machiavelli, N. (1950). *The prince and the discourses.* New York: Modern Library.

Masson, V. (1979). On power and vision in nursing. *Nursing Outlook, 27,* 782–784.

Moloney, M. (1979). *Leadership in nursing: Theory, strategies, action.* St. Louis: Mosby.

Mulder, M., Koppelaar, L., de Jong, R., & Verhage, J. (1986). Power, situation, and leaders' effectiveness: An organizational field study. *Journal of Applied Psychology, 71*(4), 566–570.

Nyberg, D. (1983). Power over power. *Teachers College Record, 84*(3), 768–773.

Peterson, G. (1979). Power: A perspective for the nurse administrator. *Journal of Nursing Administration, 9,* 7–10.

Raven, B., & Kruglanski, W. (1975). Conflict and power. In P. Swingle (Ed.), *The structure of conflict.* New York: Academic Press.

Rogers, M. (1973). Instrumental and infra-resources: The bases of power. *American Journal of Sociology, 79*(6), 1418–1433.

Russell, B. (1938). *Power.* New York: W.W. Norton.

Scheff, J. (1961). Control over policy by attendants in a mental hospital. *Journal of Health and Human Behavior, 2,* 93–105.

Shiflett, N., & McFarland, D. (1978). Power and the nursing administrator. *Journal of Nursing Administration, 8,* 19–23.

Simon, H. (1957). *Models of man.* New York: Wiley.

Stogdill, R. (1974). *Handbook of leadership.* New York: Free Press.

Thibaut, J., & Kelley, H. (1959). *The social psychology of groups.* New York: Wiley.

Wrong, D. (1968). Some problems in defining social power. *American Journal of Sociology, 73,* 673–681.

Teaching

All managers and leaders are teachers. The purpose of teaching is to facilitate learning in another person. Learning is an intrinsic experience for the receiver. It denotes an integration of knowledge, attitudes, and experience in a person's past and present (La Monica, 1985). When someone learns, change occurs in that individual. The manager's primary goal is motivating others to accomplish goals. Managers should constantly be developing strategies to change what people would normally do if uninfluenced to what they need to do to accomplish the goals of an organization. To effect this change, followers must *learn* what the task requires; managers must facilitate this learning by *teaching*. Being a teacher is a subrole of being a manager. The intent of a teacher is to facilitate learning. The focus of this chapter is to discuss the teaching methods and processes that are available to managers.

Teaching can be formal or informal. Formal processes occur when teaching programmes are explicit—planned, organized, and evaluated. Staff development, continuing education, or in-service education are all common labels for teaching units in community care organizations. Such departments predominantly run formal programmes in the following areas: orientation, ongoing education, executive development, and patient education (Donovan, 1975; Littlejohn, 1980). Teaching formal programmes becomes the responsibility of managers when teaching units and their staff are not separate components in an agency.

Incidental teaching (informal) is also done through teaching units but

TABLE 12.1 The Problem-Solving Method in Management and in Teaching

Teaching	Management
Identifying learning needs	Problem identification
Stating the teaching priorities	Problem definition
Developing programme objectives	Problem analysis
Exploring teaching strategies	Alternative solutions
Recommending a programme	Recommended action

on a much smaller scale. This type of teaching is often called coaching (Darling & McGrath, 1983; Fournies, 1978; Hersey & Blanchard, 1988; Myers, 1966; Phillips-Jones, 1982). Coaching involves the daily or almost daily reinforcement and development carried out by a manager as an employee is guided through the learning (change) process.

Managers often participate in formal educational programmes, which may draw learners from an array of units within hospitals or which may be targeted to one specific group. Usually, however, managers have greater responsibility for on-the-spot teaching of their immediate system. In this sense, more informal teaching is involved. This type of teaching can be impromptu or can be planned, organized, and evaluated. The target system is usually those people who are led by the manager, or it may be only a portion of them.

Teachers can use the problem-solving method to increase their probability for effectiveness in their teaching outcome goals. This process can be thought about quickly, as in impromptu teaching situations, or it can be applied over a period of months. Teachers involved in formal and/or informal teaching would use the same process—the detail to which each would become involved as well as the amount of time devoted to the teaching project would differ. The problem-solving method in teaching is analogous to the problem-solving method that was presented in Chapter 1. Table 12.1 compares these two methods. The five teaching areas shown in Table 12.1 are discussed separately in this chapter.

IDENTIFYING LEARNING NEEDS

Identifying learning needs is the first step in the problem-solving method. Sovie (1981) called this "investigate before you educate". The process of diagnosis is appropriate for diagnosing learning needs of others and of self—O'Connor (1978) discussed the latter in detail. A learning need is identified by the difference between what a system actually knows (actual) and what one should know in order to accomplish a goal (optimal). Figure 12.1 illustrates this point.

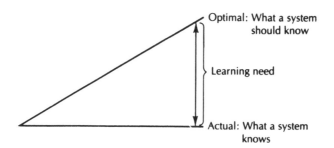

FIGURE 12.1 Identifying a learning need.

Suppose that a ward sister observed that during the past six months an increasing number of patients on chemotherapy protocols were received on the unit. The ward sister would first need to identify the system responsible for care of these patients. Then information would have to be gathered, examined, and interpreted from primary and secondary sources on whether the system had the knowledge and experience to provide quality individualized nursing care to patients on chemotherapy protocols. A comparison of the outside standard for quality care—what should be known and experienced according to experts—with what is known by the system would result in the specification of a difference that is the learning need. If no difference exists, then a learning need does not exist either. For example:

> *Actual:* A new chemotherapeutic agent is being used in treatment protocols. Nurses are used to working with clients who receive chemotherapy but the nurses are unfamiliar with the new drug and the different protocol and record-keeping system required for research purposes.
>
> *Optimal:* All nurses caring for patients on chemotherapy protocols must have knowledge and understanding of drug actions and side effects, administration regimen, special orders, nursing implications, and record-keeping systems.
>
> *Learning Need:* Knowledge and understanding in all areas of the new chemotherapeutic agent.

STATING THE TEACHING PRIORITIES

Systems of human resources most often have many learning needs. How does a manager decide what to teach first? Obviously, all learning needs cannot be priorities. Maslow's (1970) hierarchy of needs (refer to Figure 2.3) can be used to answer this question.

A health care manager should attempt to identify all of the learning needs for all followers given a specific context and period of time. The number of people who have the learning need in focus should be specified; this is the size of the system. Learning needs can then be placed into one of Maslow's five levels: physiological, safety/security, social/affiliative, esteem/recognition, and self-actualization. Table 12.2 provides a format for accomplishing this process; the procedure for stating teaching priorities is discussed more fully in the following paragraphs.

Learning needs involve two areas: (1) those needs essential to quality, individualized nursing care (areas of nursing's clinical responsibility) and (2) those which must be met for the development of the staff (teamwork). Recalling the descriptions in Chapter 4 of the needs in Maslow's (1970) hierarchy, Table 12.3 presents guidelines for classifying areas of nursing responsibility and teamwork needs with Maslow's five levels.

Once the format for stating teaching priorities has been completed, then those learning needs which are first priority—physiological needs—are immediate concerns. Second, third, and fourth priorities—safety/security, social/affiliative, and esteem/recognition—should be handled in that order. This is not to say that all physiological needs must be filled before a manager thinks of or plans for safety needs, for example. The size of the system becomes important. Small systems containing only a few people or maybe only one person with a specific learning need can be taught much more quickly and more informally than larger systems.

TABLE 12.2 Format for Stating Teaching Priorities

Learning Needs	Number of Learners (Size of the System)	Maslow's Need Level*
1. _____	_____	_____
2. _____	_____	_____
3. _____	_____	_____
4. _____	_____	_____
5. _____	_____	_____
$\downarrow$ n		

*In order of priority: (1) physiological, (2) safety/security, (3) social/affiliative, (4) esteem/recognition, (5) self-actualization.

TABLE 12.3 Maslow's Hierarchy of Needs Paralleled with Areas of Clinical Responsibility and Teamwork Needs

Maslow	Areas of Clinical Responsibility*	Teamwork Needs
Physiological	Nutrition Sleep, rest patterns Elimination Prevention of complica-tions Assurance of physiological status—health maintenance	Ongoing clinical education regarding physiological client needs Salary
Safety/Security	Comfort Exercise Personal hygiene Safety Environmental consider-ations Spiritual comfort and assistance Emotional support, coun-selling Teaching	Orientation Ongoing clinical education regarding safety/social needs of clients Working conditions Job security Company and admin-istrative policy
Social/Affiliative	Diversional activities Socializing and privacy	Ongoing clinical education regarding social/affiliative client needs Interpersonal relations—superiors, associates, and followers
Esteem/ Recognition	An amplification of what has emerged before, but considering the client's need for achievement	Ongoing clinical education regarding esteem/recognition client needs Executive develop-ment Advancement Status Job enrichment
Self-Actualization	The client can take care of self—allow it!	The system can take care of itself—let it!

*Source: La Monica, E. (1985). *The humanistic nursing process.* Boston: Jones and Bartlett.

When a large number of people require teaching in a certain area, then a more formal programme should be developed and priorities for the large programme should follow Maslow's theory. Managers, however, can meet a smaller system's needs concurrently. Also, do not forget to use other teaching resources: national, state, and local continuing education programmes; in-house programmes for people with similar needs; an associate "buddy" system (whereby two managers with the same staff needs split teaching responsibilities, and so forth). Creative use of resources is limitless.

DEVELOPING PROGRAMME OBJECTIVES

After a manager decides what is to be taught, several activities are necessary. The more formal the teaching programme, the more explicit should be these activities. Mager (1984), in his classic book, said that the goal of a programme must first be stated, followed by instructional objectives. The method to evaluate the programme's effectiveness should be directly related to the instructional objectives.

The example statement of a learning need that was presented earlier in this chapter is the goal. A description of the course content and procedures may also be given (Mager, 1984). An objective describes the desired outcome of the course, and an evaluation must elicit information on whether the desired outcome has been achieved. An objective should be observable and measurable.

The experiential exercises at the ends of Parts I, II, and III of this book contain purposes of the exercises. These purposes are more general than are terminal objectives discussed by Mager (1984). Purposes and a discussion of terminal objectives are presented so that the reader can make an informed decision on the exact type of objective that should be used in a programme. The degree of programme formality must be considered in making this choice. Applications for continuing education units (CEUs) require explicit terminal objectives and a means for evaluation; implicit objectives and evaluation criteria may only be required, for example, when reviewing colostomy care for a new graduate on the unit.

Mager's (1984)* steps for developing an instructional objective are as follows:

1. Identify the terminal behaviour by content name and specify the acceptable behaviour indicating that learning has occurred;

---

*Mager's programmed instruction on this topic is an easy-to-follow, quick-to-read, fun-to-do, and qualitative classic source for further learning.

2. Define the behaviour by stating the conditions under which the behaviour should occur; and

3. Specify acceptable performance.

For example:

Orientation Goal: To review pharmacology, dosages, and solutions.

Terminal Objectives:

1. To be able to pass a written 30-item objective pharmacology test at the conclusion of the orientation programme with 90% accuracy.

2. To be able to pass a written 25-item objective test on dosages and solutions at the conclusion of the orientation programme with 100% accuracy.

Explanation: The content names of the terminal behaviours are pharmacology in the first objective and dosages and solutions in the second objective. The condition under which the behaviour should occur is a written test at the conclusion of the orientation programme in both objectives. Acceptable performance is the accuracy level required. The evaluative test is the evaluative mechanism.

Evaluating a programme is a control process. Newman (1975) specified three types of controls—steering, yes–no, and post-action—as discussed in Chapter 7. The most frequently used method of evaluation is the post-action type, in which the evaluation occurs at the end of a programme. Leaders who run programmes over a long span of time, however, should employ a yes–no control such as a midpoint evaluation. An experienced teacher uses steering controls when evaluating a teaching approach by eliciting discussion when people question and by responding to learners' needs during a presentation.

There are many ready-made programme evaluation forms that can be applied, adapted, or used as a reference by teachers. The experiential exercises at the conclusion of Part III contain one such form.

EXPLORING TEACHING STRATEGIES

With objectives specified, the content and method(s) for achieving the objectives must be delineated—what will be taught and how it will be taught, our ever-familiar content and process.

Content

It is essential to delineate a detailed outline (at least) of the content that must be taught in order to fulfill programme objectives. This is the knowledge base. In the pharmacology example discussed in an earlier section of this chapter, the content would generally include common drug classifications and actions with details on the most commonly used drugs in each category. Specific actions, dosages, administration principles, and side effects would be discussed for the specific drugs. General principles of dosages and solutions would also be taught along with intravenous therapy procedures. The agency's medication procedure would also be content. Given these content areas, what is the best way to teach?

Learning Principles

Learning principles must be considered when deciding how to teach. The literature is replete with discussions of learning theory; a basic overview is provided in this section.

1. A learner must perceive (Bruner, 1960; Conley, 1973; Dewey, 1963, 1982; Ganong & Ganong, 1980).

2. Individual differences such as past experience, intellectual variations, and developmental maturation affect what is learned (Conley, 1973; Ginsburg & Opper, 1969; Wadsworth, 1984; Wertheimer, 1945).

3. The environment influences learning (Conley, 1973; von Bertalanffy, 1968; Watson, 1928).

4. The learner's degree of motivation affects what is learned (Conley, 1973; Hull, 1942; Maslow, 1970).

5. Behavioural reinforcement increases the probability that the desired behaviour will recur in another context (Bruner, 1960; Conley, 1973).

6. Repetition facilitates learning (Thorndike [cited in Bower & Hilgard, 1981]).

7. People learn by imitating others (Pohl, 1978).

Rogers (1969) believed that learning has a quality of personal involvement— it is self-initiated and self-reliant. He, therefore, offered the following learning principles that reflect these beliefs:

1. Human beings have a natural potential to learn.

2. Learning is greatly enhanced when learners perceive relevance in the content being taught.

3. Learning that threatens one's self-image tends to be resisted; reduction of external threats eases this effect and facilitates experience.

4. Learning is facilitated when the learner is involved in the process.

5. Self-initiated learning is most powerful—it is lasting and pervasive.

6. Learning the process of learning is most important because it allows one to be continually open to experience.

Within the framework of learning principles, a variety of instructional modes and media—teaching strategies—can be used to fulfill learning objectives.

Instructional Modes and Media

Conley (1973) distinguished modes from media by defining *modes* as types of conversations between the teacher and learner(s); *media* are devices or vehicles to amplify and/or augment various modes of teaching. Various modes and media are presented and explained (Conley, 1973).

Modes

Lecture—This mode is widely used in formal education systems and involves one-way communication from teacher to learners. It is useful when a large group has a particular learning need and is best when followed by small-group discussion to reinforce learning. Content that is in the cognitive domain is often taught by the lecture mode.

Group Discussion—This mode involves two-way communication between teacher and learners and between learner and learners. It is one of the best ways to teach content in the affective domain. Moreover, problems can be shared and support groups or teams can be facilitated. Keenan (1982) referred to this method as a "cooperative goal structure" (p. 487).

Panel Discussion—Expert panel members discuss a topic or an issue among themselves, and/or an interchange among learners and panel members may occur.

Seminar—One or two members present an issue or a problem, and the entire group participates in the discussion. A patient conference is one example of this method. The seminar is useful in self-learning peer groups.

Demonstration—Role modelling in an actual or hypothetical case is one example of demonstration. Any media can be used by the teacher to personify intended learning. Demonstration and laboratory instruction are especially useful when learning involves the psychomotor domain.

Laboratory Instruction—This mode involves learner self-discovery in a safe, low-risk environment. Simulations such as the experiential exercises in this book may be involved. The learner actually "tries on" what is being taught.

Team Teaching—Two or more professionals have responsibility for teaching a particular programme; this mode requires coordination and integration of efforts. Learners have the opportunity to hear different points of view on the same issue.

Media

Television—Closed-circuit and public television are becoming increasingly popular. Television specials on topics such as rape and life after death are also media that can be used by a teacher.

Programmed Instruction and Computer-Assisted Instruction—The learner is carried step-by-step through content, using teaching machines or books. The learner receives immediate feedback. Even though this feedback can be thought of as two-way communication, learning occurs better when group or individual discussion follows use of these media.

Motion Pictures—Films on specific content areas can amplify and demonstrate content.

Simulations—Laboratory learning and role modelling are involved in simulations. The preface of this book provides discussion of a rationale for this medium of instruction.

Pictorial Presentations and Printed Language—Pictures, figures, graphs, slides, and overhead transparencies are examples of this category.

Tape and Disc Recordings—These are most useful in seminars and group discussions. They also often augment slides, films, and other similar media.

Models—These are representations of objects needed in demonstrations, such as those used in teaching life support systems.

Different media can be used in the teaching modes. Selection should be guided by what would be most suitable given the objectives, what would be the most well received, and what is most enjoyable for the teacher. Do not overlook the latter statement—people are best at what they like to do, and there is no substitute for a teacher who enjoys what is being done. Learners catch the excitement.

RECOMMENDING A PROGRAMME

This step in the problem-solving teaching method is writing out the following in formal teaching situations and rehearsing the following to oneself in informal situations:

- Title of the programme (stems from the learning need)
- Description of the programme
- Objectives
- Outline of content
- Teaching methods: modes and media
- Faculty/teachers
- Evaluation methods
- Required textbooks and/or reading
- Bibliography
- Handouts (optional)

SUMMARY

Teaching is ubiquitous in management, and all managers and leaders are teachers. Because teachers facilitate learning in people, they change people.

The process of teaching can be informal or formal. Both types should follow the problem-solving method for teaching: identify learning needs, state the teaching priorities, develop programme objectives, explore teaching strategies, and recommend a programme. Details in each of these areas formed the basis of this chapter. All teaching must reflect knowledge and application of learning principles—what research has suggested has a high probability for facilitating learning as a product of teaching.

REFERENCES

Bower, G., & Hilgard, E. (1981). *Theories of learning* (5th ed.). Englewood Cliffs, NJ: Prentice-Hall.

Bruner, J. (1960). *The process of education.* Cambridge, MA: Harvard University Press.

Conley, V. (1973). *Curriculum and instruction in nursing.* Boston: Little, Brown.

Darling, L., & McGrath, L. (1983). Minimizing promotion trauma. *Journal of Nursing Administration, 13*(9), 14–19.

Dewey, J. (1963). *Experience and education,* New York: Macmillan.

Dewey, J. (1982). *Democracy and education: An introduction to the philosophy of education* (reprint of 1932 ed.). Darby, PA: Darby Books.

Donovan, H. (1975). *Nursing servicing administration: Managing the enterprise.* St. Louis: Mosby.

Fournies, F. (1978). *Coaching for improved work performance.* New York: Van Nostrand Reinhold.

Ganong, J., & Ganong, W. (1980). *Nursing management.* Rockville, MD: Aspen.

Ginsburg, H., & Opper, S. (1969). *Piaget's theory of intellectual development.* Englewood Cliffs, NJ: Prentice-Hall.

Hersey, P., & Blanchard, K. (1988). *Management of organizational behavior: Utilizing human resources* (5th ed.). Englewood Cliffs, NJ: Prentice-Hall.

Hull, C. (1942). Conditioning: Outline of a systematic theory of learning. In *The Psychology of Learning* (Part 2). Forty-first Yearbook of the National Society for the Study of Education. Chicago: University of Chicago Press.

Keenan, M. (1982). Collaboration in students: How can we improve it? *Nursing & Health Care, 3,* 486–488.

La Monica, E. (1985). *The humanistic nursing process.* Boston: Jones and Bartlett.

Littlejohn, C. (1980). What new staff learned and didn't learn. *Nursing Outlook, 28,* 32–35.

Mager, R. (1984). *Preparing instructional objectives* (2nd rev. ed.). Belmont, CA: D.S. Lake Pub.

Maslow, A. (1970). *Motivation and personality,* (2nd ed.). New York: Harper & Row.

Myers, S. (1966). Conditions for manager motivation. *Harvard Business Review, 44*(1), 142–155.

Newman, W. (1975). *Constructive control.* Englewood Cliffs, NJ: Prentice-Hall.

O'Connor, A. (1978). Diagnosing your needs for continuing education. *American Journal of Nursing, 78,* 405–406.

Phillips-Jones, L. (1982). *Mentors and proteges.* New York: Arbor House.

Pohl, M. (1978). *Teaching function of the nursing practitioner.* Dubuque: W.C. Brown.

Rogers, C. (1969). *Freedom to learn.* Columbus: Merrill.

Sovie, M. (1981). Investigate before you educate. *Journal of Nursing Administration, 11,* 15–21.

von Bertalanffy, L. (1968). *General system theory.* New York: Braziller.

Wadsworth, B. (1984). *Piaget's theory of cognitive and affective development* (3rd ed.). New York: David McKay.

Watson, J. (1982). *Psychological care of infant and child.* New York: Norton.

Wertheimer, M. (1945). *Productive thinking.* New York: Harper & Row.

Interviewing*

The interview is the primary procedure used in data collection—this can be for varied purposes such as gathering information on a client for the nursing care plan or gathering information from potential and hired employees. On a smaller scale, a manager can interview an employee informally regarding a situational event.

The process of interviewing is a human interaction during which information is needed and/or is shared. The interactors determine the exact process; the interview has a high interpersonal component and is also seen as a developmental procedure. Gathering data through an interview is a skill that is built on other skills. Observation, listening, and communication are particularly essential.

---

*Much of this chapter is an adaptation, replication, and expansion of the chapter on interviewing written by this author in the following source: La Monica, E. (1985). *The humanistic nursing process.* Boston: Jones and Bartlett.

WHAT IS AN INTERVIEW?

In many areas of the literature, the interview is recognized as a strategy. Kahn and Cannell (1964) conceived the interview as purposeful conversation. Schatzman and Strauss (1973) agreed with this description even though their perspectives were as field researchers in the areas of sociology and anthropology. Hein (1980) stated simply that interviewing was a human interaction during which information is requested and/or shared.

In discussion of nursing care planning, Bermosk (1966) defined the interview as a special time when the nurse focuses particular attention on the client and/or the client's system or family. Interpreting this definition in nursing management, the manager's client essentially is the employee or follower. The principles of interviewing apply in whatever situation is in focus. The eventual purpose of the interviewing process, according to Keltner (1970), is determined by the people involved in the unique process. Bermosk and Mordan (1973) believed that the interview involved sequenced, directed, and progressive changes in all participants of the interview process.

PURPOSES OF AN INTERVIEW

Perhaps the primary purpose for an interview has been explicated by Hein (1980) in discussion of nursing care planning. This author interprets Hein's original description for nursing management. In the practice of nursing management, verbal communication is used to interrelate with a potential or an actual employee with the intent of facilitating, educating, and/or restoring the person to his or her fullest potential. It is therefore a strategy for data collection to help the manager discern another's world, recognize areas requiring assistance or education, and plan an individualized programme that is aimed toward accomplishing the stated goals. Marriner-Tomey (1988) termed the interview as goal-directed communication. The following specific purposes for an interview are described. Hiring, promotion, and retention refers to employee interviewing; planning individualized care refers to client interviewing; and describing an event or collecting data refers to both.

Hiring

The interview that occurs prior to employment generally is aimed at collecting and sharing information: (1) to discern whether the person being interviewed has the behaviours necessary for success in the position; (2) to describe the position to the applicant; (3) to sell the job to the applicant; (4) to answer questions from the applicant; and (5) to ascertain the applicant's career commitment (Brydon & Myli, 1984).

The interviewer should be keenly aware of the laws governing discriminatory questions since legal action against health care institutions for unlawful pre-employment interviews is great (Poteet, 1984). Managers who must conduct interviews should check with the personnel departments in their organizations. Such offices have the guidelines and procedures readily available.

Promotion

Employees are often interviewed prior to the selection of a single person who will be promoted. In this instance, the pre-promotion interview is similar to the interview for hiring. Basically, one wishes to collect information from a candidate that could lead to the best decision regarding success in a designated position.

On the other hand, employees are interviewed upon promotion to collect information on their feelings, goals, and so forth. This type of interview can occur immediately following promotion, and/or can occur as a delayed interview one to two months following promotion in order to discover how the person feels in the new position and what, if any, particular assistance is required as a result of being in the position for a short time.

Retention

The interview that is conducted for the purposes of retention is most often called the performance evaluation. This topic will be discussed in Chapter 18.

Planning Individualized Care

This interview is often called the therapeutic interview (Bermosk, 1966). Bermosk (p. 205) described this as "a specific kind of communication which is in operation when the professional person (the nurse) focuses . . . attention on the patient (client, subject, group, family) and attends to the business of helping this person to better understand what is happening or what has happened to him at a particular moment in a particular situation . . . [The nurse] encourages him to describe his actions and to express his thoughts and feelings so as to identify needs and to establish goals which will help him to regain, maintain, or improve his health status".

Categories of information that may be obtained during the interview process refer to those areas of the PELLEM Pentagram (La Monica, 1985) (see Figure 3.1, Chapter 3, this volume):

1. Description of the happening;
2. Perceptions of the client regarding the event;
3. Behaviours of the client;
4. Attitudes and beliefs of the client;
5. Client feelings; and
6. Client values.

Questions and statements by the nurse or interviewers should have the purpose of generating information on the categorical guidelines as stated above. They should describe and elaborate, clarify, validate, substantiate, interpret, and compare. In a sense, the interviewer's comments should be levers by which the interviewee can find further self-expression.

Since the nurse manager is often the primary nurse, it is important to see the gathering of client information and the subsequent nursing care plan as an essential function in one's position. As the shortage of nursing personnel continues, as all sources predict, the nurse manager may be found to be the only professional nurse who is guiding nursing care; actual nursing care may be provided by technical nurses and other personnel. Though the above situation is definitely not the wish of this author, increasingly it has been observed as reality. As any good manager knows, contingency planning is the best way to meet demands in any situation.

Describing an Event or Collecting Data

Occasionally, situations occur in which a description is required for records, or just discussion. The purpose of this type of interview is to gather data on the attitudes, feelings, values, and perceptions of interviewees—or those involved in the situation. In a sense, the manager is collecting information so that decisions and actions can be based on a complete record of data that are considered to be valid. This type of interview is usually open-ended with the interviewer stating the situation and asking the interviewee to share what was thought to have occurred. An exit interview is another example of this type of interview.

TYPES OF INTERVIEW

The interview can be structured, semi-structured (Ivancevich, Donnelly, & Gibson, 1989), or unstructured. *Structure* implies that specific questions related to topic areas are posed by the interviewer and are asked of all people being interviewed for a specific purpose. *Semi-structure* is less rigid than the structured interview, allowing the interviewer more flexibility; only some questions are prepared in advance (Ivancevich, Donnelly, & Gibson, 1989). An *unstructured* interview relates to the fact that the interviewer's wording of questions is not specified prior to the interview. General content is identified; however, questions flow spontaneously from the interview context. Different interviewees may be asked different questions, depending on the flow of conversation and responses. The purposes of a specified interview may remain constant in all types of interviews. Also, the rule of thumb is that the more experienced the interviewer, the less structure is required in order to obtain the needed information.

Formal and *informal* are words used to further classify interviewing. Formality broadly represents the fact that time, place, and content are arranged prior to the interaction. It generally involves a longer period for interviewing than does the informal interview. Informal interviewing can be anything from a lengthy, unplanned talk over lunch to a five-minute, spontaneous interaction in a hallway.

CONTINGENCIES OF THE INTERVIEW

Schatzman and Strauss (1973) stated various contingencies that shape the interview's form and content:

1. *Expected duration:* How long is it expected to last? Will it be interrupted? Can it be extended or shortened as guided by the interaction?
2. *Single interview versus a series:* Is this the only one? Is there a series? Where in the series does this one fall?
3. *Setting:* Is this a public or a private place? What does the environment feel like? Is this feeling conducive to the interview's purpose? Is a specific conversational style more appropriate than others in this setting?
4. *Identities:* Is the interviewer an outsider or insider to the system? Can the interviewer and the interviewee be seen as part of the same group?
5. *Style of the respondent:* Is the interviewee comfortable enough to provide responses that are not overshadowed and skewed by anxiety?

In addition to these noted above, this author includes the following:

6. *Style of the interviewer*

7. *Harmony between the respondent's style and that of the interviewer.*

Steps in the Interview Process

The following guidelines are provided as a framework for conducting an interview:

1. The interviewer should do the necessary homework prior to the interview. Background information should be available for discussion. Notes on the content of the interview should be delineated. If the interview is formal, time and place should be stated. The interviewee should be instructed on what to study, bring, think about, or prepare.

2. The applicant/interviewee should be greeted. The aim is to quickly establish rapport and put the interviewee at ease. If introductions are necessary, they occur during this step.

3. The purpose(s) of the interview should be stated briefly.

4. Ground rules should be established—boundaries regarding the purpose, time limits, people involved, and so forth.

5. The next step is the exploration phase where data are collected and/or shared. Structured interview questions may be asked during this portion of the interview.

6. The interviewer should review notes to be sure that all information has been covered.

7. The interviewee should be asked if he or she has any questions. These should be answered as is feasible and within the responsibility and authority of the interviewer.

8. The interview should be closed. Follow-up, if indicated, should be specified regarding time and place—or procedure.

9. The interview should be evaluated to determine if it was successful in accomplishing its purpose(s) or unsuccessful in that the stated goals were not met.

PRINCIPLES OF INTERVIEWING

Kahn and Cannell (1964) viewed the interview as a lengthy conversation in which there are three conditions for success: accessibility, cognition, and motivation. The first requires that the information received by the interviewer be in a conscious, clear, and relevant form. It must relate to the purposes of the interview for each unique interviewee. Cognition requires that the person interviewed understand his/her role, and the reasons for data collection. Finally, motivation, or willingness to interact, is the major requirement for a successful interview.

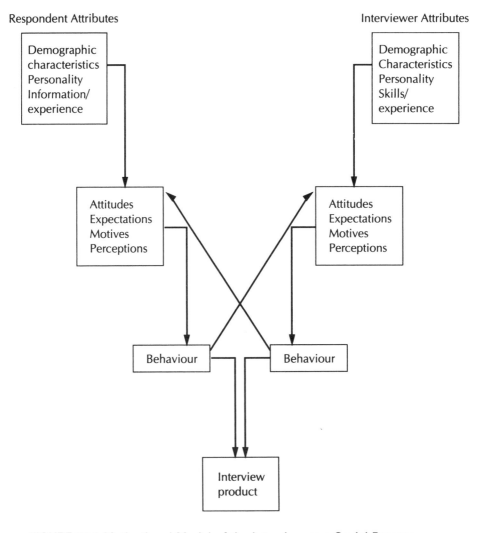

FIGURE 13.1 Motivational Model of the Interview as a Social Process

Source: *The Dynamics of Interviewing*, by R. Kahn and C. Cannell. Copyright © 1964 by John Wiley & Sons, Inc. Reprinted by permission.

Since client motivation has been observed as a paramount and necessary condition, much research by social scientists has been devoted to the area. In one example, Kahn and Cannell (1964) postulated both instrumental and intrinsic factors in their motivational framework (Figure 13.1).

It is easy to observe that the interview can and should be regarded as a complex social phenomenon. *Instrumental factors* of motivation focus heavily on the interviewee's belief that the results of the interview will have some positive effect on what happens to him/her. The second type of motivational factors, *intrinsic* (Kahn & Cannell, 1964), reflect the qualities of the interviewer. Receptiveness, warmth, understanding, and interest are all important. It is also pertinent to note that the principles of communication which were presented in Chapter 9 are also valid for a productive interview.

Certain principles for an effective interview must be integrated into interview techniques. Hein (1980, p. 26) explicated the following essentials; they are adapted for the nurse manager by this author:

1. An interview is effective to the degree that the manager creates an atmosphere that encourages and supports the employee's or potential employee's freedom of expression.

2. An interview is effective to the degree that the manager clearly establishes and understands the goals of the interview.

3. An interview is effective to the degree that the manager can relate to the follower without using value judgments.

4. An interview is effective to the degree that the manager examines, encourages, and clarifies mutual thoughts and feelings that may affect the issue and outcome.

5. An interview is effective to the degree that the manager consistently evaluates needs, goals, and the behavioural responses of the interviewee.

6. An interview is effective to the degree that the manager is able to evaluate his or her communication behaviour objectively in relation to the needs and behavioural responses evidenced by the interviewee.

7. An interview is effective to the degree that the manager employs and encourages the use of feedback in conveying, implementing, and evaluating goals.*

---

*From *Communication in Nursing Practice*, by E. Hein. Copyright © 1980 by Little, Brown and Co., Inc. Reprinted with permission.

In addition, Bermosk (1966, p. 207–210) stated other requisites:

8. The climate the manager creates within the interaction influences the substance of the interview.

9. Professional attitudes of warmth, acceptance, objectivity, and compassion are essential for effective interviewing.

10. The identification and clarification of conflicting thoughts and feelings of the participants lead toward a harmony of goals in the interview.*

The social process involved in the interview can again be noticed by studying the principles; the interpersonal facet involves the nurse interviewer, the client, and the interaction of both.

SUMMARY

It becomes clear that interviewing is a complex social process involving the principal interactors, purposes guided by principles of interviewing, and many extraneous variables that also must be considered. This chapter contained discussion of the primary purposes of an interview along with the types of interviews that can occur, depending on the preference and experience of the interviewer and the reasons for the interview. The section on interview contingencies included the generic steps of the interview process. The chapter concluded with principles of interviewing.

REFERENCES

Bermosk, L. (1966). Interviewing: A key to therapeutic communication in nursing practice. *Nursing Clinics of North America, 1,* 205–214.

Bermosk, L., & Mordan, M. (1973). *Interviewing in nursing.* New York: Macmillan.

Brydon, P., & Myli, A. (1984). After the interview: Who gets the job? *American Journal of Nursing, 84*(6), 736–738.

Hein, E. (1980). *Communication in nursing practice* (2nd ed.). Boston: Little, Brown.

Ivancevich, J., Donnelly, J. Jr., & Gibson, J. (1989). *Management: Principles and functions* (4th ed.). Homewood, IL: Irwin.

Kahn, R., & Cannell, C. (1964). *The dynamics of interviewing.* New York: Wiley.

Keltner, J. (1970). *Interpersonal speech-communication: Elements and structures.* Belmont, CA: Wadsworth.

---

*Reprinted with permission from *Nursing Clinics of North America*, by Bermosk, L. 1966, Vol. 1. No. 2.

La Monica, E. (1985). *The humanistic nursing process.* Boston: Jones and Bartlett.

Marriner-Tomey, A. (1988). *Guide to nursing management* (3rd ed.). St. Louis: Mosby.

Poteet, G. (1984). The employment interview: Avoiding discriminatory questioning. *Journal of Nursing Administration, 14*(4), 38–42.

Schatzman, L., & Strauss, A. (1973). *Field research: Strategies for a natural society.* Englewood Cliffs, NJ: Prentice-Hall.

CHAPTER 14

Assertiveness
by Patricia M. Raskin*

Although the concepts underlying assertiveness training have been gaining increasing popularity, the usefulness of the training model to the helping professions was first noted in 1949. Originally conceived as a limited form of behaviour therapy (Salter, 1961; Wolpe, 1958), assertiveness training has been found to have so many applications that it can no longer be considered as a single technique, but rather as an array of techniques designed to be effective with a large and varied number of

---

*Patricia M. Raskin, Ph.D., is an Associate Professor of Counseling Psychology at Teachers College, Columbia University, New York. She is currently Chair of the Department of Social, Organizational and Counseling Psychology. As a psychologist, she consults nationally with industry, health care systems, and educational institutions. Dr Raskin is a former coordinator of the Women's Task Force of the American College Personnel Association. She has been teaching assertiveness to various lay and professional groups since 1974.

target populations (Shoemaker & Satterfield, 1977). Most of the strategies and techniques, however, rest on three basic assumptions about human nature (Percell, 1977):

1. That feelings and attitudes relate closely to behaviour;
2. That behaviour is learned; and
3. That behaviour can be changed.

The purpose of this chapter is to define and discuss the concept of assertiveness and its application to the health care fields, especially nursing. Following a discussion of the definition and the theoretical aspects of the assertiveness paradigm, the goals and components of training are presented. The final section of the chapter is devoted to an application of assertiveness techniques.

WHAT IS ASSERTIVENESS?

It is not unusual for people to make the assumption that the words *assertive* and *aggressive* have the same meaning. According to most dictionary definitions, they are synonyms. Professionals who teach people how to be more assertive, however, make a distinction between those words. A continuum along which assertive behaviour can be rated is presented in Figure 14.1.

A *passive* communication is one in which an individual's needs, wishes, desires, or concerns are not expressed explicitly, usually because the sender believes the receiver of the message wants something different, or the sender consciously or unconsciously feels that the receiver is responsible for caretaking or mind-reading. An *aggressive* communication involves pushing one's needs, wishes, desires, or concerns onto another. In *assertive* communication, it is clear that in any given dyad there are two actors; two people may express their needs, wishes, desires, or concerns, and the opportunity exists for both to listen and respond to one another nondefensively. An assertive message is an open one that facilitates or enhances effective communication, understanding, and/or closure.

People are rarely completely passive, assertive, or aggressive; rather, messages are usually contextually bound. It is entirely possible, for

FIGURE 14.1 Assertiveness continuum

instance, that a staff member who is tongue-tied with a supervisor at work can be clear, direct, and confident with family members, children's teachers, and the mechanic at the local garage. The same supervisor, who is an effective, assertive administrator, may have difficulty returning clothing to a store, changing her mind about an order in a restaurant, or asking a family member for a favour.

WHY IS ASSERTIVE BEHAVIOUR DESIRABLE?

Both passive and aggressive messages are costly, sometimes only to the conversation in which they occur, but often to relationships as well. A passive communication leaves the sender or responder with thoughts or feelings that still need expression; this often leads to resentment or a belief that one is misunderstood or that what is said is of no consequence to the other. Even with resentment evident, its source may be unclear. A passive message is deficient in information, so it does not help another to understand the needs, wishes, desires, concerns, or limits of the sender as fully as may be possible. The hidden agenda in a passive message is often an unwillingness to take responsibility for the matter at hand, a wish to be taken care of, a set of unrealistic expectations ("If she really cared about me, she'd figure out what I need"), or an unwillingness to accept the consequences for one's own actions.

Aggressive communications have more directly observable costs to their recipients and therefore are not brought to the attention of the aggressor for some time. Aggressive behaviours tend to elicit "fight or flight" reactions; people either respond with equal or greater aggression or else they withdraw. In both cases, the aggressor ought to be sensitive to the fact that he or she is at least partly responsible for the reaction that occurs; that sensitivity, however, is exactly the trait that is in shortest supply at the moment of aggression.

Extended periods of passivity often lead to an explosion of aggression given the "right" stimulus—the straw that breaks the camel's back. In this instance, the time is long past for discussion and mediation. The statements, "I've had it up to here, and I quit", may reflect a build-up of resentment that resulted from passivity. It is clear that there is not much left to be negotiated when the person making those statements ends the discussion abruptly.

Assertive behaviour is desirable from at least two points of view: (1) It represents an open, mature, direct way of communicating that allows the other to learn about one's feelings and identify, while enhancing self-esteem (Percell, 1977), and (2) it is more likely to preserve effective interpersonal relationships than are either passive or aggressive behaviours.

ASSERTIVE BEHAVIOUR IN NURSES

The need for assertiveness training for nurses has been widely documented both in the field and in the literature (Clark, 1978, 1979; Kilkus, 1986; Marriner, 1979; Pardue, 1980). Initially, most of this documentation was limited to nurse leaders and managers. There is increasing evidence that staff nurses, particularly those in the beginning of their careers, can benefit from assertiveness training, especially since most nurses are female and are subject to all of the effects of sex-role socialization that operate to inhibit assertive behaviours (Angel & Petronko, 1983; Jakubowski-Spector, 1973). Further, when assertive behaviours are learned early in a nurse's career, the chances increase that they will develop over time. These mature behaviours enable one to be a better candidate for administrative positions and to be more effective in such positions (MacDonald, 1986).

The occupational characteristics of health care are changing (Kinney, 1985; Milauskas, 1985), thereby creating demands for greater responsibility and authority at all levels of the profession. Such demands alter both the role concept and professional self-concept of practitioners.

Super (1957) suggested that choosing a career is a means of implementing one's self-concept. Engaging in work that permits self-expression and is congruent with personal values may therefore be a function of personality and style as well as of exposure and opportunity. Although there are many reasons for choosing health care as a career, one primary motive is the opportunity to help others. Until recently, nurses, for example, have accepted the demands of unquestioning obedience, the maintenance of one's place in the hierarchy, and the dependence of subordinates on supervisors (Valiga, 1982). The historical roots of nursing have led to the widespread view of nurses as submissive handmaidens to consultants, doers rather than thinkers, and reactors rather than initiators (Keller, 1973).

It is reasonable to suggest that people attracted to the old view of nursing might have difficulty adapting to the new demands and altering their behaviour to include greater initiative, more persistence, and more autonomy in decision making. In fact, McIntyre, Jeffrey, and McIntyre (1984) found nurses to be sufficiently subassertive as a group and to be the ideal test population for their comprehensive assertion training package. Speigel, Smolen, and Jones (1985) reported that many medical students had less difficulty being aggressive with nurses than with authority figures or peers. They suggested that this finding might be interpreted in light of Hayes and Patterson's (1975) observation that medical students become domineering, while nurses become submissive early in multidisciplinary groups. There is some evidence, however, that this pattern is changing. Klein and Klein (1984) found that nursing graduates from 1980 felt more independent, felt that they had achieved more, and were more assertive than their 1974 counterparts.

It follows from the preceding paragraphs that there are several reasons assertiveness training is appealing to nurses: (1) Those nurses who are more comfortable in a reactive stance might need to become more at ease with and fluent in the skills and language of more active participation in their work; (2) those who support a professional and primary role for nurses might find the assertiveness training paradigm useful for facilitating the development of attitudes about responsible nursing behaviour as well as effective communication skills; and (3) those nursing professionals who are concerned with the public view of nursing might find a way of communicating their attitudes and expectations more clearly.

GOALS OF ASSERTIVENESS TRAINING

Alberti and Emmons (1986) pointed out that the goals of assertiveness training are to teach people how to exercise their rights, to assist them in developing an expanded repertoire of behaviours, and to help them to act in their own best interest. Because assertiveness training is a behavioural (rather than insight-oriented) method, the goals are inductive rather than deductive. There are three levels at which assertiveness occurs: techniques, response style, and lifestyle. Reinforcement occurs as one learns and practises the techniques of assertion. Making requests, saying no, accepting compliments, and expressing concern become easier, rewarding the individual with increased self-respect and improved interactions. In turn, this may lead to an assertive response style, in which being assertive becomes more natural and is characterized by open verbal and nonverbal expression. At the most complex cognitive level, one may develop an assertive lifestyle, one that includes both intra- and interpersonal awareness. If assertiveness training "takes" at this level, the end result is quite similar to the goals of many forms of humanistic psychotherapy: ease in interpersonal relationships; congruence among thoughts, feelings, and behaviours; and a willingness to accept responsibility for one's actions as well as to accept the consequences of those actions.

COMPONENTS OF ASSERTIVENESS

Assertive behaviours can be broadly separated into two components: verbal and nonverbal. In order for a communication to be categorized as assertive, both components must be present. It is entirely possible that an individual says all the right words, for example, "I'd like the sweater back that you borrowed", but does so in either such an aggressive way (hands on hips, eyes glaring, edge to the voice) or in such a passive way (small voice, downcast eyes, pleading tone) that the receiver of the message is either offended or uncomfortable. In order for a message to be truly assertive, the words and the music behind the words have to go together. People have learned, for instance, that tenderness is not expressed in a loud tone of voice, that intimate conversations do not take place between two people who are 15 feet apart, and that anger is not expressed with a smile. As a matter of fact, when the words and the music do not go together, it is difficult to know what to believe. Confusion results, and the natural response of the listener to this mixed message is avoidance, withdrawal, anger, or some other form of interpersonal distance.

Nonverbal Components

Serber (1977) suggested that the nonverbal components of behaviour are:

> Loudness of voice,
> Fluency of spoken words,
> Eye contact,
> Facial expression,
> Body expression, and
> Distance from person with whom one is interacting (p. 69).

Loudness of Voice. Neither screaming nor whispering is assertive. Tone of voice does not depend on the content of the message sent. An assertive tone should be loud and firm so that it is heard clearly; it should not, however, be so loud that it is assaultive to the ear of the receiver.

Fluency. Fluency of spoken words also does not depend on the content of the message. People who use too many pauses or "filler" words such as *uh, er, huh, you know, like,* and so forth, are likely to be perceived as hesitant, whereas people who speak too quickly are often experienced as overwhelming. A moderate, unbroken rate of speech is assertive.

Eye Contact. It is impossible to be assertive when not looking at the intended receiver of one's message. Without eye contact, there is no way of gauging a response, and the receiver of a message is forced to intrude on the sender in order to give feedback about the communication. Staring or glowering, of course, are intrusive by their very nature. Assertive eye contact means that one is able to look at the receiver's face more or less continuously without such intensity that the receiver's gaze is challenged.

Facial Expression. People who giggle when angry or frown when saying loving, affectionate words sabotage the content of their messages. When people are angry, they do not smile; when expressing appreciation, they do. Although facial expression is hard to measure or describe, most people have been socialized to be capable of choosing congruent facial expressions for the meaning of their words. It is often a signal of discomfort or anxiety when one is unable to get the words and music together; since congruence and anxiety are mutually exclusive reactions, being congruent may help to reduce the anxiety.

Body Expression. Like facial expression, how one stands, sits, or moves conveys a complex series of attitudes. A person who is slouching can be perceived as hostile, uninterested, or frightened. Crossed arms may give the impression that one is guarded, armed, or unreceptive. Hands on hips may indicate a combative, patronizing attitude, while a rigid, wooden posture can indicate fear. People who are assertive in their body expression seem relaxed but do not slouch, stand straight without being rigid, and use their hands and shoulders to embellish their conversation without being too forceful or abrupt.

Distance. How far away one stands from the person while interacting varies from culture to culture and individual to individual. The term *bubble* has been applied to the invisible boundary that people use to protect themselves from intrusion (Sommer, 1969). In southern Europe, for example, one may become uncomfortably aware of how close people stand when engaging in a conversation. It is natural for Americans to back away in order to feel more comfortable—to protect their bubble. Although the example just given is of a cultural difference rather than interpersonal style, it is possible to experience new European friends as aggressive or intrusive. The other extreme involves too much distance. A meaningful interpersonal dialogue usually does not occur at a distance of five feet. People who are assertive in their distance from others stand close enough so that not much can pass between them and their receiver (like another person, for instance) but not so close they break the receiver's bubble.

Verbal Components

What is said is just as important as how one says it. It is unlikely, for instance, that someone who makes an unclear statement or request will get an appropriate response. It may not be that the listener is unresponsive, but rather that the message is too ambiguous for a lucid answer. Cooley and Hollandsworth (1977) suggested three verbal components of assertive statements:

1. Saying "no" or taking a stand;
2. Asking favours or asserting rights; and
3. Expressing feelings.

Saying no. Assertive statements can be either initiations or reactions. There are ways to say no assertively in response to another's request or demand. Many people feel backed into a corner when asked to do something that they do not want to do. "I just couldn't say no" is a common complaint. The reasons people cannot or will not say no vary; some are afraid of the other's anger or disapproval; some are afraid of hurting others' feelings; some are afraid of rejection; and some feel that to say no would violate their self-concept as "nice". Nevertheless, everyone wants to or needs to refuse a favour or a request from time to time; if saying no is uncomfortable, one may unintentionally become aggressive or overjustify a refusal. A crucial aspect of saying no assertively is that the refusal be understood and believed. Saying too much makes one less convincing while saying too little may seem rejecting. The object is to say no firmly and uncompromisingly while acknowledging the other's right to ask. Saying no assertively means that one can refuse a request and give a reason for refusing the request while indicating that the other person has been heard: "I appreciate your need to change shifts with me, but I can't on Thursday because I already have plans."

Taking a Stand. This component of assertion may be either an initiation or a response to a situation. The key elements in this area are the clarity of one's position, the self-respect with which such a position is stated, and an understanding of the other's position: "I know that you believe that Mrs Lloyd is recovering; I'm not convinced, however, that she's ready for discharge, and I will not support her release."

Asking Favours. Many people believe that they do not have the right to ask for a favour. This is not true. People do not have the right to get everything they request, but permission to ask is unnecessary. If one has trouble asking for favours, it sometimes means that more meaning may be attached to a refusal than is appropriate in the circumstance: "If he says no to this, it means he doesn't love me." Or it may mean that one will feel guilty and obligated for asking: "If she lends me her car, I'll have to do whatever she wants whenever she wants it done." When asking for favours, being assertive means stating the problem clearly and making a specific request. How long to persist with the request is a matter of judgement; the request should end with either its being granted or with the understanding of why it cannot or would not be granted. One should not end a request before this point has been reached.

Asserting Rights. In our society, no human being has the right to take advantage of another; every human being has the right to speak. Differences in power between two individuals do not alter those fundamental rights, although sometimes the less powerful member of the dyad may feel the need to remind the more powerful member that this is the case, and, of course, the consequences of power inequities need to be considered. The key components of asserting one's rights are similar to those in asking favours: stating the problem, making a specific request for resolution or change, and persisting until one has effectively communicated a point. "I understand that you sometimes need me to work later than usual. I don't like it when you simply expect that and don't check with me. If you give me some advance notice, I'm sure I'll be able to accommodate you most of the time."

Expressing Feelings. Although feelings often appear to be obvious from nonverbal behaviour, people may have no idea of another's feelings unless they are expressed in words. A colleague may not be aware of making a peer angry, and a friend may be blind to the pain that laughing at a neighbour's handwriting caused that person. Part of being assertive is expressing emotions such as anger and affection. "I appreciate your saying that" is a more assertive way of responding to an expression of gratitude than "it's nothing" or "it's just my job", which belittles both the sender and the receiver of the message of thanks.

APPROPRIATE USES OF ASSERTIVENESS TECHNIQUES

As discussed earlier, few people are completely nonassertive (passive) or aggressive. Most people vary in assertiveness from situation to situation, and the degree of intimacy shared with others accounts for some of this variation as well. It is possible to be appropriately assertive with one's spouse and to become quite passive with one's mother-in-law. Alternately, being assertive with strangers may be easy, and cancelling a date with a friend because of a whim to stay home may seem out of the question. Even at work, people may have a range of responses like being direct with a supervisor and being unable to give followers explicit directions on assignments.

One of the more common differences in assertiveness within rather than between individuals has to do with "managing up" versus "managing down". In the workplace, this is often compounded when authority figures are male and subordinates are female. When the component of unequal training or education is added, one may see how being assertive can be potentially confusing and difficult.

Being Assertive with Authority Figures

Many people have been raised to respect their elders and obey their parents. Although unchallenged in childhood when dependent on parents and teachers, those attitudes are not appropriate dicta for self-directed adults who bear sole responsibility for their lives. It is unlikely that parents, for instance, can rescue a subordinate from a tyrannical superior; further, it is unlikely that the authority figure's attitudes will change simply because a subordinate wants them to. Subordinates need to help the supervisor to understand that they are not doormats or children or passive troops, ready to blindly follow orders. Although most supervisors know this, some are not as adept as others in interpersonal skills. Being assertive with supervisors may be the only way that subordinates express the right to be treated as adults, even though supervisors have position power—more responsibility and authority. Of course, tact and understanding of the supervisor's role responsibilities are essential in asserting oneself.

Being Assertive with Followers

People learn how to be managers and parents by watching role models. If fate looked kindly and provided such modelling by assertive leaders, managers, parents, and helping professionals, effective interpersonal skills would be perpetuated. Fate is not always so benevolent, however, and in moments of stress, it is easy to "pass on" the aggressive or manipulative behaviours that were learned in the past. If people can be assertive with superiors, there is less angry residue that can spill on to contacts with supervisees, patients, and children; moreover, there is less likelihood of forgetting that others less powerful have a right to determine their own responses also. An illustration of this "domino theory" of aggression can be seen in the following example:

> Mrs Roy is perceived by some as a whining, complaining patient. She has been calling with various complaints and requests every ten minutes since the shift began. Responding to her for the fourth time, you feel annoyed that other responsibilities are not being carried out. Your supervisor, meeting you on your way out of Mrs Roy's room, snaps at you because a second-year resident snapped at her because another patient was neglected. You remain silent with your supervisor, secretly cursing Mrs Roy and the resident. The next time Mrs Roy calls for attention, it takes you 20 minutes to respond, and when in her room, you seem gruff, uncaring, and irritated.

The irony in the above situation is that everyone (except perhaps Mrs Roy) perceives a problem and wants it solved. Assertion in this circumstance is breaking the cycle of smouldering anger and serial accusation. On the fourth response to Mrs Roy, an assertive statement might be: "I understand that you are uncomfortable and unhappy, but I have other patients to care for, and I will not be back for a while. What is the most important thing that I can do for you right now?" The supervisor might be responded to by saying: "It seems like the staff shortage is getting to all of us. It doesn't help when you snap at me." By being assertive, considerably more control over both the situation and personal feelings can be exercised without resentment of the supervisor or of the patient. Each of them is also given a chance to respond further.

MONITORING ONE'S OWN ASSERTIVENESS

Two mechanisms give feedback about assertiveness: internal and external feedback mechanisms.

Internal Feedback Mechanisms

Nonassertion (passivity) can be felt in the body and is usually experienced as tension in the stomach, chest, throat, shoulders, and/or neck. There may also be a sense of shame attached. There may be a wish to strike back, with an equal sense that to do so is too risky. Aggressive anger is often felt as internal rage with a wish to overpower the target of aggression.

External Feedback Mechanisms

The receiver of nonassertive or aggressive messages provides feedback to the sender. Senders who act like victims are likely to be either attacked or ignored. Victims of aggression, however, probably respond by withdrawal and passive resistance; occasionally the response is a counterassault. No one is assertive all of the time. If one has the feeling of losing contact with another through aggression, that person might say something like: "I think I just ignored your feelings—I'm sorry. Can we talk about what just happened?" Alternatively, if hindsight makes one aware of nonassertion in an encounter, one can respond assertively later. For example, "I was really upset yesterday when you yelled at me. I understand that you were frustrated, but I'd rather talk out our difficulties then be shouted at."

ASSESSING AND APPLYING ASSERTIVENESS TECHNIQUES

Because assertiveness training has been so popular for so long, there are many assessment devices to help you determine whether or in what domains you could benefit from assertion training. Good general sources for that purpose can be found throughout *The Assertive Woman* (Phelps & Austin, 1987) and *Your Perfect Right* (Alberti & Emmons, 1986). One of the best ways to improve your skills is to practise through role playing in groups. You can find practice situations anywhere, of course, but there are some particularly useful vignettes reproduced in the experiential exercises in this part of the book. Practising these with colleagues is a practical way to get feedback about your strengths and weaknesses in assertive communication.

A FINAL NOTE

Although assertiveness can be taught and can be seen as simply another skill to be learned, the ramifications of not being assertive go much deeper than simply choosing not to use a new technique. Health care is a demanding profession, one in which others such as patients, nurses, doctors, administrators and families often assume that they have the right to define each other's identities and roles. For example, patients and their families are likely to misunderstand the nurse manager's role in coordinating care; patients and families may not understand the unique interdependent relationship among nurses and doctors; and patients are also likely to be at their most anxious and least level-headed state of mind when faced with illness. Responses of others cannot be controlled and it is not feasible to educate all of those people who may misperceive the roles of health care professionals. However, one can exert control over one's own behaviour. Despite difficult and trying working conditions, frustration can at least be reduced if health care professionals express feelings and thoughts directly, adequately, responsibly, and with accountability.

SUMMARY

Assertiveness in an interaction between two people means that both express their needs, wants, and concerns; both people listen and respond to the other nondefensively. An assertive message is different from a passive or an aggressive communication. Assertive behaviours have verbal and nonverbal components. Nonverbal components include loudness of voice, fluency of spoken words, eye contact, facial and body expressions, and spatial relations between interactors. Verbal aspects include saying no, asking favours, expressing feelings, asserting rights, and taking a stand on an issue.

REFERENCES

Alberti, R.E., & Emmons, M.L. (1986). *Your perfect right: A guide to assertive living* (5th rev. ed.). San Luis Obispo, CA: Impact.

Angel, G., & Petronko, D.K. (1983). *Developing the new assertive nurse: Essential for advancement.* New York: Springer.

Clark, C. (1978). *Assertive skills for nurses.* Wakefield, MA: Contemporary Publishing.

Clark, C. (1979). Assertiveness issues for nursing administrators and managers. *Journal of Nursing Administration, 9,* 20–24.

Cooley, M., & Hollandsworth, J. (1977). A strategy for teaching verbal content of assertive responses. In Alberti, R.E. (Ed.) *Assertiveness: Innovations, applications, issues.* San Luis Obispo, CA: Impact.

Hayes, S., & Patterson, M. (1975). Interaction between students in multidisciplinary health teams. *Journal of Medical Education, 50,* 473–475.

Jakubowski-Spector, P. (1973). Facilitating the growth of women through assertive training. *The Counseling Psychologist, 4,* 75–86.

Keller, N. (1973). The nurse's role: Is it expanding or shrinking? *Nursing Outlook, 21,* 236–240.

Kilkus, S.P. (1986). Adding assertiveness to the nursing profession. *Nursing Success Today, 3*(8), 17–19.

Kinney, C.K.D. (1985). A reexamination of nursing role conceptions. *Nursing Research, 34*(3), 170–176.

Klein, C.P., & Klein, S. (1984). Emerging independence in nursing graduates: An analysis of traditional-nontraditional value patterns. *Sex Roles, 10*(11/12), 993–1002.

MacDonald, J. (1986). Time for a change. *International Nursing Review, 33*(6), 187.

Marriner, A. (1979). Assertive behavior for nursing leaders. *Nursing Leadership, 2,* 14–20.

McIntyre, T.J., Jeffrey, D.B., & McIntyre, S.L. (1984). Assertion training. The effectiveness of a comprehensive cognitive-behavioral treatment package with professional nurses. *Behavioral Research and Therapy, 22*(3), 311–318.

Milauskas, J. (1985). Will nursing assert itself? *Nursing Administration Quarterly, 9*(3), 1–15.

Pardue, S. (1980). Assertiveness for nursing. *Supervisor Nurse, 11,* 47–50.

Percell, L. (1977). Assertive behavior training and the enhancement of self-esteem. In Alberti, R.E. (Ed.) *Assertiveness: Innovations, applications, issues.* San Luis Obispo, CA: Impact.

Phelps, S., & Austin, N. (1987). *The assertive woman: A new look.* (2nd ed.). San Luis Obispo, CA: Impact.

Salter, A. (1961). *Conditioned reflex therapy* (2nd ed.). New York: Capricorn.

Serber, M. (1977). Teaching the nonverbal components of assertiveness training. In Alberti, R.E. (Ed.) *Assertiveness: Innovations, applications, issues.* San Luis Obispo, CA: Impact.

Shoemaker, M., & Satterfield, D. (1977). Assertion training: An identity crisis that's coming on strong. In Alberti, R.E. (Ed.) *Assertiveness: Innovations, applications, issues.* San Luis Obispo, CA: Impact.

Sommer, R. (1969). Studies in personal space. *Sociometry, 22,* 247–260.

Spiegel, D.A., Smolen, R.C., & Jones, C.K. (1985). Interpersonal conflicts involving students in clinical medical education. *Journal of Medical Education, 60,* 819–829.

Super, D.E. (1957). *The psychology of careers.* New York: Harper & Row.

Valiga, T.M.G. (1982). *The cognitive development of and perceptions about nursing as a profession of baccalaureate nursing students.* Unpublished doctoral dissertation. New York: Teachers College, Columbia University.

Wolpe, J.E. (1958). *Psychotherapy by reciprocal inhibition,* Stanford, CA: Stanford University Press.

Group Dynamics

Group dynamics involves the study and analysis of how people interact and communicate with each other in face-to-face small groups. The study of group dynamics provides a vehicle to analyse group communications with the intent of rendering the groups more effective (Davis & Newstrom, 1985; La Monica, 1985).

Chapter 15 begins with a discussion of the purposes for studying group dynamics, followed by details of what can be observed in groups. One area for observation, group roles, is presented in a separate section. Processing group behaviours is then discussed, with common health care groups concluding the chapter.

PURPOSES FOR STUDYING GROUP DYNAMICS

According to general system theory (von Bertalanffy, 1968, 1975), a system is more than a sum of its parts. It involves pooling the energy of a group of human and material resources toward goal accomplishment. (Refer back to Chapter 2 for a thorough discussion of general system theory.) Contemporary management practices apply this theory. It follows, therefore, that a manager's best bet is to motivate the group to work together toward goal accomplishment. The more effectively a group works as a team, the higher the probability for cost-effective services. Because fostering teamwork is one of the purposes of a manager's communications, studying group dynamics is an important facet of organizational work (Baker, 1980; Weeks, Barrett, & Snead, 1985). What a system (group) accomplishes has as much to do with the goal as it does with how well the group works as a team.

Lippitt and Seashore (1980) delineated more specific purposes for studying group dynamics. The manager's goal is to develop an effective team by facilitating:

1. A clear understanding of purposes and goals;

2. Flexibility in how a group accomplishes goals;

3. Effective communication and understanding among members—on personal feelings and attitudes as well as task-related ideas and issues;

4. Effective decision-making strategies that secure commitment of members to important decisions;

5. An appropriate balance between group productivity and individual satisfaction;

6. Group maturation so that leader responsibilities can be shared according to the group's ability and willingness;

7. Group cohesiveness while maintaining the needed measure of individual freedom;

8. Use of members' different abilities;

9. How a group is solving its own problems; and

10. A balance between emotional and rational behaviour—steering emotions into productive teamwork.

WHAT TO OBSERVE IN GROUPS

The literature contains discussions of many aspects in group behaviour that can be studied (Charrier, 1980; Clark, 1987; Lippitt & Seashore, 1980;

Marram, 1978; Sampson & Marthas, 1981). The labels attached to these aspects differ. Dimensions of group behaviour that are discussed in this chapter are: goals, background, participation, communication patterns, cohesion and membership, climate, norms, and decision-making procedures. Group roles will be discussed in the section that follows the present one.

Group Goals

It has been stated repeatedly in this book that groups must have a goal. Sometimes the goal is formal, and sometimes it is informal, such as having a complaint session to let off steam. These goals represent the tasks of the group. How the group as a team accomplishes these tasks is group behaviour.

Group Background

The history and traditions of the group bear directly on the life of the group as it seeks to accomplish its immediate task (Lippitt & Seashore, 1980). Traditions, norms, procedures, and activities should be studied in terms of how they affect the present. Positive aspects of past group behaviour (aspects that a manager considers as having the probability to facilitate task accomplishment) should be fostered. Strategies to counteract previous negative dimensions must be specified and implemented.

Group Participation

A manager's goal should be to facilitate the fullest possible participation of the system's human resources. Recalling von Bertalanffy's (1968) assumption of an open system—a group is more than a sum of its parts (Chapter 2)—the more energy that members put into teamwork, the more output will result from the group. The manager has to apply motivation theory to accomplish this most important aspect of group behaviour.

Communication Patterns

This area involves the social organization of the group. The primary reasons for studying communication patterns are to draw out member issues and focus on task issues more effectively. Areas that should be discussed are: who is talking with whom, what is said, how it is said, nonverbal behaviour, and who is listening to whom (La Monica, 1985; Lippitt & Seashore, 1980).

Communication Networks. Various communication networks have effects on variables such as speed of performance, accuracy, job

| Circle | Chain | Wheel |

FIGURE 15.1 Classic communication networks.

satisfaction, flexibility, and so forth. Figure 15.1 shows three classic communication networks. Obviously many other patterns can exist.

Bavelas and Barrett (1951) and Leavitt (1951) suggested that the circle network resulted in slow group speed, poor accuracy, no informal leader, very good job satisfaction, and fast flexibility to change. The chain resulted in speedy performance, good accuracy, increased likelihood that a leader would emerge, poor job satisfaction, and slow flexibility to change. The wheel, called such because all communications are channelled through the centre person, obviously has a pronounced leader. Performance is speedy and accuracy is good with this network; however, job satisfaction tends to be poor and flexibility to change is slow. Even though the initial research on communication networks was done early, more recent studies corroborated the findings presented (Cohen, 1962; Mears, 1974; Shaw, 1954a, 1954b). It was underscored by Davis and Newstrom (1985) that groups naturally solve their assigned problem as efficiently as possible using networks that are necessary. One network, therefore, is as good as another, depending on the system.

Transactional Analysis (TA). Transactional analysis is another method that can be used to study behaviour between and among people. It was developed by Berne (1972, 1978) and led into popularity by Harris (1982), James and Jongeward (1971, 1978), and Jongeward (1976).

According to TA, people have three ego states—parent, child, and adult. The parent state is the evaluative part of us all. It is our conscience, which provides the home for values, rules, standards, and so forth. The two kinds of parent states are nurturing parent and critical parent.

The child ego state is emotion-laden and contains the "natural" impulses and attitudes that are usually identified in children. The child ego state can be categorized as happy and destructive.

The adult is the rational, reality-oriented ego state. The adult solves problems and makes decisions by balancing the child ego state and the parent ego state against the realities of the environment at a specific time and place. Figure 15.2 shows the three ego states with subcategories.

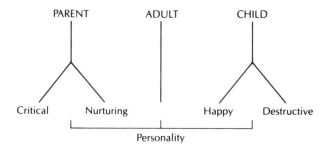

FIGURE 15.2 Transactional analysis: Ego states.

All three ego states exist in people at different times. A problem occurs when one or two of the ego states dominate. Parent-dominated people tend to believe that their answers are right; they know what is right and wrong. Adult-dominated people are always working. Child-dominated individuals are often selfish in a group and not inclined to be rational and to think outside of self.

Transactions can be complementary or crossed, as seen in Figure 15.3. A principle in complementary styles is that responses can be expected. Crossed transactions result in communication breakdowns because responses are usually inappropriate and confusing. Figure 15.4 shows various transactions with examples of each.

Group Cohesion and Membership

Lippitt and Seashore (1980) saw group cohesion as the "attractiveness of the group to its members" (p. 4). Cohesion involves the willingness of members to accept group decisions and whether group activities are grounded on commitment to a common goal or on likes and dislikes of persons for each other. Subgroups may form in groups (often called "cliques"). They are usually based on friendship or common needs. If group desires are split among members, two or more factions within a group may develop. Ideally, a group should work together while members maintain their individuality (Lippit & Seashore, 1980).

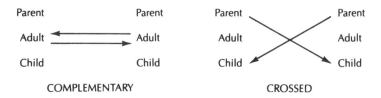

FIGURE 15.3 Types of transactions.

PARENT-TO-PARENT COMPLEMENTARY

Coordinator to ward sister:
"Primary nursing is the best
model of nursing care delivery."
Response: "I certainly agree."

CHILD-TO-CHILD COMPLEMENTARY

Associate to associate: "I'm tired
of always being interrupted by you!"
Response: "Well, next time don't
talk so much!"

PARENT-TO-CHILD COMPLEMENTARY

Supervisor to staff nurse: "Come
to my office at 9 AM tomorrow."
Response: "Yes. [Silence] Did I do
something wrong?"

CROSSED TRANSACTION

Supervisor to nurse's aide: "You
should not be doing this
procedure by yourself."
Response: "I have been doing this
for five years, and I am in a
hurry at the moment. I have
work to do."

ADULT-TO-ADULT COMPLEMENTARY

Head nurse to orderly: "Would you
please turn Mr Robinson in Room 246."
Response: "Yes, as soon as I get
Mr Jones back in bed."

FIGURE 15.4 Examples of crossed and complementary transactions.

Group Climate

The climate of the group refers to the tone and atmosphere that is created by the group. Are members competitive, tense, polite, friendly, flat, energetic, and/or enthusiastic, for example? Creating a positive group climate is important because enthusiasm and energy are catching and tend to snowball in growth. Unfortunately, the converse—a negative climate—also is catching and grows (La Monica, 1985).

Group Norms

Group norms involve standards or ground rules. The beliefs of the group's majority usually set the norms—"what behaviour should or should not take place in the group" (Pfeiffer & Jones, 1972, p. 24). Norms may be explicit, implicit, or operating outside of the members' awareness. A manager should seek to facilitate awareness and frequent examination of group norms.

Group Decision-Making Procedures

The procedures used by a group to make decisions should be studied. Schein (1969) discussed six ways in which groups make decisions:

1. *Decision by lack of response (the "plop").* This occurs when members suggest decisions without due discussion of issues and alternatives; the group simply bypasses the ideas. Then one idea is suggested, and the group immediately decides that it is the best. There are usually hidden attitudes operating, which are often a lack of commitment to the goal and/or feelings of powerlessness on the part of members. Results of this type of group decision-making procedure are negative feelings about self and other group members.

2. *Decision by authority rule.* Authority is delegated to someone in a position of power—the leader. This type of group decision making is fine if the leader communicates that he or she will make the decision but needs advice. If the leader, however, communicates that the group can decide on a course of action and then concludes the session by ignoring the group's suggestions, then the group may feel duped— rightfully so. Such action results in many negative feelings toward the leader, with harmful long-range effects.

3. *Decision by majority rule.* One or more people use pressure tactics to railroad a decision in this decision-making style. The balance of members are left feeling impotent, helpless, and "out-of-breath". They may wonder what happened.

4. *Decision by majority rule: voting and/or polling.* This is the most common style of group decision making. The position of each group member on the issue is requested either formally (by voting) or informally (by polling). A member can be for or against an issue or resolution or can abstain from making a decision. The best group procedure is to state the issue and then facilitate group discussion on all sides of the issue; decision by voting and/or polling follows. If the group must

implement the decision—that is, they must individually do something in order for the goal to be attained—then group decision by majority rule is not best. Decision by consensus would be better than a majority ruling, because it is more probable that group members will be committed to the decision and less probable that the decision or task will be undermined during implementation.

5. *Decision by consensus.* This is a psychological state in which group members see rationale in the decision and agree to support it. This operates even though some members may be more or less committed than others; there even may be a minority vote.

6. *Decision by unanimous vote.* This method, though desirable, is rarely attained in organizations. It is demanded in jury trials but consensus is usually sufficient in management situations.

The roles that the leader and members play in a group also bear observation. They are discussed in the following section.

GROUP ROLES

Understanding the roles that members play in a group can increase effectiveness in group endeavours. Equally important is members' awareness of how they perceive their roles, juxtaposed or consonant with how others perceive their roles. The role of the formal leader is discussed first, followed by a list of common roles that all group members (including the formal and informal leader[s]) can play. It should be noted that members may be observed in one or more roles during a particular group session.

Role of the Formal Leader

The formal leader's behaviour in a group can range from almost complete control to delegation, or almost complete control by the group. It follows that the functions required to propel a group toward its goal can be assumed by the leader or can become the responsibility of the members.

The precise dimensions of the formal leader's role are decided after the system is diagnosed (see Chapter 4), and an appropriate leader behaviour is selected based on the system's diagnosis (see Chapter 5). Recalling that a leader can behave in any of four styles, the roles that a leader plays in group decision making fit into these same four Ohio State leadership styles (Stogdill & Coons, 1957):

- High structure and low consideration   (LB1)
- High structure and high consideration   (LB2)
- High consideration and low structure   (LB3)
- Low structure and low consideration   (LB4)

Group decision making should only be a leader's option in LB2, LB3, and LB4. In other words, a system that is immature (requiring LB1) should not be involved in group problem solving because the group requires knowledge and experience first—discussion about the issue comes later. Group problem solving is a consideration intervention because it involves two-way communication: leader to followers and followers to leader.

When LB2 is required, given the system's diagnosis, consideration and structure should be high. When LB2 is required, however, the system is only beginning to move toward maturity. The leader should not, therefore, relinquish too much control to the group. In LB3, greater control should be shifted from the leader to the group, and in LB4, when the group is mature in relation to carrying out the task, the leader can delegate to the group and leave the group alone to solve problems and make decisions.

The types of management decision styles discussed in Chapter 6 (Vroom, 1973; Vroom & Jago, 1988; Vroom & Yetton, 1973) can be applied to make more precise how a leader should behave in a group. The reader can refer back to Table 6.1 and Figure 6.1 for a refresher on these styles.

Roles of Group Members

In order for group goals to be accomplished, two categories of functions must be performed in the group: task functions and maintenance functions. Task functions relate to what the group must accomplish, while maintenance functions are concerned with how the group carries out its task. These activities can be controlled variously by the leader in accordance with the requirements of the group for leader behaviour. Given that, members can assume different roles. Figure 15.5 portrays the relationship between leader behaviour and group roles.

Benne and Sheats (1948) identified three major categories of group roles. Although different labels may be used in current literature, the basics remain the same. A partial list of the roles is provided (La Monica, 1979, pp. 280–281*), and a complete list can be obtained from the original source.

---

*Reprinted by permission from La Monica, Elaine L., *The Nursing Process: a Humanistic Approach*, pp. 280–281. Copyright © 1979 by Addison-Wesley Publishing Company, Inc., Menlo Park, Calif.

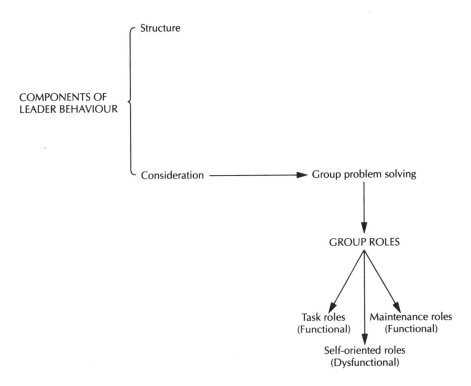

FIGURE 15.5 Relationship between leader behaviour and group roles.

Task Roles. These relate to the task with which the group is involved:

1. *Initiator*—Introduces new ideas or procedures; tries to establish movement toward the goal.

2. *Information seeker*—Tries to obtain needed information or opinions; points out gaps in information; asks for opinions; responds to suggestions.

3. *Evaluator*—Tries to determine where the group stands on an issue; tests for consensus; evaluates progress.

4. *Coordinator*—Points out relationships among ideas or procedures; pulls ideas together and builds on the contributions of others; takes things one step further.

5. *Procedural technician*—Expedites group work by performing routine tasks, distributing material, and so forth.

6. *Recorder*—Writes down ideas, decisions, and recommendations; keep minutes.

Maintenance Roles. These are oriented toward the functioning of the group as a whole unit, building group-centred attitudes, and strengthening productivity:

1. *Encourager*—Offers warmth and support to another's contribution; accepts what each member says.

2. *Harmonizer*—Mediates the differences between and among members; attempts to reconcile disagreements.

3. *Compromiser*—Seeks a middle position position between opposing viewpoints.

4. *Standard setter*—Tries to bring to awareness the norms and standards of the group.

5. *Gatekeeper*—Keeps communication channels open; facilitates participation of all members; keeps track of time.

Self-Oriented Roles. These roles involve attempts by members to satisfy their own needs through the group and are usually not directed toward effective group work. Self-oriented roles are often seen as dysfunctional.

1. *Aggressor*—Deflates the status of others; attacks the group, its individual members, or the task; displays envy toward the contributions by taking credit for them.

2. *Blocker*—Negative, stubborn opposer who reintroduces issues that have been previously decided upon.

3. *Recognition seeker*—Works in myriad ways to call attention to self; boastful and self centred.

4. *Playboy*—Displays lack of interest by being cynical or humorous on important issues.

5. *Dominator*—Asserts authority or superiority over others by manipulating the group; flatters, interrupts, or gives authoritative directions.

6. *Help seeker*—Calls attention to self and seeks a sympathetic response from the group.

PROCESSING GROUP BEHAVIOUR

Processing group behaviour involves giving feedback to the group on how it functioned. The intent is to increase shared understanding about the behaviour, feelings, and motivations of individuals; to facilitate development of a growth relationship by building trust and fostering openness among members; and to increase awareness of how people affect others. Criteria for feedback are found in Chapter 9. The criteria should be applied both to one-to-one and group interactions.

Time should be allotted at the conclusion of meetings to process how the group worked on its task. Group process observation sheets are provided for this purpose in the experiential exercises at the conclusion of Part III. These forms are arranged from simple to complex, and they should be used for learning in that order as group members mature in processing their group behaviour.

COMMON HEALTH CARE GROUPS

There are numerous situations in which a health care manager must facilitate group problem solving. This portion of the chapter includes discussion of the common health care groups: staff support groups, teaching conferences, procedure conferences, patient conferences, directive conferences, and self-help groups.

Staff Support Groups

Scully (1981) described the purpose of staff support groups as helping people to help themselves. It has been documented that helpers who are aware of and accepting toward their own feelings will more probably be able to form a helping relationship with another than helpers who are unaware (Rogers, 1961). A ladder effect is operative: if a manager is satisfied with self, there is greater likelihood that the manager will be open to establishing a productive relationship with followers. If followers are then satisfied with their work responsibilities, there is greater chance that they will be more open to giving to their clients.

Health care professionals need support. Since health care is a profession of human service, it mandates constant giving—thinking about others. Moreover, health care professionals must give to many people in a short span of time. They must listen to others, feel with others, and respond to others' needs. This is giving, and carers must be replenished. Otherwise the human tendency is to withdraw when drained, which is counterproductive. Peer support is the best type of help that managers can engender among staff members. Conferences can be in areas of stress management, conflict resolution, team building, and/or any issue that is a priority in the group.

Teaching Conferences

A teaching conference involves a skill or a process that is taught to staff members. This type of conference is analogous to a staff development or a continuing education programme, but is generally on a smaller scale.

A ward sister who wishes to apprise followers of the outcome of primary nursing on an experimental unit would use a teaching conference. Another example is Marram's (1978) referral to a group dynamics session whose purpose is to increase skill and knowledge in group decision making. Facilitating group leadership experiences for students by having them co-lead a conference (Browne, 1980) would also be considered a teaching conference even though two purposes for the conference would probably exist.

Procedure Conferences

A procedure conference is similar to a teaching conference, but the teaching conference is concerned with skill and knowledge (content) from the domain of helping, which includes patient care, and the procedure conference usually refers to topics of policies and procedures in a specific organization. Alerting staff to a revised informed consent procedure for a hospital is one example of a topic for this type of conference.

Patient Conferences

Problem-oriented care of a patient is discussed and evaluated in a patient conference (Douglass & Bevis, 1979). All persons (the team) involved in the care of the patient and family discuss the care plan, solve problems, explain, gain confidence, or evaluate (La Monica, 1985). The leader of this conference should facilitate multidisciplinary sharing of expertise and perceptions concerning the diagnoses. Decisions that result from a patient conference are generally more patient-centred, valid, and creative than decisions of one professional.

Directive Conferences

Directive conferences most often occur at the beginning and end of shifts; occasionally a midshift direction conference is called. The overall purposes of this type of conference are to make assignments and receive reports.

Assigning. Assignments are made at a shift's beginning for communicating job assignments, specifying areas of responsibility, and giving pertinent information regarding patient care. A manager may make general announcements during this conference.

Assignments generally are made according to one of four basic methods for delivering nursing care: the case method, the functional method, team nursing, or primary nursing. "Case management" is a combination of the original case method model and primary nursing. Table 15.1 contains descriptions of the basic methods with the values and disadvantages of each.

TABLE 15.1 Nursing Care Delivery Models: Descriptions, Values, and Disadvantages

Description	Values	Disadvantages
Case Method/Management		
The complete care of one or more clients is assigned to a nurse for a period of time. In the early case method, care was for a shift. In typical case management, the nurse may carry the assigned clients for the entire length of stay and maybe, even in the home care agency.	1. The nurse can better see and attend to the total needs of clients due to the time and proximity of interactors. Coordination of all aspects of care is the responsibility of the nurse: physical, emotional, medical regimen, teaching, and all other aspects. 2. Continuity of care can be facilitated with ease. 3. Client/nurse interaction/ rapport can be developed due to the intensity of time and proximity of those involved. 4. Client may feel more secure knowing that one person is thoroughly familiar with the needs and the course of treatment.	1. Many clients do not require the intensity of care inherent in this type of service. 2. The method must be modified if nonprofessional health workers are to be used effectively. 3. There are not enough nurses to fill the demand of this model; cost-effectiveness must be considered. 4. It is difficult for all levels of professional and technical nurses to share expertise in the process of planning care.

(continued)

TABLE 15.1 (*continued*)

Description	Values	Disadvantages
	5. Educational needs of clients can be closely monitored.	
	6. Family and friends may become better known by nurses and more involved in the care of the client.	
	7. Work load can be equally divided among available staff.	
	8. Nurses' accountability for their functions is built-in.	
Functional Method		
Selected functions (vital signs, medications, and so forth) are assigned to staff members who are qualified to carry out these functions for patients on a unit for a given period of time.	1. One person can become particularly skilled in performing assigned tasks; this method can be efficient and economical.	1. Client care may become impersonal, compartmentalized, and fragmented.
	2. The best utilization may be made of a person's aptitudes, experience, and desires.	2. There is a tremendous risk for diminishing continuity of care.
	3. Less equipment is needed, and what is available is usually better cared for when used only by a few personnel.	3. Staff may become bored and have little motivation to develop self and others. Work may become monotonous.
	4. This method saves time	4. The staff members are accountable for the taxk; only the nurse in charge of the unit has accountability for

TABLE 15.1 (*continued*)

Description	Values	Disadvantages
	because it lends itself to strict organizational protocol.	the individual, whole clinet.
	5. The potential for development of technical skills is amplified.	5. There is little avenue for staff development, except as it relates to tasks.
	6. There is a sense of productivity for the task-oriented nurse.	6. Clients may tend to feel insecure, not knowing who is their own nurse.
	7. It is easy to organize the work of the unit and staff.	7. Only parts of the nursing care plan may be known to personnel.
		8. It is difficult to establish client priorities and operationalize the care plan that reflects the same.
		9. It is only safe when the ward sister can coordinate the activities of all members of the staff and make certain that nothing essential in client care is overlooked or forgotten. This is a tremendous responsibility for one person who probably has to think of approximately 30 or more clients, plus the staff.

(*continued*)

TABLE 15.1 (*continued*)

Description	Values	Disadvantages
Team Nursing		
Total care of a group of patients is the responsibility of a team of professionals and nonprofessionals who work together to give comprehensive, quality, individualized nursing care. There is no protocol for how the work gets assigned; the team leader assigns the care of patients to those qualified to carry out specific tasks.	1. It includes all health care personnel in the group's functioning and goals. 2. Feelings of participation and belonging are facilitated with team members. 3. Work load can be balanced and shared. 4. Division of labour allows members the opportunity to develop leadership skills. 5. Every team member has the opportunity to learn from and teach colleagues. 6. There is a variety in the daily assignments. 7. Interest in clients' well-being and care is shared by several people; reliability of decisions is increased. 8. Nursing care hours are usually cost-effective. 9. The client is able to identify personnel who are responsible	1. Establishing the team concept takes time, effort, and constancy of personnel. Merely assigning people to a group does not make them a "group" or "team". 2. Unstable staffing patterns make team nursing difficult. 3. All personnel must be educated in client-centred nursing care. 4. The team leader must have complex skills and knowledge: communication, leadership, organization, nursing care, motivation, and other skills. 5. There is less individual responsibility and independence regarding nursing functions.

TABLE 15.1 (*continued*)

Description	Values	Disadvantages
	for his or her care.	
	10. All care is directed by an RN.	
	11. Continuity of care is facili- tated, especially if teams are constant.	
	12. Barriers be- tween profes- sional and nonprofessional workers can be minimized; the group effort prevails.	
	13. Everyone has the opportunity to contribute to the care plan.	
Primary Nursing*		
A professional nurse has 24-hour responsibility for the care of assigned patients [or cases] —all aspects of the nursing process are directed by the primary nurse.	1. There is oppor- tunity for the nurse to see the client and family as one system.	1. The nurse may be isolated from colleagues.
	2. Nursing ac- countability, responsibility, and indepen- dence are increased.	2. There is little avenue for group planning of client care.
	3. The nurse is able to use a wide range of skills, knowl- edge, and expertise.	3. Nurses must be mature and independently competent.
	4. The method potentiates creativity by the nurse; work satisfaction may increase signifi- cantly.	4. It may be cost- ineffective even though recent articles indicate otherwise.
		5. Staffing patterns may necessitate a heavy client load.

(*continued*)

TABLE 15.1 (*continued*)

Description	Values	Disadvantages
	5. The scene is set for increased trust and satisfaction in the client and nurse.	

*The usual procedures of the case method of nursing care delivery and primary nursing overlap into what is currently identified as case management.

Source: Reprinted and adapted by permission from La Monica, Elaine L., *The Nursing Process: A Humanistic Approach*, pp. 369–373. Copyright © 1979 by Addison-Wesley Publishing company, Inc., Menlo Park, Calif.

Remember, there is no best model of health care delivery, even though literature currently abounds with announcements that boast the benefits of primary nursing and case management (Deiman, Noble, & Russell, 1984; Kasch, 1986; McClure, 1984; Mutchner, 1986; Zander, 1985, 1987, 1988). Though these models definitely enhance the professional base for practice, in essence, any model for delivering health care is *only* as effective as is the competency of the staff who function within the model. This point was recently documented by Shukla (1981) in a study comparing primary and team nursing.

The needs and care of patients are priority considerations when making out assignments: what is involved; how long it takes; and what skills, knowledge, and experience are required in order to meet the needs. Then the abilities of the staff must be matched to the requirements of the patients so that members of the team are functioning according to their qualifications. Members who need to learn a particular treatment or skill should be assigned to work with another person who has that expertise.

Mechanically, assignments should be written out so that members have copies during the conference and can make notes. Responsibilities should be explicit.

Reporting. Verbal reports are made at the end of work shifts; in some agencies, these reports are tape-recorded. Pertinent information about the patients is communicated to those continuing patient care in inpatient facilities and to those in charge of outpatient facilities. Listening is the most important function of the leader in this type of conference. Douglass and Bevis (1979, p. 163) further stated that report conferences have four goals: (1) to report information about patients, (2) to give reactions to situations, (3) to evaluate care, and (4) to update care plans.

Self-Help Groups

Self-help groups are generally composed of nonprofessionals who organize and operate themselves around specific topics. These groups range from informal ones to organized ones such as Alcoholics Anonymous and Parents Without Partners. Self-help groups are concerned with self-care and self-improvement (Maloney, 1979). The principal force behind self-help groups is peer support. People with common problems pool their resources to help and receive help from one another. In one sense, staff support groups discussed earlier can be thought of as self-help groups— only composed of members who are professional.

Professional nurses, as well as other helpers, are often involved in self-help groups. Marram (1978, p. 39) saw the role of the nurse as: (1) verifying the success of individuals and the group, (2) identifying and referring people to the groups, and (3) providing knowledge to the group as a resource person and a teacher. Self-help groups are also often organized and led by agency staff around particular needs of their clientele.

SUMMARY

Group dynamics involves the study of how people interact with each other in small groups. The goal of study is to render the groups more effective. The more effectively a group works as a team, the higher is the probability for cost-effectiveness of the services. Studying group dynamics is, therefore, an essential aspect of the manager's responsibilities— fostering team maturity. Areas of group behaviour that require observation and study include the following: goals, background, participation, communication patterns, cohesion and membership, climate, norms, and decision-making procedures. Group roles are other important areas in group dynamics. The formal leader's behaviour can range from almost complete control to delegation or almost complete control by the group. How a manager behaves specifically is governed by the maturity level of the system in relation to the system's ability to carry out the task.

Task functions and maintenance functions are performed in group problem-solving activities. Group members can assume various functional and dysfunctional roles in each of these categories. Processing group behaviour involves giving the group feedback on how it functioned.

Health care professionals must facilitate group problem solving in a variety of informal and formal situations. Among the most common formal situations are the following groups: staff support groups; teaching conferences; procedure conferences; patient conferences; directive conferences—assigning and reporting; and self-help groups.

REFERENCES

Baker, K. (1980). Application of group theory in nursing practice. *Supervisor Nurse, 11*, 22–24.

Bavelas, A., & Barrett D. (1951). An experimental approach to organizational communication. *Personnel, 27*, 366–371.

Benne, K., & Sheats, P. (1948). Functional roles of group members. *Journal of Social Issues, 4*, 41–49.

Berne, E. (1972). *What do you say after you say hello?* New York: Bantam Books.

Berne, E. (1978). *Games people play.* New York: Ballantine.

Browne, S. (1980). Group leadership experiences for students. *Nursing Outlook, 28*, 166–169.

Charrier, G. (1980). Cog's ladder: A model of group growth. In M. Berger, D. Elhart, S. Firsich, S. Jordan, & S. Stone (Eds.) *Management for nurses: A multidisciplinary approach* (2nd ed.). St. Louis: Mosby.

Clark, C. (1987). *The nurse as group leader* (2nd ed.). New York: Springer.

Cohen, A. (1962). Changing small-group communication networks. *Administrative Science Quarterly, 6*, 443–462.

Davis, K., & Newstrom, J. (1985). *Human behavior at work: Organizational behavior* (7th ed.). New York: McGraw-Hill.

Deiman, P., Noble, E., & Russell, M. (1984). Achieving a professional practice model: How primary nursing can help. *Journal of Nursing Administration, 14*(7), 16–21.

Douglass, L., & Bevis, E. (1979). *Nursing management and leadership in action.* St. Louis: Mosby.

Harris, T. (1982). *I'm OK—You're OK.* New York: Avon.

James, M., & Jongeward, D. (1971). *Born to win: Transactional analysis with gestalt experiments.* Reading, MA: Addison-Wesley.

James, M., & Jongeward, D. (1978). *Born to win.* New York: NAL Pub.

Jongeward, D. (1976). *Women as winners: Transactional analysis for personal growth.* Reading, MA: Addison-Wesley.

Kasch, C. (1986). Establishing a collaborative nurse-patient relationship: A distinct focus of nursing action in primary care. *Image, 18*(2), 44–47.

La Monica, E. (1979). *The nursing process: A humanistic approach.* Menlo Park, CA: Addison-Wesley.

La Monica, E. (1985). *The humanistic nursing process.* Boston: Jones and Bartlett.

Leavitt, H. (1951). Some effects of certain communication patterns on group performance. *The Journal of Abnormal and Social Psychology, 46*, 38–50.

Lippitt, G., & Seashore, E. (1980). *Group effectiveness: A looking-into-leadership monograph.* Fairfax, VA: Leadership Resources.

Maloney, E. (1979). A perspective on groups in the health field in the 1980s. In E. La Monica. *The nursing process: A humanistic approach.* Menlo Park, CA: Addison-Wesley.

Marram, G. (1978). *The group approach in nursing practice.* St. Louis: Mosby.

McClure, M. (1984). Managing the professional nurse: Part II. Applying management theory to the challenges. *Journal of Nursing Administration, 14*(3), 11–17.

Mears, P. (1974). Structuring communication in a working group. *The Journal of Communication, 24*, 71–79.

Mutchner, L. (1986). How well are we practicing primary nursing? *Journal of Nursing Administration, 16*(9), 8–13.

Pfeiffer, J., & Jones, J. (Eds.). (1972). *The 1972 annual handbook for group facilitators.* La Jolla, CA: University Associates.

Rogers, C. (1961). *On becoming a person*. Boston: Houghton Mifflin.

Sampson, E., & Marthas, M. (1981). *Group process for the health professions*. New York: Wiley.

Schein, E. (1969). *Process consultation: Its role in organization development*. Reading. MA: Addison-Wesley.

Scully, R. (1981). Staff support groups: Helping nurses to help themselves. *Journal of Nursing Administration, 11*, 48–51.

Shaw, M. (1954a). Some effects of problem complexity upon problem solution efficiency in different communication nets. *Journal of Experimental Psychology, 48*, 211–217.

Shaw, M. (1954b). Some effects of unequal distribution of information upon group performance in various communication nets. *The Journal of Abnormal and Social Psychology, 49*, 547–553.

Shukla, R. (1981). Structure vs. people in primary nursing: An inquiry. *Nursing Research, 30*, 236–241.

Stogdill, R., & Coons, A. (Eds.). (1957). *Leader behavior: Its description and measurement*. Research Monograph No. 88, Columbus, Bureau of Business Research, Ohio State University.

von Bertalanffy, L. (1968). *General system theory*. New York: Braziller.

von Bertalanffy, L. (1975). *Perspectives on general system theory: Scientific-philosophical studies*. New York: Braziller.

Vroom, V. (1973). A new look at managerial decision-making. *Organizational Dynamics, 1*, 66–80.

Vroom, V., & Yetton, P. (1973). *Leadership and decision-making*. Pittsburg: University of Pittsburgh Press.

Vroom, M., & Jago, A. (1988). *The new leadership: Managing participation in organizations*. Englewood Cliffs, NJ: Prentice-Hall.

Weeks, L., Barrett, M., & Snead, C. (1985). Primary nursing: Teamwork is the answer. *Journal of Nursing Administration, 15*(9), 21–26, 34.

Zander, K. (1985). Second generation primary nursing: A new agenda. *Journal of Nursing Administration, 15*(3), 18–24.

Zander, K. (1987). Nursing case management: A classic. *Definition, 2*(2), 1–3.

Zander, K. (1988). Managed care within acute care settings: Design and implementation via nursing case management. *Health Care Supervisor, 6*(2), 24–43.

Conflict Resolution

Every human being has a unique set of drives, goals, and needs that are constantly seeking satisfaction. Earth contains all of these individuals who move in various directions across time and space on their journeys. If these journeys could be thought of as self-contained capsules that floated around other capsules, then each would be autonomous, and humans could not be considered sociologically; general system theory would not be viable.

In a sense, people are capsules, but needs are met by being dependent and interpendent on other capsules and independent of other capsules. If all people and their capsules desired complementary things, that is, what one wanted to obtain the other wished to give, and what one wanted to keep the other did not want, then systems could exist with total integration. Such harmony, however does not exist in reality. Conflict exists in the absence of harmonious total integration. Conflict always exists, therefore, even though it may be suppressed. People simply do not think, believe, and desire the same things.

Conflict is an absolute; a manager must learn to facilitate effectively the resolution of conflict among people in order to accomplish goals, which is the content of this chapter. The chapter begins with definitions of conflict, followed by discussion of the types and causes of conflict. These content areas set the stage for the conflict process and strategies for resolving conflict. Productive and destructive outcomes of conflict are the final topics.

DEFINITIONS OF CONFLICT

Deutsch (1969) defined conflict as a clash or a struggle that occurs when one's balance among feelings, thoughts, desires, and behaviour is threatened. This disturbance results in incompatible behaviour that interferes with goals. Douglass and Bevis (1979) stated that conflict is a struggle between interdependent forces. This struggle can be within an individual (intrapersonal conflict) or within a group (intragroup conflict) (Nielsen, 1977).

Since conflicts exist, a manager has the power to move the conflict to a constructive or a destructive resolution. In the constructive approach, the outcomes of an encounter result in individual and/or group growth, heightened awareness and understanding of self and others, and positive feelings toward the outcomes of the interaction. Destructive resolutions result in an expansion of the conflict and negative feelings toward self and/or others.

TYPES OF CONFLICT

Conflict arises within, between, and among people out of differences in facts, definitions, views, authority, goals, values, and controls. Conflict in an organization can be structurally categorized as vertical or horizontal (Marriner, 1979a). Vertical conflict involves differences between superiors and followers. It often results from poor communication and a lack of shared perceptions regarding expectations of appropriate behaviour for one's own role and/or that of others. Horizontal conflict is line-staff conflict and has to do with domains of practice, expertise, authority, and so forth. It is often interdepartmental strife.

Conflict can be further broken down into types as shown in Table 16.1. Examples are provided for each type of conflict.

CAUSES OF CONFLICT

Health care literature is replete with discussions of the predisposing factors of conflict (Coombs, 1987; Douglass & Bevis, 1979; Filley, 1980;

TABLE 16.1 Types of Conflict

Conflict*	Description*	Example
Intrasender	Same sender, conflicting messages	The same supervisor demands high-quality care, refuses to fire incompetent staff members, and refuses to recruit additional staff.
Intersender	Conflicting messages from two or more senders	Top nursing management stresses the need to adopt primary nursing as the nursing care model; followers believe that they can achieve individualized, quality nursing care using the team method.
Interrole	Same person belonging to conflicting groups	Nursing director belongs to a community-based consumer group seeking to consolidate obstetrical and paediatric services in a geographic locality by having all obstetrics shared between two of four hospitals and all paediatrics shared between the other two hospitals. The same nurse is also an employee of one hospital that is fighting to keep both services.
Person-role	Same person, conflicting values (cognitive dissonance)	A nurse believes that patients should receive individual attention in a clinic by one nurse who follows them from visit to visit. Requirements of the position and the system for delivering care make achieving such a goal infrequent if not impossible.
Interperson	Two or more people acting as protagonists for different groups	The director of nursing competes with other directors for new positions.
Intragroup	New values from outside are imposed on an existing group	Continuing education (CE) is mandated by the state for continuing

TABLE 16.1 (*continued*)

Conflict*	Description*	Example
		nursing licensure. The rural health care agency has no funds to send staff nurses to CE programmes, and staff nurses, who are underpaid but satisfied, cannot afford to support their own CE.
Intergroup	Two or more groups with conflicting goals	The nursing department demands that the operating and recovery room nurses organizationally come under nursing. The surgery department, composed of consultants, believes that they should control nurses in these areas.
Role ambiguity	A person is not aware of the expectations others have for a particular role	A newly hired nursing supervisor has no position description and has no previous experience as a supervisor.
Role overload	A person cannot meet the expectations of others for a role	A newly qualified registered nurse is expected by a nursing director to be in charge of a 40-bed acute-and-chronic-medical unit on the night shift.

*Source: Columns 1 and 2 from Marriner, A., Conflict theory. *Supervisor Nurse, 10*, 12–16. Copyright 1979 by S-N Publications, Inc. Reprinted by permission.

Marriner, 1982; Nielsen, 1977; Silber, 1984). Edmunds (1979) cited the following nine general factors that seem to account for all possible causes:

Specialization—A group that assumes responsibility for a particular set of tasks or area of service sets itself apart from other groups. Intergroup conflict often results.

Multitask Roles—The nursing role requires that one be a manager, a skilled care giver, a human relations expert, a negotiator, an advocate, and so forth. Each subrole with its tasks requires different orientations that can cause conflict.

Role Interdependence—A role of nurse practitioner in private practice would not be as complicated as one being a part of a multidisciplinary health care team. In the latter, the individual domains of practice have to be discussed with others who may compete for certain areas.

Task Blurring—This results from role ambiguity and failure to designate responsibility and accountability for a task to one individual or group.

Differentiation—A group of people may occupy the same role but the attitudinal, emotional, and cognitive behaviours of these people toward their role differs. This engenders conflict, especially in problem-solving and decision-making activities.

Scarcity of Resources—Competition for money, patients, and positions are an absolute source of interperson and intergroup conflict.

Change—Whenever change occurs, conflict is not far behind. As change becomes more apparent and/or threatening, the probability and depth of conflict increases proportionately.

Conflict Over Rewards—When people are differentially rewarded, conflict is often a result unless they were involved in developing the reward system.

Communication Problems—Ambiguities, perceptual distortions, language failures, and incorrectly used communication channels all can cause conflict.

Conflict exists within people and within groups; the causes of conflict, though stated generally, are unique. The next portion of the chapter contains a discussion of the conflict process.

THE CONFLICT PROCESS

Filley (1980), drawing from the early works of Corwin (1969), Fink (1968), Pondy (1967, 1969), Walton and Dutton (1969), and Schmidt (1973) depicted the following six steps to the conflict process, shown in Figure 16.1:

1. *Antecedent conditions* are causes of conflict and were discussed in the previous section of this chapter.
2. *Perceived conflict* is the recognition of conditions that exist between parties or within self that can cause conflict. Perceived conflict is logical, impersonal, and objective.

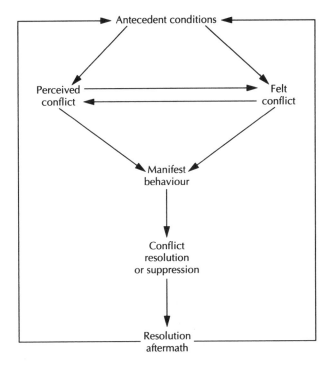

FIGURE 16.1 The conflict process.

Source: From *Interpersonal Conflict Resolution* by Alan C. Filley. Copyright © 1975 Scott, Foresman and Company. Reprinted by permission.

3. *Felt conflict* is subjective because people feel the conflict relationship. These feelings are often described as threat, hostility, fear, and/or mistrust.

4. *Manifest behaviour* can take the forms of aggression, non-assertion, assertion, competition, debate, or problem solving. Perceived and/or felt conflict generally result in action—actual overt behaviour.

5. *Conflict resolution or suppression*, the next step in the conflict process, brings the conflict to an end either by agreement among those involved or through the defeat of one party. In competitive conflict, rules specify the outcome.

6. *Resolution aftermath* is the legacy left at the end of this cycle —feelings, beliefs, awards, and so forth. Sometimes these leftovers are called consequences. Since conflict is experienced, learning takes place within an individual and both negative and positive learning can become antecedent conditions for conflict in another time and place.

RESOLVING CONFLICT

Now that one has an understanding of how conflict works, what can a manager do, to facilitate positive conflict resolution? Authors within and outside of the management profession offer myriad ideas on helping groups to resolve conflict. This author does not believe in one or two best ways to resolve or prevent conflict. An array of suggestions from the literature and experience are offered so that learners can choose what they believe to be best in a unique situation. All strategies are useful to have accessible in one's repertoire, available for use given diagnosis of the system including the environment. Two formal approaches for preventing conflict are discussed first—contingency contracting and management by objectives. A subsection of less formal approaches will then follow.

Contingency Contracting

Contingency contracting (Homme, 1970) is one leadership strategy that can be employed to lead followers developmentally toward self-management. This has potential for preventing conflict between leaders and followers because control will be given to followers based on their abilities to handle it effectively toward goal accomplishment. Control issues, as almost everyone is aware, can range in strength from relatively benign to positively lethal. This strategy is based on theory—what people need to reach maturity as they work toward goal accomplishment.

According to Homme (1970), a manager controls (1) what followers are supposed to do (the task) and (2) what reward(s) followers will receive for doing it (the reinforcement). Five types of contingency contracts are delineated, and an application in nursing for each is provided.

Leader Control. The task and the reinforcement are determined by the manager. The manager presents the contract; the follower accepts the contract and performs.

> Example: The nursing director formulates a policy, prepares a memorandum or directive, and presents it to the supervisors.

Partial Control by Follower. The follower assumes joint control over the reinforcement, and the manager retains full control over the task, or the follower assumes joint control over the task, and the manager retains full control over the reinforcement.

> Example: A ward sister prepares a survey questionnaire on which there are two alternative procedures. The nursing staff is requested to elect the procedure of choice. Upon tabulation of the responses, the

procedure of choice is apparent. A directive is then sent to all staff stipulating the procedure that will become policy.

Equal Control by Leader and Follower. The manager and follower assume equal control over the task and reinforcement, or the manager retains control over one of the two areas, and the follower assumes control over the other area.

> Example: A nursing director requests that the nursing administrative staff develop a policy on a specific issue. The policy is formulated by a subgroup within the administrative staff. It is then taken back to the administrative conference, which is composed of all members in nursing administration, and voted upon.

Partial Control by Leader. The follower has full control over the task or reinforcement and shares joint control with the manager over the other.

> Example: In order to resolve a specific patient care problem, the team nurses, the ward sisters and the charge nurses brainstorm and list all possible procedures that could resolve the situation at hand. The list is sent to all patient care staff on the unit; each staff member is asked to select the procedure that he or she believes is best. The procedure that becomes policy is based on a majority vote.

Follower Control. Both the task and the reinforcement are determined by the follower.

> Example: Followers are aware of the required holiday coverage on a unit. They meet by themselves and jointly decide the staffing schedule. It is then given to the ward sister.

Hersey and Blanchard (1988) integrated contingency contracting into situational leadership theory. This author adds the Ohio State model of leadership (Stogdill & Coons, 1957). Figure 16.2 presents this integration. Given the relationships shown in Figure 16.2, the following suggestions can be made (Hersey & Blanchard, 1988):

1. *Leader-control contracting* is appropriate when the system is at R1 level of maturity (low maturity), and LB1 (high structure/task and low consideration/relationship) is indicated.

2. *Partial-control-by-follower contracting* would be used by a leader when the system is at R2 (moderate maturity), and LB2 (high structure/task and high consideration/relationship) is required.

FIGURE 16.2 Contingency contracting, situational leadership theory, and the Ohio State model of leadership.

Source: This figure was adapted from one presented by Paul Hersey, & Kenneth H. Blanchard, *Management of Organizational Behavior: Utilizing Human Resources*, (5th ed.), © 1988, p. 443. Reprinted by permission of Prentice Hall, Inc, Englewood Cliffs, NJ.

3. *Equal-control-by-leader-and-follower contracting* should be used when a system is at R2-3 (moderate maturity), and the leader behaviour style is consistent with LB2 and LB3 (high structure/task and high consideration/relationship or high consideration/relationship and low structure/task).

4. *Partial-control-by-leader contracting* parallels with R3 (moderate maturity) and LB3 (high consideration/relationship and low structure/task).

5. *Follower-control contracting* should be used with a highly mature system (R4) when LB4 (low structure/task and low consideration/relationship) is indicated.

A manager can now employ contingency contracts in strategies for accomplishing goals. These should be based on the system diagnosis and resultant identification of a leader behaviour style that has the highest probability for motivating a system to accomplish a goal.

Management by Objectives

Management by objectives (MBO) is a participative approach for developing and sharing performance expectations among staff members at all levels in an organization. The concept was developed by Drucker (1954, 1985a, 1985b, 1985c) and also advanced by Odiorne (1965, 1979) and Humble (1967). The concept has received a wealth of attention in the literature, both in the disciplines of business and nursing (Cain & Luchsinger, 1978; Golightly, 1979; Odiorne, 1975; Palmer, 1973; Skarupa, 1971).

MBO is defined by Odiorne (1965, 1979) as a process whereby superiors and their followers jointly identify and set goals, define individual areas of responsibility, plan strategies and designate tasks for achieving goals, and measure and evaluate success. The MBO approach, when effectively implemented, enables expectations between followers and superiors to be public. Potential conflict is thereby reduced because goals are negotiated between involved parties, and then a contract is set; mutual commitment is, therefore, gained. MBO can provide a framework for achieving organizational goals and employee satisfaction (Olsson, 1968). Odiorne (1965) graphically portrayed the entire cycle of MBO, as shown in Figure 16.3.

Even though the attention MBO has received in the literature might lead someone to suggest that MBO is a managerial plus, the concept has received major criticisms (Ford, 1979; Hersey & Blanchard, 1988; Levinson, 1970). MBO is participatory in nature—equal control by superiors and followers. Not all followers are mature enough in their position to be able to set realistic objectives for themselves. Hersey and Blanchard (1988) pointed out that the role a superior will play in helping the follower to accomplish the set objectives is not clearly defined in MBO. Further, if a leader behaviour style is in the contract, it can tie a manager to one way of behaving, which may not be appropriate for all tasks. Ford (1979) asserted, among other important issues, that companies using MBO may overlook opportunities that develop after objectives were set.

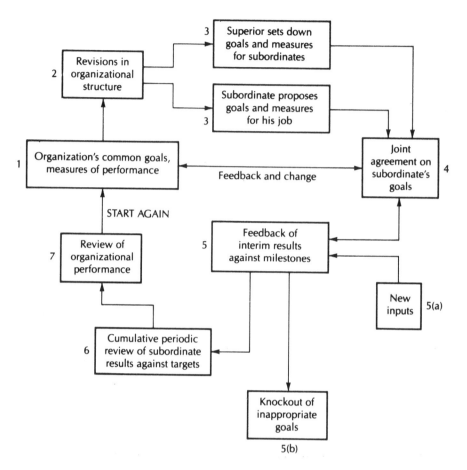

FIGURE 16.3 Cycle of management by objectives.

Source: Odiorne, G., *Management by Objectives: A System of Managerial Leadership.*
Copyright © 1965 by Pitman Publishing Corporation. Reprinted by permission of
Pitman Learning, Inc, Belmont, Calif.

Given the positive and negative points regarding MBO, it should be
employed by the leader if appropriate given the needs of the system or the
individual follower.

Other Ways to Resolve Conflict

Nielsen (1977) suggested an approach called creative conflict resolution
that is composed of six phases, similar to the problem-solving method:

1. Problem recognition with desire to solve it.

2. Concentrated effort to solve the problem through routine behaviour.

3. A period of frustration due to failure of customary actions, resulting in withdrawal.

4. An incubation period to reformulate the problem into a new perspective—redefinition.

5. Tentative solution to the newly defined problem.

6. A final solution.

One of the benefits of the creative approach is that conflict is given time to breathe and change. Forcing conflict resolution often has the effect of heightening the energy in the direction of greater conflict.

Marriner (1979b) suggested three ways of dealing with conflict. Win–lose methods include use of position power, mental or physical power, silence, majority rule, and railroading. Lose–lose strategies include compromise, bribes for accomplishing unpleasant tasks, arbitration, and use of general rules instead of looking at issues qualitatively. Win–win strategies focus on goals, emphasizing consensus and integrative approaches to decision making. The steps to win–win strategies follow the problem-solving method.

Edmunds (1979) underscored what Marriner (1979b) suggested and added that the most constructive way to handle conflict involves verbal rather than nonverbal communication—talking out rather than acting out. This author believes that both behaviours are important; verbal communication is often best when it precedes nonverbal communication—talk it out and then act on the basis of what has been discussed.

Assertive confrontation as a way to resolve conflict is discussed by Hughes (1979), Haw (1980), and Nichols (1979). Express opinions, feelings, and ideas directly and honestly in a way that does not insult, degrade, or humiliate others. Group-processing activities and giving and receiving feedback are other useful ways for resolving potential and present conflict. Davis and Newstrom (1985) suggested employee counselling as another way to resolve conflict, especially individual conflict. Thomas and Kilmann (1977) identified five conflict resolution modes: accommodating, avoiding, competing, compromising, and collaborating.

OUTCOMES OF CONFLICT

Conflicts result in outcomes that can be productive to the growth of an individual or an organization. Conversely, conflict can be extremely destructive (Kramer & Schmalenberg, 1978; Lewis, 1976; Myrtle & Glogow, 1978; Nielsen, 1977).

Deutsch (1969, 1973) identified four primary factors that determine the outcome of conflict: the issue, power, responsiveness to needs, and communication. The discussion follows that provided by Kramer and Schmalenberg (1978).

The Issue

In destructive conflict, the issue is amplified, broadly defined with the addition of tangential items, and emotionally charged. In constructive conflict, the issue is focused and kept to a manageable size. Only peripheral issues that relate to the main point are discussed, and the process of choice is action rather than reaction.

Power

In destructive power, situations are maintained or changed through threats and coercion. Competition is the climate with a resultant winner and loser. Constructive power involves finding an acceptable solution that may be a compromise or a new one; personal needs and views are not imposed on others.

Responsiveness to Needs

Only one's own needs are considered in destructive conflict. As time goes on, one becomes surer that one's beliefs and behaviours are right. Constructive conflict resolution is characterized by solutions that respond to the needs of all participants in the conflict.

Communication

Mutual distrust, misperception, and escalated emotional charges make up a destructive conflict course. Constructive resolution involves open and honest dialogue, sharing individual concerns, and listening with the desire to understand others. The intent is to get the problem out in the open so that it can be dealt with effectively.

Conflict is beneficial in an organization, providing that the leader is skilled in facilitating constructive conflict resolution. When different opinions on an issue are voiced and when problems are aired, it shows that people are involved and care. The opposite of love is not hate; the opposite is indifference. With both love and hate there is energy—those about whom one cares have the power to engender hate. Indifference is empty. Energy derived through effective conflict resolution can be used positively toward goal accomplishment. Nielsen (1977) said that conflict is "the root of personal and social change" (p. 153). It stimulates problem solving and the resultant creative solutions, it can be enjoyable, and it permits the development of a personal identity.

SUMMARY

Conflict is a clash or a struggle that occurs when one's balance among feelings, thoughts, desires, and behaviour is threatened. The struggle can be within an individual or within a group. Leaders can move the conflict to destructive or constructive outcomes.

Structurally, conflict can be vertical, involving differences between superiors and followers, or it can be horizontal as in line-staff relationships. Nine types of conflict are noted in the literature: intrasender, intersender, interrole, person-role, interperson, intragroup, intergroup, role ambiguity, and role overload.

Causes of conflict are unique and compounded. General causes, however, are cited and discussed. These refer to areas such as specialization, multitask roles, role interdependence, task blurring, differentiation, scarcity of resources, change, rewards, and communication. The process of conflict starts with antecedent conditions that move to perceived and/or felt conflict. Behaviour follows with the conflict either being resolved or suppressed.

Constructive conflict resolution is an important aspect of managerial responsibility. An array of approaches, including contingency contracting and management by objectives, is discussed. There is no best method for facilitating conflict resolution. A manager must have knowledge of possible strategies together with knowledge of the processes of managing and leading people; the best strategy given the unique environment must then be chosen and implemented.

REFERENCES

Cain, C., Luchsinger, V. (1978). Management by objectives: Applications to nursing. *Journal of Nursing Administration, 8*, 35–38.

Coombs, C. (1987). The structure of conflict. *American Psychologist, 42*(4), 355–363.

Corwin, R. (1969). Patterns of organizational conflict. *Administration Science Quarterly, 14*, 507–521.

Davis, K., & Newstrom, J. (1985). *Human behavior at work: Organizational behavior* (7th ed.). New York: McGraw-Hill.

Deutsch, M. (1969). Conflict: Productive and destructive. *Journal of Social Issues, 25*, 7–41.

Deutsch, M. (1973). *The resolution of conflict: Constructive and destructive processes.* New Haven: Yale University Press.

Douglass, L., & Bevis, E. (1979). *Nursing management and leadership in action.* St. Louis: Mosby.

Drucker, P. (1954). *The practice of management.* New York: Harper & Row.

Drucker, P. (1985a). The discipline of innovation. *Harvard Business Review, 64,* 67–72.

Drucker, P. (1985b). *Effective executive.* New York: Harper & Row.

Drucker, P. (1985c). *Managing in turbulent times.* New York: Harper & Row.

Edmunds, M. (1979). Conflict. *Nurse Practitioner, 4,* 42, 47–48.

Filley, A. (1975). *Interpersonal conflict resolution.* Morristown, NJ: Scott, Foresman.

Filley, A. (1980). Types and sources of conflict. In M. Berger, D. Elhart, S. Firsich, S. Jordan, & S. Stone (Eds.). *Management for nurses: A multidisciplinary approach* (2nd ed.). St. Louis: Mosby.

Fink, C. (1968). Some conceptual difficulties in the theory of social conflict. *Journal of Conflict Resolution, 13,* 413–458.

Ford, C. (1979). MBO: An idea whose time has gone? *Business Horizons, 22,* 48–55.

Golightly, C. (1979). MBO and performance appraisal. *Journal of Nursing Administration, 9,* 11–20.

Haw, M. (1980). Conflict resolution and the communication myth. *Nursing Outlook, 28,* 566–570.

Hersey, P., & Blanchard, K. (1988). *Management of organizational behavior: Utilizing human resources* (5th ed.). Englewood Cliffs, NJ: Prentice-Hall.

Homme, L. (1970). *How to use contingency contracting in the classroom.* Champaign, IL: Research Press.

Hughes, E. (1979). Helping staff to manage conflict well. *Hospital Progress, 60,* 68–71, 83.

Humble, J. (1967). *Management by objectives.* London: Industrial Education and Research Foundation.

Kramer, M., & Schmalenberg, C. (1978). Conflict: The cutting edge of growth. *Nursing Digest, 5,* 59–65.

Levinson, H. (1970). Management by whose objectives? *Harvard Business Review, 48,* 125–134.

Lewis, J. (1976). Conflict management. *Journal of Nursing Administration, 6,* 18–22.

Marriner, A. (1979a). Conflict theory. *Supervisor Nurse, 10,* 12–16.

Marriner, A. (1979b). Conflict resolution. *Supervisor Nurse, 10,* 46, 49, 52–54.

Marriner, A. (1982). Comparing strategies and their use: Managing conflict. *Nursing Management, 6,* 29–31.

Myrtle, R., & Glogow, E. (1978). How nursing administrators view conflict. *Nursing Research, 27,* 103–106.

Nichols, B. (1979). Dealing with conflict. *The Journal of Continuing Education in Nursing, 10,* 24–27.

Nielsen, H. (1977). Resolving conflict. In K. Claus, & J. Bailey, *Power and influence in health care.* St. Louis; Mosby.

Odiorne, G. (1965). *Management by objectives: A system of managerial leadership.* Belmont, CA: Pitman.

Odiorne, G. (1975). Management by objectives: Antidote to future shock. *Journal of Nursing Administration, 5,* 27–30.

Odiorne, G. (1979). *MBO II: A system of managerial leadership for the 80s.* Belmont, CA: D.S. Lake Pub.

Olsson, D. (1968). *Management by objectives.* Palo Alto, CA: Pacific Books.

Palmer, J. (1973). Management by objectives. *Journal of Nursing Administration, 3,* 55–60.

Pondy, L. (1967). Organizational conflict: Concepts and models. *Administrative Science Quarterly, 12,* 296–320.

Pondy, L. (1969). Variances of organizational conflict. *Administration Science Quarterly, 14,* 449–506.

Schmidt, S. (1973). *Laterial conflict within employment service district offices.* Unpublished doctoral dissertation. University of Wisconsin, Madison.

Silber, M. (1984). Managing confrontations: Once more into the breach. *Nursing Management, 15*(4), 54–58.

Skarupa, J. (1971). Management by objectives: A systematic way to manage change. *Journal of Nursing Administration, 1,* 52–56.

Stogdill, R., & Coons, A. (Eds.). (1957). *Leader behavior: Its description and measurement* (Research Monograph No. 88). Columbus: Bureau of Business Research, Ohio State University.

Thomas, K., & Kilmann, R. (1977). Developing a forced-choice measure of conflict-handling behavior: The "MODE" instrument. *Education and Psychological Measurement, 37,* 309–325.

Walton, R., & Dutton, J. (1969). The management of interdepartmental conflict: A model and review. *Administrative Science Quarterly, 14,* 73–84.

Time Management

People plan within a boundary of time, look on the past over a span of time, and set goals for the future that are to be met within a period of time. Time can facilitate goal accomplishment, and it can be an oppressive force in finishing tasks. It can make people nervous in one context and can relax those same people in another context. Life is run on a time schedule—in some instances the schedule is philosophical, and in other instances it is concrete. For example, one has six months to live or one has a whole lifetime. Is there any philosophical difference in these statements? Clocks, calendars, watches, seasons, holidays, birthdays, and so forth, all point to time—the unidirectional process of growth.

Managers should attend particularly to time because it costs money to an organization—efficiency pays off. Life without wasted time is impossible. A manager, however, can increase the probability that time will be used efficiently by following some general guidelines that have been primarily developed by Cooper (1971), Dayton (1983), Drucker (1967), Lakein (1973), Mackenzie (1972), McCay (1959), Oncken and Wass (1974), and Webber (1981). Applications of the time management concept have recently been observed in literature from the helping professions (Brown, 1980; Byrd, 1977, 1980; Eliopoulos, 1984; Ferri, 1987; McGee-Cooper, 1986a, 1986b, 1986c, 1986d; Marriner, 1979; Rutkowski, 1984; Schwartz & Mackenzie, 1979; Smith & Besnette, 1978; Volk-Tebbitt, 1978; Wiley, 1978).

Every person has all the time there is, yet few people have enough time (Mackenzie, 1972). Since no manager is going to get more time, the time one has must be used more efficiently. Believe it or not, this is possible. The philosophy of time will be discussed first in this chapter followed by the time management process. Time-managing techniques are discussed in the concluding part of the chapter. The intent is to help managers to learn how to get "a little more" out of the time given.

PHILOSOPHY OF TIME

Time has been defined by Arnold (cited in Volk-Tebbitt, 1978) as a system of references for understanding and describing the occurrence and sequence of events. It is also a resource (Mackenzie, 1972) that cannot be stockpiled or accumulated—it cannot be turned on or off. According to Drucker (1967), time is so important that unless it is managed, nothing else can be managed.

Classifying Activities

Activities are either time wasters or time consumers. The Health Care Management Team of the Minnesota Hospital Association (Volk-Tebbitt, 1978) said that a time waster is an activity that has a lower payoff than an alternate activity that could be done during a particular time period. Drop-in visitors, unproductive meetings, telephone interruptions, and so forth, are examples of time wasters.

Lakein (1973) viewed a time-consumer activity as complex and/or difficult with high payoffs. He classified activities as As, Bs, and Cs. Cs are activities that no one asks about; they are trivial and have little or no payoff. If a memo is received, then the activity is a B—moderately important with moderate payoff. Activities receiving an A are important— calls get received on them, and people come to visit and inquire about them. As have a high payoff. Lakein (1973) claimed that people spend 80% of their time doing C activities and only 20% doing As. Yet A priorities make the difference. This factual philosophy leads into the Pareto Principle.

The Pareto Principle

The Pareto Principle, named after the 19th century Italian economist and sociologist Vilfredo Pareto, stated that a relatively small number of items, tasks, or behaviours in a group are significant ones (Mackenzie, 1972). Juran (1964) labelled these items as the "vital few" and the balance of items as the "trivial many". The Pareto Principle is a way of explaining that normally the trivial many situational problems use 80% of the group's time in producing 20% of the positive results. In contrast, the vital few situations or problems use 20% of the expended time to produce 80% of the positive results.

Applying the principle to nursing, suppose the goal of increasing patient satisfaction with nursing care were sought. The nursing system, above average in readiness on this task, required LB3—high consideration and low structure. They identified 20 interventions that could be made to increase patient satisfaction. When the Pareto Principle is applied, 4 of the 20 would generally account for 80% of the change in patients when the interventions were implemented and evaluated. The rest of the interventions would reap little payoff in terms of cost effectiveness. The time used in low-payoff activities—time wasters—could be channelled into higher-payoff interventions connected to solving another problem, which is also of high priority but on a different level. Figure 17.1 portrays this priority process.

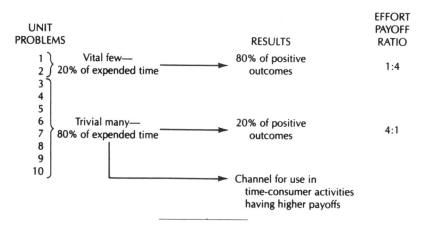

FIGURE 17.1 Priority process using the Pareto Principle.

The primary goal of time management is to make activities count, to the degree that is possible. This goal is achieved by controlling time so that the least amount of effort produces the greatest positive outcomes—making the 1:4 (effort:payoff) ratio shown in Figure 17.1 even better with less effort and better results.

Kinds of Time

A manager has two categories of time: specialty time and managerial time (Graf, 1979; Mackenzie, 1972). Specialty time involves those responsibilities which are accomplished alone. This does not exclude the need of input from others, as required by the task. It simply means that when the activity is to be done, it is usually done by the manager. A nurse supervisor might see staffing, mapping out long-term goals, and/or preparing the agenda for the next ward sisters' meeting as specialty items. Keep in mind that the inclusion of activities into either category is relative to the unique system and its particular needs.

Managerial time is time that is shared with or given to others in a system— it involves some level of interaction between or among people. Managerial time can be subdivided into response time and discretionary time. Response time generally involves such activities as speaking on the telephone to a caller or returning a call, having office visits, attending meetings, and making rounds. Discretionary time has to do with activities that suggest or ask for a response but the leader has the option of deciding whether or not to actually behave in accordance with the request. Time may be better used in another activity.

Specialty and managerial time contain activities that can be prioritized according to Lakein's (1973) ABC system, described earlier in this chapter. There is no formula for the ratio of managerial time to specialty time in a manager's position. This is purely according to the environment that includes the unique manager, system, and tasks. One general rule of thumb, however, is that the more generally mature the system is, the greater opportunity the manager has to corner specialty time. Obviously, the opposite is also true—the more generally immature the system is, the fewer options the manager has to corner specialty time.

THE TIME MANAGEMENT PROCESS

The time management process is another extension of the problem-solving method, as shown in Table 17.1. Perusing Table 17.1 and thinking about the focus of this chapter can lead to the conclusion that the problem-solving method pertains to managing others toward cost effectiveness, whereas the time management process focuses on managing the self so that the ratio of effort to payoff is high. The processes are

TABLE 17.1 The Time Management Process and the Problem-Solving Method

Time Management Process*	Problem-Solving Method
Analyzing the present situation ◄━━━━━━━━► Problem identification (Where I am now?)	
Developing relevant assumptions (What conditions will most likely exist within the time span of the plan?) ◄━━━━━━━━► Point of view	
Establishing objectives (What do I want to achieve?) ◄━━━━━━━━► Problem definition and/or goal statement ➤ Problem analysis	
Developing alternatives (What ways might I attain objectives?) ◄━━━━━━━━► Alternative solutions	
Making a decision ◄━━━━━━━━━━━━━━► Recommended action	
Implementing the decision	
Establishing review and control procedures	

*Source: Column 1 is taken from Mackenzie, R.: *The Time Trap: Managing Your Way Out*, New York, McGraw-Hill, 1972, pp. 44–45.

parallel while the content and subjects differ. All the previously discussed principles of managing, goal setting, motivation, and so forth apply in this chapter also.

A person must first look at his or her present situation (the actual) on personal and professional (specialty and managerial) grounds. One should pose and answer the question of where one is on important areas. Then, given reasonable projections of what environmental conditions will exist at different slices of time—one month, one year, five years, and whenever—ask where would one like to be on those same areas. What comes out of this thinking, as the reader of this book already knows, is the problem/goal. The objectives, which flow from the goal, describe the desired outcome. (Refer to Chapter 12 on teaching for further discussion on goals and objectives.)

Once objectives have been designated, they must be arranged on the basis of priorities. One useful way of doing this is according to Lakein's (1973) ABCs. Or ponder each objective with the questions: "How much effort will be involved in fulfilling this objective, and what is the expected payoff?" Then assign priorities according to least effort/most payoff (high priority) down to most effort/least pay-off (low priority). A scale of one to five (low to high) can be used if finer quantification in this process is sought. Then attack the top priorities—just two or three.

Develop alternative strategies for accomplishing these objectives.

These strategies are concerned with how the objectives will be attained. The goals and objectives themselves are what is to be attained. Again, develop an effort/payoff ratio for each solution and pinpoint the best strategy for action. Implement it and evaluate it by comparing intent with results. Evaluation can range from completely subjective to very objective. The need for formality of the evaluation phase can be assessed by looking at the effort against the possible payoff. As a side note, formal evaluations are costly in terms of effort. They may, however, be worth it. Consult a book on evaluation procedures and evaluation research such as Thorndike and Hagen (1977) should formal evaluation controls be indicated.

Now, does all of this seem simple? Do not be fooled. Parasites eat and piranhas nip away at our time, and the concept called time management is most useful because readers on the topic can receive myriad helpful hints on controlling parasites and piranhas. The next portion of this chapter is devoted to discussing these techniques. The content is not inclusive—many more tips are available in time management literature and from personal experiences.

TIME MANAGEMENT TECHNIQUES

This section presents an array of techniques for attacking parasites and piranhas (Lakein, 1973; Mackenzie, 1972). Each topic is discussed separately.

Personal Commitment to Improving

How many psychiatrists does it take to change one 60-watt light bulb? The answer is "only one, but the light bulb has to be willing"—corny but true. Brown (1980) termed personal commitment to time saving as the *sine qua non*. So examine yourself. Those who care should read on. Those who discover unwillingness should try to discern why it exists and work on changing from unwillingness to willingness—then read on. McConnell (1983) underscored that in order to become an effective manager of others, a leader must first become an effective manager of self—through personal effort.

Deciding What Not to Do

A requisite for success, according to Nunlist (cited in Mackenzie, 1972) is refusing to do the unimportant. "They must learn to forget the unnecessary and to ignore the irrelevant" (p. 55). Then do a fantastic job on the essentials.

Learning to Say No

Read the book entitled *When I Say No, I Feel Guilty* by Smith (1985). Someone always has a priority—essential—that another must do. In a hospital, the "someones" abound. The manager must sort out the important from the unimportant, or high-payoff tasks from low-payoff tasks, and say no to the latter tasks and yes to the former ones —without feeling and probably communicating guilt or some other self-defeating emotion.

Recording How Time is Used

The "Time Analysis Worksheet" (Brown, 1980) that is found in the exercises at the conclusion of this part is one way to find out how time is used—where it goes. This raises consciousness of one's own behaviour by making the abstract concrete. The "Time Log", also found in the exercises, can be used for the same purpose.

Planning Use of Time

List responsibilities, choose priorities, and schedule for their accomplishment. Develop a daily, weekly, and/or monthly "to do" list. Check off progress; this is self-reinforcement for further accomplishment. Do not let minutia intrude on the list but also allow for some flexibility, especially in the longer-term lists.

Fire Fighting Versus Fire Prevention

Graf (1979) explained fire fighting as responding to whatever comes up, like applying oil to the squeaky wheel. It is necessary when planning is poor. Fire prevention involves contingency planning—looking ahead and asking, "What can be done today to avoid problems in the future?" Of course, preventing fires can become a parasite in and of itself. So invest enough energy in this area to make the payoff worthwhile.

Prime Time

Most people have a certain portion of a day that they know is their "prime time". During this period, people are at their best, and work is usually easiest to accomplish. Find out what this block of time is and use it—hang a "do not disturb" sign outside the door, refuse calls, do not schedule meetings, and so forth. This is probably the time when 80% of work gets accomplished, so protect it.

Programming Blocks of Time

Graf (1979) pointed out that "one of the best ways to complete big projects is to program large blocks of time for the effort" (p. 17). Otherwise, the task will be broken up into smaller pieces and much time will be wasted getting oriented to where one was at the end of the last session.

Organizing the Workspace

Arrange the environment to make life easier. Make the office space fit your individual personality—from the colour of the walls to the arrangement of furniture or addition of plants to anything else that is pleasing. Keep the desk uncluttered; keep only the project in immediate focus on it. Any other material on the desk may become a distractor. Have tools such as pencil sharpeners, staplers, and so forth handy. Eliminate the need to get up and wander around—time gets wasted both from the short journey and from re-entry.

Memoitis

Oh, the memoranda that infest offices! Mackenzie (1972) reported an estimate that puts the paperwork cost of running the US economy at a sum equal to about one-seventh of the total yearly output of goods and services. Memos are part of this mountain.

Memos are to remind, to clarify, and to confirm (Mackenzie, 1972). They involve one-way communication. Use them only when essential. In many instances, a phone call is the better bet.

Learn to scan memos received for a quick assessment of their importance. If it passes the best of "reading worthiness", then read it fully. If not, throw it immediately in a conveniently placed wastebasket. Take a speed-reading course if possible.

Blocking Interruptions

Common courtesy is always necessary but it should not be confused with a need to extend carte blanche to telephone calls or to visits (Mackenzie, 1972). A manager can extend the "open door policy" when it is decided that the door should be opened—definitely not during one's prime time.

Drop-in visitors should be discouraged. Simply say once, "I would like to talk with you at a time when I am not involved in a project. We can schedule an appointment at. . . .:" A drop-in-type person usually gets the message after the first or second such interchange. Confer with drop-in visitors standing up and outside one's office, if possible. This is a barrier to the visitor's discourteous intrusion. Consider the intruder who "knows it is not regular office hours but just needs one minute for a 'quick' question". The scene might go like this.

> That one-minute intrusion minimally involves the following, without exaggeration: (1) thinking about what you were doing ends; (2) your mind switches gear to contain anger at the disruption first and then to think about what the intruder is asking; (3) time to respond coherently, masking flaming anger; (4) listening to the almost sure second and third questions and/or comments of the intruder; (5) responding again when secretly vowing not to let this situation be repeated, maybe even blaming your secretary; (6) bidding farewell and emphasizing that it would be a pleasure to talk again—simply make an appointment or come in during regular office hours; (7) getting coffee to calm your nerves; and (8) sitting down trying to recall what you were doing prior to the intrusion and where you were on the matter. This intrusion costs at least 30 minutes, ignoring the nonquantifiable cost to your nervous system.

The telephone is another piranha because it can ring anytime, and sometimes just the ring is intrusive. If possible, have a secretary screen calls on the following basis: "immediate response is required" and "delayed response is required". Handle the immediate calls and arrange telephone hours to return other calls. When available, have a secretary place the calls and then transfer them to the caller.

Managing Meetings

"Parkinson's Second Law stated that people tend to devote time and effort to tasks in inverse relation to their importance" (adapted from Mackenzie, 1972, p. 107). Mackenzie (1972) offered several pages of rules for getting more out of meetings; here are a choice few together with beliefs of this author:

1. Start on time; give warning only the first time.
2. End on time.
3. Develop an agenda and circulate it to the attendees prior to the meeting.
4. Only those needed should attend a meeting.
5. Gather information prior to a meeting; summarize it during the meeting.
6. Stick to the agenda; avoid interruptions; squelch side-trips around or away from the agenda.

7. Limit the amount of time for a particular agenda; place the meeting so that the intended gets accomplished.

8. Arrange for a comfortable environment but not so plush that people would rather be there than somewhere else.

9. Items that involve one-way communication by their nature should be typed and distributed—not verbally announced. The latter simply wastes time.

10. Have a secretary take and distribute the minutes of the meeting within one week from the date of the meeting. Minutes should record the issues and the decisions. Brief reports of the points of discussion may be included. When minutes are verbatim accounts of the meetings, the secretary wastes time and so do all the readers.

Managing People

Time management books, such as those in the references at the end of this chapter, include a portion on delegating. The focus is to alert the manager that managers lead people to accomplish goals. Therefore, managers should delegate work to others.

As the reader is aware by now, managers must use a variety of styles to help followers mature in relation to accomplishing a task. Depending on the system's level of maturity at a certain time and place, the manager must appropriately either tell, sell to, participate with, or delegate to followers. Managers must examine themselves in order to discern whether they use different leader behaviour styles because the system needs them or because of their own needs. When a system's maturity indicates, the push is always toward delegation because then the manager has freed time for other managerial and/or specialty tasks. It behoves managers to examine themselves and to give followers the leadership they need, pushing them toward maturity. This is a responsibility of managers, and in terms of time management it is a reward of management.

Springing the Time Trap

In *The Time Trap*, Mackenzie (1972) included an appendix on time wasters he has most commonly encountered, their causes, and their possible solutions. The list is not exhaustive but certainly can help. Table 17.2 presents his work.

TABLE 17.2 How to Spring the Time Trap

Time Waster	Possible Causes	Solutions
Lack of planning	Failure to see the benefit	Recognize that planning takes time but saves time in the end.
	Action orientation	Emphasize results, not activity.
	Success without it	Recognize that success is often in spite of, not because of, methods.
Lack of priorities	Lack of goals and objectives	Write down goals and objectives. Discuss priorities with subordinate.
Overcommitment	Broad interests	Say no.
	Confusion in priorities	Put first things first.
	Failure to set priorities	Develop a personal philosophy of time. Relate priorities to a schedule of events.
Management by crisis	Lack of planning	Apply the same solutions as for lack of planning.
	Unrealistic time estimates	Allow more time. Allow for interruptions.
	Problem orientation	Be opportunity-oriented.
	Reluctance of subordinates to break bad news	Encourage fast transmission of information as essential for timely corrective action.
Haste	Impatience with detail	Take time to get it right. Save the time of doing it over.
	Responding to the urgent	Distinguish between the urgent and the important.
	Lack of planning ahead	Take time to plan. It repays itself many times over.
	Attempting too much in too little time	Attempt less. Delegate more.
Paperwork and reading	Knowledge explosion	Read selectively. Learn speed reading.

TABLE 17.2 (*continued*)

Time Waster	Possible Causes	Solutions
	Computeritis	Manage computer data by exception.
	Failure to screen	Remember the Pareto Principle. Delegate reading to subordinates.
Routine and trivia	Lack of priorities	Set and concentrate on goals. Delegate nonessentials.
	Oversurveillance of subordinates	Delegate; then give subordinates their space. Look to results, not details or methods.
	Refusal to delegate; feeling of greater security dealing with operating detail	Recognize that without delegation it is impossible to get anything done through others.
Visitors	Enjoyment of socializing	Do it elsewhere. Meet visitors outside. Suggest lunch if necessary. Hold stand-up conferences.
	Inability to say "no"	Screen. Say no. Be unavailable. Modify the open-door policy.
Telephone	Lack of self-discipline	Screen and group calls. Be brief.
	Desire to be informed and involved	Stay uninvolved with all but essentials. Manage by exception.
Meetings	Fear of responsibility for decisions	Make decisions without meetings.
	Indecision	Make decisions even when some facts are missing.
	Overcommunication	Discourage unnecessary meetings. Convene only those needed.
	Poor leadership	Use agenda. Stick to the subject. Prepare concise minutes as soon as possible.

(*continued*)

TABLE 17.2 (*continued*)

Time Waster	Possible Causes	Solutions
Indecision	Lack of confidence in the facts	Improve fact-finding and validating procedures.
	Insistence on all the facts—paralysis of analysis	Accept risks as inevitable. Decide without all facts.
	Fear of the consequences of a mistake	Delegate the right to be wrong. Use mistakes as a learning process.
	Lack of a rational decision-making process	Get facts, set goals, investigate alternatives and negative consequences, make the decision, and implement it.
Lack of delegation	Fear of subordinates' inadequacy	Train. Allow mistakes. Replace if necessary.
	Fear of subordinates' competence	Delegate fully. Give credit. Ensure corporate growth to maintain challenge.
	Work overload on subordinates	Balance the work load. Staff up. Reorder priorities.

Source: Reprinted, by permission of the publisher, from *The time trap: Managing your way out*, by R. Alec Mackenzie, © 1972 by AMACOM, a division of American Management Associations, pp. 173–176. This list is adapted from "Troubleshooting Chart for Time Wasters," in R. Alec Mackenzie, *Managing time at the top*. New York, The President's Association, 1970.

SUMMARY

The concept of time is a constant phenomenon. Each person has all the time there is, and no one ever has enough time. The intent of applying time management techniques is to get "a little more" out of the time given.

Time is a system of references for understanding and describing the occurrence and sequence of events. Activities can be classified as time wasters or time consumers, which are relative terms. The Pareto Principle is a way of explaining how 20% of one's time involved in time consumers produces 80% of positive outcomes. Eighty percent of expended time in activities that are time wasters result in 20% of positive outcomes. The trick/goal is to have the least amount of effort produce the greatest positive outcomes.

Managers have specialty time for themselves and managerial time spent interacting in some form with others. The time management process parallels the problem-solving method. It can be used to guide a manager toward goal fulfillment in professional and personal areas.

Time management techniques were discussed in the last part of the chapter. The intent of these techniques is to offer a manager a potpourri of interventions against the parasites and piranhas of time. It is essential that each person recognize his or her inherent potential to waste and to save time—his or her own as well as another's.

REFERENCES

Brown, D., (1980). *The use of time: A looking-into-leadership monograph.* Fairfax, VA: Leadership Resources.

Byrd, E. (1977). Time management. *American Rehabilitation, 2,* 24–26.

Byrd, E. (1980). Irrational ideas in the management of time. *Journal of Applied Rehabilitation Counseling, 11,* 46–49.

Cooper, J. (1971). *How to get more done in less time.* Garden City, NY: Doubleday.

Dayton, E. (1983). *Tools for time management: Time saving tools for managing your life* (rev. ed.). Grand Rapids, MI: Zondervan.

Drucker, P. (1967). *The effective executive.* New York: Harper & Row.

Eliopoulos, C. (1984). Time management: A reminder. *Journal of Nursing Administration, 14*(3), 30–32.

Ferri, R. (1987). In search of the excellent one-minute megatrend . . . or how to tolerate the five minute burden. *American Journal of Nursing, 87,* (1), 109–110.

Graf, P. (1979). *Ten techniques for improving time management.* Unpublished manuscript.

Juran, J. (1964). *Managerial breakthrough: A new concept of the manager's job.* New York: McGraw-Hill.

Lakein, A. (1973). *How to get control of your time and your life.* New York: Peter H. Wyden.

Mackenzie, R. (1972). *The time trap: Managing your way out.* New York: AMACOM (A Division of the American Management Association).

Marriner, A. (1979). Time. *Journal of Nursing Administration, 9,* 16–18.

McCay, J. (1959). *The management of time.* Englewood Cliffs, NJ: Prentice-Hall.

McConnell, C. (1983). Supervisor, manage yourself. *The Health Care Supervisor, 1*(3), 57–68.

McGee-Cooper, A. (1986a). Time management—Part II: Rewriting obsolete work rules. *AORN Journal, 44,* 409–414.

McGee-Cooper, A. (1986b). Time management—Part III: Making the time for joy. *AORN Journal, 44,* 599–602.

McGee-Cooper, A. (1986c). Time management—Part IV: Decontaminating work and play time. *AORN Journal, 44,* 809–813.

McGee-Cooper, A. (1986d). Time management—Part V: Energy engineering. *AORN Journal, 44,* 977–982.

Oncken, W., & Wass, D. (1974). Management time: Who's got the monkey? *Harvard Business Review, 52,* 75–80.

Rutkowski, B. (1984). The nursing approach to better time management. *Nursing Life, 4*(5), 54–57.

Schwartz, E., & Mackenzie, R. (1979). Time-management strategy for women. *Journal of Nursing Administration, 9,* 22–26.

Smith, H., & Besnette, F. (1978). Effective time management: The forgotten administrative and nursing supervisor art. *Hospital Topics, 56,* 32–37.

Smith, M. (1985). *When I say no, I feel guilty.* New York: Bantam.

Thorndike, R., & Hagen, E. (1977). *Measurement and evaluation in psychology and education* (4th ed.). New York: Wiley.

Volk-Tebbitt, B. (1978). Time: Who controls yours? *Supervisor Nurse, 9,* 17–22.

Webber, R. (1981). *Time and management.* Nutley, NJ: Moffat.

Wiley, L. (1978). The ABCs of time management. *Nursing 78, 8,* 105–112.

Performance Appraisal

Performance appraisal is one method for a manager to control what is occurring in the organization. It is a way to compare the outcomes of individual and group behaviours toward goal accomplishment with the initiatives that were planned. Further, it is the way most managers formally and informally guide employees in their professional development within an organization.

The literature is replete with articles on the topic of performance appraisal. There are authors who have developed objective performance appraisal systems (Ganong & Ganong, 1983; Richards, 1984; Stalker, Kornblith, Lewis, & Parker, 1986); others have studied the process for conducting the performance appraisal (Meyer, 1984; Rothwell, 1984; Stull, 1986); and investigators have studied the effects of feedback and other processes on employee development (Lachman, 1984; Pearce & Porter, 1986). There is literature on the factors that should be included in various criterion-referenced performance appraisals (Johnson & Luciano, 1988; Lampe, 1986; McCloskey & McCain, 1988) and then there is discussion about whether performance appraisals really work in producing the desired outcomes (Momeyer, 1986; Zemke, 1985).

Even though discussions about performance appraisals from both managers and followers always involve some degree of hesitation, anxiety, and even pain, the performance appraisal seems here to stay—in one form or another. The purpose of this chapter, therefore, is to discuss the general reasons for the performance appraisal, principles of appraisal, tactics for appraising, and classic methods used in conducting the performance appraisal.

PURPOSES OF THE PERFORMANCE APPRAISAL

There are two general purposes for the performance evaluation: judgemental purposes and developmental purposes (Ivancevich, Donnelly, & Gibson, 1989).

Judgemental Purposes

When performance appraisals are accomplished for the purposes of determining salary standards and salary increases and/or awarding merit increases, then they are being carried out for judgemental purposes. Other reasons in this area include selecting qualified individuals for promotions and/or transfers and demoting or terminating employment due to unsatisfactory performance (Rowland & Rowland, 1985). Performance appraisals that are done for judgemental purposes carry the highest stakes and necessarily result in the most anxiety from both the rater and the ratee.

Developmental Purposes

Developmental purposes are predominantly educative and involve coaching the employee to gain professionally through working within organizational goals. Self-learning and personal growth are both involved (Ivancevich, Donnelly, & Gibson, 1989). Rowland and Rowland (1985) described specific examples such as the following: identifying talent in the organization; determining training and development needs of individuals or groups; improving interpersonal relationships among group members; establishing standards of performance and gaining acceptance of those standards; providing employee recognition; discovering employee aspirations and reconciling them with the goals of the organization; team building; and giving employees feedback.

PRINCIPLES OF PERFORMANCE APPRAISAL

There are certain principles of performance appraisal that must be met in order for an appraisal to be useful in any purpose.

First, the appraisal must contain content that is *relevant* to the individual being appraised in a particular setting (Ivancevich, Donnelly, & Gibson, 1989). This answers the question, "What is to be appraised?" In other words, the content of the appraisal must encompass a valid sample of the behaviours or traits that are seen as important in a specified position. The affective, the cognitive, and the psychomotor areas involved in carrying out specified responsibilities in a position must be represented. Therefore, the appraisal should be based on a position analysis and a resultant position description for a given level of expertise. In typical clinical career ladders, for example, there are different position descriptions for the role of staff nurse with two years of experience, then from two to five years of experience, and so forth. At each level of experience, an employee ought to be able to achieve excellence.

Second, the *criteria* that will be used to appraise performance should be stated and *standards* should be specified whenever possible. The criteria may be stated in a paper-and-pencil rating scale by a follower or maybe a paper-and-pencil self-report or a test, for example. The standard is the minimally acceptable level of performance, such as 90% passing rate on a test or writing care plans on all patients within 24 hours of their admission. It is important that the criterion method be reliable, that is, that it be stable over time and between/among raters. If two raters rated the same person and had the same information, would their ratings be very similar? If a criterion method is said to be reliable, both raters would have similar scores. This same principle applies when the same rater is rating at two different intervals. If no change has occurred, then the score should be similar; in contrast, if the employee has grown or learned, then the score on the criterion should show improvement.

Third, a performance appraisal should be able to *discriminate* between excellent, good, and poor performance (Ivancevich, Donnelly, & Gibson, 1989). Any purpose for which an appraisal is done should involve identification of areas requiring further development and areas that just need to continue in the effective vein with possibly some enrichment.

Last, any performance appraisal must be *practical* (Ivancevich, Donnelly, & Gibson, 1989) or in measurement terminology, it must have *utility*. There are many organizations and people in those organizations that spend tremendous amounts of time developing, testing, and implementing extremely lengthy performance appraisals. In contemporary health care and nursing practice, one must evaluate the effort/payoff ratio in such an endeavour. Sometimes people develop a criterion-referenced appraisal over such a long period of time that the content is no longer valid given the requirements of the position—which seem to change quickly in current practice. Further, the longer the appraisal forms, the less likely managers are going to find time to complete them.

TACTICS OF PERFORMANCE APPRAISAL

The process of the performance appraisal can be paralleled with the problem-solving method that was presented, discussed, and applied in Part I of this book. Table 18.1 contains a comparison of these processes. The performance appraisal process noted is a blend by this author of

TABLE 18.1 Comparisons of Processes: Problem-Solving and Performance Appraisal

Problem-Solving Process	Performance Appraisal Process
1. Identify the problem	Define the job requirements—expectations
	Define the standards (benchmarks) of performance for a particular role
2. Designate the system	Specify the employee qualifications
3. Diagnose the system (self and others)	Review the objectives set by manager and employee
	Review the performance records
	Tentatively complete the appraisal form
4. Choose leader behaviour	Conduct the appraisal
5. Specify alternative solutions	Co-develop a performance improvement plan using Management by Objectives or goal setting
6. Recommend an action	Agree on a plan of action
7. Implement the plan	Provide on-the-job coaching or daily reinforcement and development activities
8. Evaluate the results	Provide ongoing feedback on performance

information contained from many sources. Operationally, it identifies the steps for planning, conducting, and following up on the evaluation.

Who Should Appraise?

Ivancevich, Donnelly, & Gibson (1989) identified five possible parties who could appraise or rate another person: a supervisor, peers, the ratee, subordinates of the ratee, or raters outside of the organizational environment. In most cases, employees should be rated by their immediate supervisor, since this person has the greatest opportunity to observe the individual's behaviour against organizational objectives.

Who Should be Appraised?

Most organizations appraise employees at all levels of the organization—from the bottom of the organizational chart right to the top managerial levels. Education and development can occur anywhere and people require feedback as a stimulus to develop further in specified directions.

When Should Appraisals Occur?

There is no rule; however, most organizations appraise older or tenured employees about once or twice a year. New employees are appraised about six weeks to two months after being hired and employees at various stages of development may be appraised more or less often than twice a year, depending on the objectives set during the previous appraisal. Progressive discipline procedures are examples of appraisals that may occur as often as every two weeks. An appraisal should contain a progress note at the bottom that is written by the appraiser; it should designate when the next appraisal will occur and the objectives for the period of time until that date.

The Appraisal Interview

The appraisal interview is a way of providing formal feedback to the employee. This author recommends that both rater and ratee complete the appraisal form or make notes relative to each criterion. Following discussion in the interview, a record can be made by the appraiser that reflects information from all involved.

In addition to the principles and discussion in Chapter 13 on interviewing, Ivancevich, Donnelly, and Gibson (1989) provided guidelines for preparing and conducting an appraisal interview. Their thoughts can found in Table 18.2.

TABLE 18.2 Guidelines for Preparing and Conducting an Appraisal Interview

Preparing for the interview:

1. Hold a group discussion with employees to be appraised and describe the broad standards for their appraisals.
2. Discuss your employees with your own manager and several of your peers.
3. Clarify any differences in language between the formal written appraisal and the interview.
4. If you are angry with an employee, talk about it before the interview, not during the interview.
5. Be aware of your own biases in judging people.
6. Review the employee's compensation plan and be knowledgeable about his or her salary history.
7. If you already have given the employee a number of negative appraisals, be prepared to take action.

Conducting the interview:

1. Focus on positive work performance.
2. Remember that strengths and weaknesses usually spring from the same general characteristics.
3. Admit that your judgment of performance contains some subjectivity.
4. Make it clear that responsibility for development lies with the employee, not with you (the rater).
5. Be specific when citing examples.

Source: Ivancevich, J., Donnelly, J. Jr., & Gibson, J. (1989). *Management: Principles and functions* (4th ed.). Homewood, IL: Irwin, p. 534.

Research Findings on Performance Appraisal

The following insights regarding performance appraisal seem important for the appraiser and the appraisee to keep in mind. With the exception of the first finding presented, Kreitner and Kinicki (1989) synthesized these results from several sources including Hedge and Kavangh (1988) and Landy and Farr (1980).

- Kraiger and Ford (1985) found that appraisers typically rate same-race appraisees higher. In a meta-analysis involving 74 studies and 17,159 individuals, white supervisors, favoured white subordinates. Similarly in a meta-analysis of 14 studies and 2,248 people, black supervisors favoured black subordinates. These findings support the findings of Hornstein (1976) in his research on prosocial and antisocial behaviour in similar and dissimilar groups.

- No consistent gender bias was found.
- The more experienced rater and the higher performance manager tended to result in higher-quality appraisals. Training and development had positive effects of appraisal quality.
- Peer ratings and self-evaluations tended toward leniency when compared with ratings from a supervisor.

PERFORMANCE APPRAISAL METHODS

There are many methods that can be used to appraise a person. The ones used predominantly in health care systems will be presented and discussed.

Graphic Rating Scales

This is the most widely used method of appraising performance and involves having behaviour statements or traits each rated on a continuum that may be quantitative or qualitative. The Likert-type scale that moves from 1 (poor) to 5 (excellent), for example, is a quantitative scale. Occasionally, qualitative adjectives may be used such as poor, average, and excellent to describe numbers. Graphic rating scales can be used by superiors in rating subordinates, or they may be used in self-reports or ratings by peers. When the quantitative scale is used, an overall appraisal score can be derived by adding all the individual scores and dividing it by the number of items.

In graphic rating scales, it is important to understand that the greater the number of quantitative intervals, the greater the chance that the intervals will not be stable across raters. In other words, if two raters are observing the same person in the same context and have been given the same information, their ratings will be more similar as the number of rating possibilities decreases.

Critical Incidents

These are examples of good and bad performances that are written down soon after occurring. In a sense, they are a diary of significant events in the work performance of an employee. Critical incidents should focus on work-related behaviour and not personality traits (Kreitner & Kinicki, 1989).

Written Essays

This is a narrative description of one's perception of another's work-related performance or it may actually be written as a self-report. This is the most subjective of the appraisal techniques since something liked (the halo effect) or something disliked (the horn effect) often runs through and flavours the entire essay. Furthermore, they are usually written long after the actual behaviour has been observed; hence, they are subject to the distortion caused by time.

Goal Setting

This method employs Drucker's (1954, 1985a, 1985b, 1985c) Management by Objectives or modifications of the method. In Management by Objectives, results are emphasized rather than activities. Objectives are mutually set between supervisor and follower and a time period during which the goals are to be met is specified. When the date is reached, then another discussion takes place in which actual results are compared with expected outcomes and a new set of objectives is formulated.

In practice, a manager can also designate activities into the plan so that the follower will have a map on how to attain the stated goals. This author recommends that goal setting be included in any of the other types of performance appraisals. In a sense, there should be a portion of the appraisal report that is open for writing objectives that are expected to be met within a given period of time. All unsatisfactory performances should have at least one objective that is intended for alleviating the unsatisfactory performance. Enrichment activities and areas of talent should be amplified in this section also.

Rankings

This technique involves ranking employees on a particular dimension of work performance (Kreitner & Kinicki, 1989). If there are several dimensions on which employees are to be ranked, then their rankings can be summed to provide an overall ranking for each employee. In health care systems, this type of appraisal is usually not evident formally. However, many supervisors have this ranking system readily available in their own thought processes.

Behaviourally Anchored Rating Scales

This type of rating scale is similar to the graphic scale, only at each point there are behavioural statements that define what each ranking represents. This method usually results in greater rater interreliability of the appraisal.

A PERSONAL NOTE ON APPRAISALS

It is possible to spend a lifetime developing a rating scale that is both reliable and valid. That is, the scale rates consistently across raters and among items (reliability), and measures a sample of behaviours that adequately represents the responsibilities in a given position (validity). Both of these concepts must be evaluated—a judgement is made that the reliability and validity of an appraisal form are adequate given the purposes for which the appraisal is used.

The amount of time that a manager has in a health care organization for the purposes of conducting performance appraisals varies greatly. However, it is safe to say that the process of appraisal is among many equally important responsibilities. It therefore should not be a totally time-consuming activity, expending a great amount of effort for an important but moderate payoff.

This author always suggests that the time spent in developing the performance appraisal form and establishing reliability and validity of the instrument should be a careful and planned consideration. It has been observed that such a great amount of time is spent on developing reliability and validity tests that by the time the developer/researcher concludes that it should be implemented, the behaviours of practice have changed—which renders the instrument invalid.

Make performance appraisals short and specific. Develop the part of the appraisal that points people in directions for growth. The end of the appraisal should have room for the appraiser's notes—goals for the next appraisal time period with specific ways that the goals will be attained. Then comments could be made in a continuous record, thereby documenting growth. Be clear on what is acceptable and unacceptable behaviour—and then, what is exceptional or distinguished. So often, managers use a rating scale that moves from 1 (poor) to 5 (excellent). It is difficult to know the differentiation between a rating of 2 or 3 and 3 or 4. And furthermore, is such a fine discrimination really important in charting the growth of an individual over the next six months or a year? This author advises that the appraisal be kept short, simple, educative, and positive—for both the appraiser and the employee being appraised.

SUMMARY

Performance appraisal was presented as a process that may have both judgemental and development/educative purposes. Principles of performance appraisal were presented followed by specific tactics that the appraiser should understand. The performance appraisal process was compared with the problem-solving method. The chapter concluded with various methods that are used in performance appraisal programmes, especially in health care environments.

REFERENCES

Drucker, P. (1954). *The practice of management.* New York: Harper & Row.
Drucker, P. (1985a). The discipline of innovation. *Harvard Business Review, 64,* 67–72.
Drucker, P. (1985b). *Effective executive.* New York: Harper & Row.
Drucker, P. (1985c). *Managing in turbulent times.* New York: Harper & Row.
Ganong, J. & Ganong, W. (1983). *Performance appraisal for productivity: The nurse manager's handbook.* Rockville, MD: Aspen.
Hedge, J., & Kavangh, M. (1988). Improving the accuracy of performance evaluations: Comparisons of three methods of performance appraiser training. *Journal of Applied Psychology, 73*(1), 68–73.
Hornstein, H. (1976) *Cruelty and kindness.* Englewood Cliffs, NJ: Prentice-Hall.
Ivancevich, J., Donnelly, J. Jr. & Gibson, J. (1989). *Management: Principles and functions* (4th ed.). Homewood, IL: Irwin.
Johnson, J. & Luciano, K. (1988). Managing by behavior and results—Linking supervisory accountability to effective organizational control. *Readings from JONA: Readings in nursing administration.* Philadelphia: Lippincott.
Kraiger, K., & Ford, J.K. (1985). A meta-analysis of ratee race effects in performance ratings. *Journal of Applied Psychology, 70*(1), 56–65.
Kreitner, R., & Kinicki, A. (1989). *Organizational behavior.* Homewood, IL: Irwin.
Lachman, V. (1984). Increasing productivity through performance evaluation. *Journal of Nursing Administration, 14*(12), 7–14.
Lampe, S. (1986). Getting the most out of needs assessments. *Training, 23*(10), 101–104.
Landy, F., & Farr, J. (1980). Performance rating. *Psychological Bulletin, 87*(1), 72–107.
McCloskey, J., & McCain, B. (1988). Variables related to nurse performance. *Image: Journal of Nursing Scholarship, 20*(4), 203–207.
Meyer, A. L. (1984). A framework for assessing performance problems. *Journal of Nursing Administration, 14*(5), 40–43.
Momeyer, A. (1986). Why no one likes your performance appraisal system. *Training, 23*(10), 95–98.
Pearce, J., & Porter, L. (1986). Employees responses to formal performance appraisal feedback. *Journal of Applied Psychology, 71*(2), 211–218.
Richards, R. C. (1984). How to design an objective performance-evaluation system. *Training, 21*(3), 38–43.
Rothwell, W. (1984). How to conduct a real performance audit. *Training, 21*(6), 45–49.

Rowland, H., & Rowland, B. (1985). *Nursing administration handbook* (2nd ed.). Germantown, MD: Aspen.

Stalker, M., Kornblith, A., Lewis, P., & Parker, R. (1986). Measurement technology application in performance appraisal. *Journal of Nursing Administration, 16*(4), 12–16.

Stull, M. (1986). Staff nurse performance: Effects of goal-setting and performance feedback. *Journal of Nursing Administration, 16*(7 & 8), 27–30.

Zemke, R. (1985). Is performance appraisal a paper tiger? *Training, 22*(12), 24–32.

CHAPTER 19

Job Stress
by Philip I. Morgan, PhD

Job stress is one of the most common, yet least recognized or understood problems facing managers today. Some of this stress is relatively harmless. However, excessive stress can cause major problems. The purpose of this chapter is to discuss stress, the symptoms, various definitions, types of stress and finally its management.

SYMPTOMS OF STRESS

Excessive stress has "costs" to both the organization and to individual employees. The "costs" to the organization include: decreased productivity, worker motivation, and morale; and increased conflicts, slow-downs, strikes, sabotage, absenteeism, and turnover. It can also be extremely costly for organizations to rehire and train replacements for the overstressed employees who leave the company.

The "costs" of job stress to individuals can be physical, psychological, and behavioural. Physical symptoms include dizziness, sweating, backache, and fatigue. Individuals may feel easily agitated, constantly tired, or inattentive. These physical symptoms may lead ultimately to heart disease, high blood pressure, ulcers, and a variety of other ailments. Psychologically, stress can lead to dissatisfaction with one's personal life, low self-esteem, and resentment toward the job. It also results in other psychological states, such as nervous tension, irritability, and ultimately depression and "burnout". Behavioural symptoms include indecisiveness, procrastination, and general inability to concentrate.

In an attempt to cope with the resulting tension, further behavioural changes may become evident, such as chain-smoking or overindulgence in alcohol or drugs which may further provoke physical illnesses. The effects of job stress, therefore, represent a vicious cycle.

DEFINITION OF STRESS

Ivancevich and Matteson (1982) defined stress as "the interaction of the organism with its environment". Hellriegel and Slocum (1976) defined it as "an adaptive response to an external situation that results in physical, psychological and/or behavioural deviations for organizational partici-pants". Selye (1978), who did much of the pioneering work on stress, defined it as a "nonspecific (adaptive) response of the body to any de-mand made upon it". According to Selye, whether the problem is pro-voked by an argument or trying to cope with overwork the effect is the same—we feel stressed and some adaptation is required in order to adjust to this stress. Selye called this defensive adaptation reaction to stress the General Adaptation Syndrome (GAS). (General because several parts of the body are affected by stressors; adaptation because the stressor stimu-lates bodily defences in an attempt to cope with the stress; and syndrome because several symptoms or reactions are produced simultaneously.)

Selye (1978) identified *three* stages to the GAS as *alarm, resistance,* and *exhaustion.* In the alarm state the stress evokes a "fight or flight" response as the body mobilizes to meet the threat imposed by the stressor. The brain causes biochemical messages to be sent to the respiratory, blood, and muscular systems, causing breathing, heart rate, and blood pressure to increase, muscles to tense and contract, and pupils to dilate. Addition-ally, blood sugar, adrenalin, and cholesterol levels increase.

If exposure to stress lasts for any length of time the second stage, *resistance,* is activated. Here the individual begins to resist the stressor to the extent that stress becomes compatible with adaptation and resistance may increase above the norm. At this point the individual begins to be generally overwhelmed by feelings of fatigue, anxiety, and tension.

Finally, prolonged exposure to stress to which the body has become somewhat adjusted may result inevitably in all of the available energy being used up and the individual reaches the third stage of *exhaustion*. Because individuals only have finite reserves of energy with which to fight stress, once the resources dry up the individual can become seriously ill, especially if any additional stress is experienced. According to Selye, the GAS places excessive wear and tear on the body each time it is activated. The result is general lassitude, ageing, and illness, especially if it reaches the exhaustion stage (Selye, 1978).

However, it should be emphasized, not all stress is negative. Selye distinguished between two types of stress: "eustress", which is the positive, creative, and motivating side to stress, and "distress", which is the negative, debilitating aspect of stress. For example, an intensity in the level of arousal increases performance, but when arousal becomes excessive, performance deteriorates and functioning becomes disrupted. As Albrecht (1979) noted, "Stress is a natural part of human functioning . . . We must learn to tell the difference between a reasonable degree of stress and too much stress . . . a zero stress condition is impossible." Thus, moderate or "eustress" helps us to reach peak performance, while too much stress causes inactivity.

The well-documented, inverted-U-shaped relationship indicates that low to moderate stress levels stimulate the body's ability to perform (McGrath, 1976). Conversely, too much stress causes poor performance by placing too many demands on the individual (see Figure 19.1). The same pattern may also describe stress reactions over time in addition to changes in intensity so that even moderate stress levels may have an enervating

FIGURE 19.1 Relationship between Stress and Job Performance: Underload/ Overload Continuum.

effect on performance as the individual is gradually worn down. For example, a nurse manager may be able to "psych" him/herself up to make a single presentation in front of a large group at a professional conference. However, even moderate stress experienced by staff continuously over time in a busy hospital emergency room can seriously impair performance. This is why it is usually a good idea to rotate staff in this situation so that unnecessary stress is avoided.

Rather than trying to eliminate stress altogether, therefore, one must strive to achieve our optimum stress level. The problem remains of trying to determine what is our optimum level since the effects of stress differ for each individual. A first step is to identify the causes of job stress.

CAUSES OF STRESS

Many factors contribute to job stress and, although many of them are interrelated, for discussion purposes they can be divided into two groups: organizational and individual stressors.

Organizational Stressors

The organization itself is the single greatest external source of employee stress. This stress may be due to organizational policies (unfair or arbitrary performance reviews, inequities in pay structure, and rigid rules and procedures); organizational structures (line-staff conflicts, centralized decision making, highly specialized functional divisions); or organizational processes (poor communication, inadequate feedback, ambiguous goals, and inappropriate management styles).

Also, the physical work setting itself may be highly stressful due to the type of work performed. For example, casualty departments and intensive care units are typically extremely stressful to staff.

Additionally, high degrees of work specialization may result in alienation and a lack of identification with the hospital or the job because employees are too far removed from the patient. Also, occupational frustrations can originate from poor career development and guidance, poor communication, and problems with bureaucratic procedures (Beech, Burns, & Sheffield, 1982).

The process of organizational change itself is often a major source of stress for employees. Change is usually associated with technological developments that may result in the restructuring of jobs or tasks. Restructuring poses further threats of relocation and possible financial insecurity through redundancy, resulting in feelings of poor self-esteem and depression. Even promotion can be a major source of stress for individuals. Finally, retirement can have a devastating effect on an individual's identity and sense of self-worth (Beech, Burns, & Sheffield, 1982).

The list of organizational stressors is obviously not exhaustive and could easily be expanded. The point is that the identification and initiation of coping strategies needs to be a continuous activity because stressors are likely to change.

Individual Stressors

French and Capland (1972) identified *eight* major causes of personal job stress:

1. Role ambiguity
2. Role conflict
3. Role overload and underload
4. Organizational territoriality
5. Responsibility for people
6. Poor relations with others
7. Lack of participation
8. Occupational differences.

Role ambiguity arises out of being given insufficient information to perform a job satisfactorily. Role conflict can develop when roles and responsibilities directly clash with each other. The problem of role overload can be either quantitative or qualitative. Quantitative overload occurs when there is too much work to do in a given period of time. This can mean long hours, unrealistic deadlines, or frequent interruptions that lead to an inability to complete tasks. Qualitative overload relates to job complexity and arises when the work exceeds the technical or intellectual competence of an individual. Role underload can also be a stressor. This is where a job fails to provide meaningful stimulation or adequate reinforcement leading to boredom. Selye would classify this as deprivational stress (Beech, Burns, & Sheffield, 1982, p. 3). (For a full discussion of role conflict, see La Monica's Chapter 16.)

Problems of occupational differences are commonly evidenced from a variety of factors. Role territoriality refers to the fact that one may have to work where one feels one doesn't belong. Responsibility for people can be either too much or too little; poor interpersonal relations may result in too little trust and support being shown from others. Lack of participation means being excluded from decision making, and occupational differences refers to factors inherent in the job which create stress.

Poor employee–management relationships are also a source of stress. Feelings of being unacceptable or discriminated against, and perceived failures of our superiors to recognize our expertise all affect our sense of well-being. This coupled with a feeling of powerlessness or lack of control over the work situations can elicit stress responses in employees (Allen, 1982).

STRESS AND LIFE EVENTS

Stress is cumulative. While one stressor in itself may be relatively unimportant, when added to an already high level of stress it may severely impair the individual's ability to cope. If this is the case it would seem reasonable to try to identify which factors individuals consider more stressful than others. To test this proposition, Holmes and Rahe (1967) developed an instrument called the Social Readjustment Rating Scale (SRRS). In all, the researchers identified 43 life events which, after careful analysis, they ranked in order of mean values. For example, they found that specific life events, such as the death of a family member, divorce, moving house were considered by respondents to be highly physiologically and psychologically stressful and so were given a high rating, whereas "minor violations of the law" was considered less stressful and so was given a low rating.

When the mean values for the items are totalled for individuals who have taken the SRRS, the researchers suggested that respondents who reported life change units totalling 150 points or less, in general, reported good health the following year, whereas 50% of the people who reported scores of between 150 and 300 points generally became seriously ill in the following year. The significance of this research for managers is that employees bring these and many more personal problems to the work situation with them. Therefore, for a complete understanding of the effects of job stress, consideration must be given to these personal factors. (Ruch and Holmes (1971) later modified and updated the scale based on further research to include additional stressors.)

Despite Holmes and Rahe's claims, other researchers have not found the correlations between the number of life change events and illness to be very high (Monroe, 1983; Perkins, 1983). This has led researchers to conclude that some other important factors, such as psychological or personality variables, may have a mediating effect on the harmful effects of job stress.

STRESS AND PERSONALITY

While we are all generally subject to the same types of pressures and stressors, individual reactions to them appear to vary considerably. What one person finds overstressful may not be to another, and vice versa.

Researchers have, therefore, concentrated their attention on trying to identify those factors that affect an individual's ability to cope with stress. For example, there is a growing body of research to suggest that one's personality is related to ability to handle stress. Friedman and Rosenman (1980) identified two personality types, Types A and B, which, because of their associated behaviour patterns, tend to modify stressful situations. According to the researchers, Type A personalities experience a feeling of chronic time urgency and feel competitively driven. They are aggressively involved in an incessant and constant struggle to achieve more and more in less and less time. They are often unable to cope with leisure time and become obsessed with measuring success in terms of how much material wealth they acquire.

Type Bs are the opposite. They don't feel any time pressure or impatience, nor do they feel a need to discuss their accomplishments with others; they tend to play and relax for fun rather than feel the need to be competitive or demonstrate their superiority. Moreover, they feel no guilt at being able to do so.

Considerable evidence has been unearthed linking Type A personalities and their behaviour with heart attacks. For example, Mathews (1982), and Rosenman, Friedman, and Strauss (1964) have all linked Type A personalities with cardiopulmonary heart disease (CHD). According to Caplan, Cobb, and French (1975), Type As are supposedly three times more likely to contract heart disease than Type Bs. Matteson and Ivancevich (1980) in a review of the literature reported that most studies found that Type As are approximately twice as likely to contract CHD as Type Bs. In a classic longitudinal study conducted by Rosenman, Friedman, and Strauss (1964, 1966, 1967) over 3000 men were rated either Type A or B by psychiatrists using intensive interviews. Two and a half years later Type A men, aged 39–49 and 50–59, had 6.5 and 1.9 times respectively more incidence of CHD than Type B men. They also had high levels of serum cholesterol. After four and a half years, Type As had significantly more incidents of acute myocardial infarction and angina pectoralis (Mathews, 1982). Ragland and Brand (1988) followed 257 men identified as both Type A and B personalities for a period of 13 years. They found Type As were 58% more likely to die than Type Bs from heart disease.

Stress is also a highly subjective phenomenon often related to a person's self-perception and *self-esteem*. One is familiar with the low self-esteem student who is plunged into the depths of depression because of a poor grade while another student with a positive self-concept, receiving the same grade, may shrug it off. In the first case the bad grade is seen by the student as further evidence of what he or she assumes is his or her incompetence, whereas in the second case the student realized that the grade was due to a lack of study; this student's self-esteem remains intact. Low self-esteem has also been linked to stress-related illnesses. For example, Kasl and Cobb (1970) found a significant correlation between self-esteem and coronary heart disease risk factors among men who had recently lost their jobs.

Another personality factor linked to job stress is locus of control. *Locus of control* is a concept used to refer to the degree to which a person feels able to control his or her life. Rötter (1966), who did much of the early research, was able to divide people into "externals" or "internals" by means of a questionnaire he devised. According to Rötter, *internals* believe that they are largely in control of their lives and their fate. *Externals* believe that what happens to them is largely due to outside forces such as fate, luck, chance, or other people.

Gemmill and Heisler (1972) studied 133 managers in three corporations to determine the amount of perceived stress they experienced and their degree of job satisfaction. Education level, length of time in career, managerial level, and number of positions held were also considered. The researchers found that "internals" reported experiencing less stress and higher levels of job satisfaction than "externals". Stress and job satisfaction were found to be correlated; those managers who perceived their job as less stressful reported greater job satisfaction (Gemmill & Heisler, 1972). Perceived stress was found to be unrelated to any other factors, such as education level, managerial level, education, length of time in career and number of positions held.

In another study, Anderson, Hellriegel, and Slocum (1977) investigated 99 owner-managers whose business had been destroyed by a hurricane. They found the same basic relationship between perceived stress and belief in the control over one's fate; "internals" perceived much less stress than "externals". However, on a more cautionary note, some evidence suggests that "internals" may be overly optimistic in their assessment of their abilities. For example, often things *are* due to luck and chance and there is some evidence to suggest that internals may be overly rigid in believing they can control everything in their environment. For this reason, they may be unrealistic in overestimating their own ability to take charge of their situation.

A MODEL OF STRESS

To summarize to this point, stress may be defined as:

> An adaptive response, mediated by individual personality and psychological differences in response to environmental conditions (stressors) that place excessive demands on the individual.

To enable one to better understand the relationship between stressors, stress symptoms, and moderators, a simple model may be useful (see Figure 19.2). From the model it can be seen that at the organizational level,

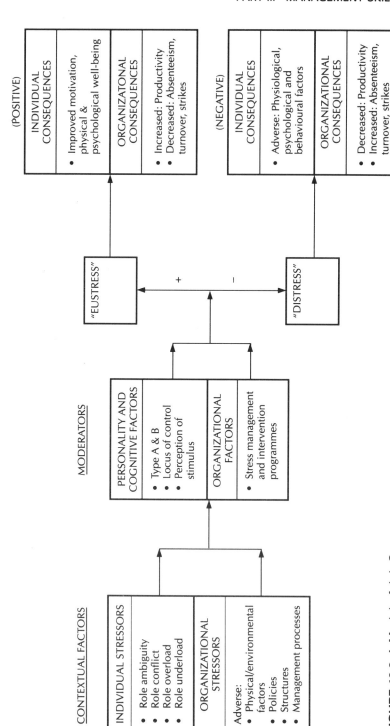

FIGURE 19.2 A Model of Job Stress.

physical stressors (noise, heat, temperature, pollution, etc.) together with company policies (lack of participative decision making, management style, and organizational structure) when combined with individual stressors, such as role conflict, role ambiguity, work overload and underload, may provoke unnecessary tension and stressful situations. These pressures are mediated by on organization's stress management or intervention strategies and by individual psychological and personality variables (Type A and B personalities, locus of control, perception of the stimulus, etc.). This situation may provoke either "eustress" leading to positive outcomes or "distress" leading to less positive outcomes. If the stress level is optimal, then high levels of performance may be expected with beneficial consequences for both the individual and the organization in the form of improved morale and increased productivity. If the stress is too severe, "distress" results with undesirable psychological and physical consequences for the individual. This may lead to inappropriate coping behaviour in the form of substance abuse. The net result is that performance is severely impaired and productivity reduced. It is at this stage that stress management strategies need to be implemented to remedy the situation.

STRESS MANAGEMENT

Stress management interventions can also be discussed in terms of two levels: personal and organizational.

Personal Interventions

At the personal level, since stress involves emotional and physical responses, individual coping strategies need to address both aspects. The importance of good nutrition and exercise in combating the physical effects of stress is widely accepted. Good nutrition influences one's mood and provides the body with food for energy and healing. The recommendation is to eat moderate amounts of a balanced diet, containing natural foods while limiting drug usage. Additionally, exercise promotes mental well-being, while increasing flexibility, strength and endurance. Twenty minutes of aerobic exercise is recommended three times a week. Exercise may take a variety of forms but must be strenuous enough to increase heart rate, and must be tailored to an individual's health and physical condition.

Emotional coping involves letting go of frustration and fear through positive thinking, relaxation, play, and support systems. Positive thinking emphasizes optimism and should be proactive. Proactive thinking involves managing one's time, planning for the future, setting goals and priorities and knowing when to withdraw strategically (Jenner, 1986). Relaxation is generally thought of as a passive activity and includes a variety of techniques to choose from. Whichever technique works for an individual should be practised daily. Play is any behaviour that is generally spontaneous, relaxing, entertaining, or fun. Playfulness can heal wounded self-esteem, unload tension, and revive a person's sense of humour. The ability to play and relax correlates with productivity. Finally, the importance of support networks has been emphasized. This includes being active and accepting in personal relationships. Without support, people suffer loneliness, depression, and a sense of hopelessness. Other approaches individuals may adopt include relaxation, meditation, and biofeedback techniques. Both relaxation and meditation techniques produce a "relaxation response" as an antidote to the GAS. It has been reported by Benson (1975) and others that muscle tension, heart rate, and blood pressure decrease while breathing slows when people engage in regular exercise. Advocates of transcendental meditation (TM) report similar benefits, which in addition to the benefits described above, include improved concentration and energy enabling one to accomplish more work in less time (Benson, 1975).

Biofeedback processes involve monitoring certain internal bodily functions so as to control them. Technology now enables people to "read" various changes in heart rate, blood pressure, and brain wave patterns normally unavailable to the senses, and to respond to them so that stress levels can be reduced. The ability to gain insights into the effects stress has on bodily processes can lead to significant beneficial changes. Preliminary results from experiments have been encouraging.

Organizational Interventions

According to Smith *et al.* (1986), among the interventions that may be introduced at the organization level to help manage stress the most successful are those that attempt to do the following:

1. To recreate a social, psychological, and organizational environment in the workplace to encourage individual autonomy and participation by managers in their jobs.

2. To build bridges between the workplace and home by enabling, for example, a manager's wife to express her views about the consequences of his work on family life and to be involved in the decision-making process that affects all family members.

3. To utilize the social and interactive skills training that help to clarify role and interpersonal relationship difficulties within organizations.

4. To create an organizational climate to foster mutual interpersonal communication, openness, and trust among managers and employees.

Individuals work to have certain needs satisfied. These needs include: income, purposeful physical and mental activity, opportunities for social contact, improved feelings of competence and self-esteem. Since an organization expects its employees to be responsible to organizational goals and demands it follows that the organization has an obligation to respond to employee needs. The relationship between an organization and its employees is one of exchange so consequently a process of mutual accommodation has advantages for both. Organizational programmes like stress management training help to foster the satisfaction of employee needs which in turn will promote the achievement of corporate objectives.

Wright (1975) suggested that "the responsibility for maintaining health should be a reflection of the basic relationship between the individual and the organization for which he works; it is in the best interests of both parties that reasonable steps are taken to live and work sensibly and not too demandingly".

Organizational interventions can take many forms and some organizations, particularly in the private sector, now offer a variety of health and fitness courses for their employees as gradually the benefits of maintaining a healthy workforce become evident. Some organizations offer general stress management programmes aimed at increasing employees' general health; others are more specific and aimed at particular problems, such as alcohol or drug abuse; while other programmes take a clinical approach and are aimed at taking preventive measures to protect the general working population. The clinical approach generally follows the traditional medical model of diagnosis, treatment, screening, and prevention. In the diagnostic stage a person with a problem asks for help and a health unit employee attempts to diagnose the problem. In the treatment phase an appropriate intervention is recommended accompanied by counselling and supportive therapy, or the person may be referred to an outside professional. Further periodic screening is then provided to enable early detection and correction of any further problems or complications. Finally, prevention in the form of education and persuasion is provided to convince the high-risk employee to do something to prevent the recurrence of health problems.

Prevention and change at an organizational level are more efficient than teaching large groups of people to cope with excessively high stress levels or undertaking therapeutic intervention for these large groups. Employee uncertainty, ambiguity, and feelings of helplessness can be lowered by reducing environmental stressors. This can be accomplished by job redesign and job enrichment, clarifying performance evaluation standards, decentralizing authority, and improving communication networks. Simply redesigning physical surroundings can reduce stress. Teaching problem-solving approaches such as time management, proactive planning, career assessment, and assertiveness techniques can also lessen dysfunctional behaviours related to stress (Mallinger, 1986). Social support and team-building activities can also play a role in decreasing organizational stress. Finally, stress management training can be instituted either commercially by contracting with private employee assistance programmes or internally through corporate training programmes.

Whether a stress management programme is commercial or corporate, certain basic principles should be followed for its design. Already identified are the needs and sources of stress that produce them. These employee and organizational needs should be considered along with organizational resources when structuring the programme. Coercion won't force people to change, so for any programme to be successful there must be a high level of self-motivation and participation. This can be accomplished by getting employees involved, encouraging experimentation, reinforcing changed behaviour, and providing top-down organizational support (Kindler, 1984).

Training objectives will dictate the context of the programme, but the basic goals should relate to knowledge and skill acquisition, and feedback. Knowledge acquisition should develop employees' awareness of stress and how it affects their lives both positively and negatively. Skill acquisition will help to identify specific techniques employees can initiate to prevent negative stress reactions or to dissipate these reactions more productively. Feedback provides participation with specific information relating to their current level of stress, certain behavioural patterns, and personal orientation. All of this information is important and will serve as a basis for more effective stress management (Ivancevich & Matteson, 1982).

What becomes clear is that any stress management programme is actually an ongoing problem-solving effort in which long-range goals are established and achieved through a series of steps. The steps can last for any period of time, and during this time, change is attempted and evaluated. If necessary, a new plan can then be established and instituted (Weigel & Pinsky, 1982). A word of caution is necessary here since there are situations which may develop with individuals where this process will not be helpful. It is important, therefore, to identify these instances and to refer such persons to appropriate therapy.

There is a real dearth of information in the literature on actual cost/benefit analysis of stress management programmes. Two reasons may be proposed for this. One is that the identification and measurement of all proper costs and benefits is rather nebulous. Second, there is a problem of expressing all costs and benefits in terms of a common denominator and then translating this information into monetary values (Starr & Byram, 1985).

Regardless of the inadequate substantiating data it seems obvious that stress reduction will benefit an organization financially. Development of skills that help to reduce a person's level of illness accomplishes two things. One is a reduction in medically related costs for the employer. Second, there is an increase in productivity which not only benefits the organization but will help to improve the individual's feelings of self-worth.

STRESS: A FINAL WORD

Obviously, being able to manage stress effectively can contribute considerably to organizational effectiveness. Dubrin (1974) summarized the key points made in this chapter when he suggested the following:

1. *Practice good management*—Use common sense and generally accepted management principles. Ensure authority-responsibility relationships are clarified, and place people in positions for which they are neither under- nor overqualified.

2. *Create meaningful jobs*—Stress is reduced when people are more committed to their work. Job commitment is closely related to an individual's perception of the importance of his or her job.

3. *Modify the organization structure*—Make sure the structure facilitates the accomplishments of organizational goals and does so in the simplest way possible.

4. *Strengthen personal qualifications*—Resistance to stress can be improved by staying in good physical health, taking positive or constructive action, maintaining interactions with other people, or being involved in a creative experience or meaningful work.

Finally, the following is a summary of some key points of things to do to avoid excessive stress in managing yourself and others.

First, in *managing yourself:*

1. Manage your time effectively. Develop a system of prioritizing and rating your work.

2. Learn when to say "no". If you feel that you cannot do any more work (role overload) explain to your superior that, while you know that the new work is important, you have other priorities to work on.

3. Build supportive relationships.

4. Clarify expectations (role ambiguity). If any aspects of your work are unclear, ask to have them explained by your superior, and set goals and objectives for yourself.

5. Ask for challenging work (role underload) if you feel undervalued by the kind of work you do.

6. Find time to relax. Set aside time in the week for exercise and relaxation. You will return to work refreshed.

The following are some suggestions for *managing others* effectively:

1. Examine your management style. Perhaps your manner of managing and communicating may cause unnecessary stress in subordinates.

2. Clarify expectations for subordinates, explaining fully their areas of responsibility and authority. Also, explain in detail how they may be expected to be evaluated.

3. Reward effective performance. Subordinates need to be encouraged in their work. Failure to reward desirable behaviours causes stress and may eventually cause work performance to drop off altogether.

4. Develop a supportive climate by promoting openness and trust among subordinates. When appropriate, encourage two-way communication by giving and receiving feedback.

5. Play a coaching role. Develop subordinates' abilities by discussing problem areas with them, and by providing further training and promotion opportunities.

SUMMARY

Stress is a complex process involving physical, psychological, and behavioural factors. These manifest themselves in the form of symptoms that affect individual health and organizational productivity. Stress is defined as an adaptive response, mediated by individual personality and psychological differences in response to environmental conditions (stressors) that place excessive demands on the individual.

Selye's General Adaptation Syndrome (GAS) was described as an aid to understanding stress. This consists of three stages, *alarm, resistance,* and *exhaustion,* each of which has progressively severe symptoms associated with it. A distinction is made between "eustress" (the positive side of stress which promotes optimal performance) and "distress" (the negative aspects of stress that lead to illness). Causes of job stress, both personal and organizational, were outlined. Type A and B personalities, locus of control, and perceptual variables all appear to serve a mediating role in modifying the effects of job stress. Many researchers have found a direct relationship between personality, stress symptoms, and illness. For example, the relationship between Type A personality and heart disease identified by Rosenman *et al.* seems well established.

Personal and organizational stress management interventions were described as a means of reducing unnecessary job stress for individuals in work situations. The chapter concluded with some specific recommendations on how managers can effectively manage excessive stress in themselves and others.

REFERENCES

Albrecht, C. (1979). *Stress and the manager*. Englewood Cliffs, NJ: Prentice-Hall.

Allen, R. D. (1982). Occupational stress and perceived organizational effectiveness in formal groups: An examination of stress level and stress type. *Personnel Psychology, 35,* 359–370.

Anderson, C. R., Hellriegel, D., & Slocum, J. W. Jr. (1977). Managerial response to environmentally induced stress. *Academy of Management Journal, 20,* 260–272.

Beech, H. R., Burns, L. E., & Sheffield, B. F. (1982). *A behavioural approach to the management of stress*. New York: John Wiley and Sons.

Benson, H. (1975). *The relaxation response*. New York: William Morrow.

Caplan, R. D., Cobb, S., & French, J. R. P. (1975). Relationships of cessation of smoking and job stress: personality and social support. *Journal of Applied Psychology, 60*(2), 211–219.

Dubrin, A. J. (1974). *Fundamentals of organisational behaviour*. New York: Pergamon Press, 103–132.

French, J. R. P., & Caplan, R. D. (1972). Organisational stress and individual strain. In A. J. Marrow (ed.), *The failure of success*. New York: American Management Academy, 30–66.

Friedman, M., & Rosenman, R. H. (1980). *Type A behaviour and your heart*. New York: Alfred A. Knopf.

Gemmill, G. R., & Heisler, W. J. (1972). Fatalism as a factor in managerial job satisfaction, job strain and mobility. *Personnel Psychology, 25,* 241–250.

Hellriegel, D., & Slocum, J. W. (1976). *Organisational behaviour: contingency views*. St Paul: West Publishing.

Holmes, T. H., & Rahe, R. H. (1967). Social readjustment scale. *Journal of Psychosomatic Research, 2,* 213–218.

Ivancevich, J., & Matteson, M. (1982). The how, what and why of stress management training. *Personnel Journal*. October, 772.

Jenner, J. R. (1986). On the way to stress resistance. *Training and Development Journal*, May, 113.

Kasl, S. & Cobb, S. (1970). Blood pressure changes in men undergoing job loss: a preliminary report. *Psychosomatic Medicine*, January–February, 19–38.

Kindler, H. S. (1984). Time out for stress management training. *Training and Development Journal*, June, 64.

McGrath, J. E. (1976). Stress and behaviour in organizations. In M. D. Dunnett (ed.), *Handbook of industrial and organizational psychology*. Chicago: Rand McNally.

Mallinger, M. A. (1986). Stress management: an organisational and individual responsibility. *Training and Development Journal*, February, 16.

Mathews, K. A. (1982). Psychological perspectives on the Type A behavior pattern. *Psychological Bulletin*, March, 293–323.

Matteson, M. T. & Ivancevich, J. M. (1980). The coronary-prone behaviour pattern: a review and appraisal. *Social Science and Medicine*, July, 337–351.

Monroe, S. M. (1983). Major and minor life events as predictors of psychological distress: further issues and findings. *Journal of Behavioural Medicine*, June, 189–205.

Perkins, D. V. (1983). The assessment of stress using life events scales. In L. Goldberg and S. Breznitz (eds.), *Handbook of Stress*. New York: Free Press, 230–231.

Ragland, D. R., & Brand, R. J. (1988). Type A behavior and mortality from coronary heart disease. *New England Journal of Medicine, 318*(2), Jan, 65–69.

Rosenman, R. H., Friedman, M. & Jenkins, C. D. (1967). Clinically unrecognized myocardial infarction in the Western collaborative group study. *American Journal of Cardiology, 19*, 776–82.

Rosenman, R. H., Friedman, M. & Strauss, R. (1964). A predictive study of CHD. *Journal of the American Medical Association, 189*, 15–22.

Rosenman, R. H., Friedman, M. & Strauss, R. (1966). CHD in the Western collaborative group study. *Journal of the American Medical Association, 195*, 86–92.

Rötter, J. B. (1966). Generalized expectances for internal versus external control of reinforcement. *Psychological Monographs, 80* (609), 1–28.

Ruch, L. O., & Holmes, T. H. (1971). Scaling of life changes: Comparison of direct and indirect methods. *Journal of Psychosomatic Research, 15*, 224.

Selye, H. (1978). *The stress of life*. New York: McGraw-Hill.

Smith, M., Beck, J., Cooper, C. L., Cox, C., Ottaway, D., & Talbot, R. (1986). *Introducing organizational behaviour*. London: Macmillan.

Starr, A., & Byram, G. (1985). Cost/benefit analysis for employee assistance programs. *Personnel Administrator*, August, 59.

Weigel, R., & Pinsky, S. (1982). Managing stress: a model for the human resource staff. *Personnel Administrator*, February, 58.

Wright, H. B. (1975). *Executive ease and dis-ease*. Epping: Gower Press.

Zimbardo, P. G. (1979). *Psychology and life*. Glenville, Ill.: Scott, Foresman.

CHAPTER 20

Total Quality Management
by Philip I. Morgan, PhD

There has been growing concern in the National Health Service (NHS) to improve aspects of health care since the early 1980s when the Griffiths Report (NHS Management Inquiry, 1983) placed explicit emphasis on quality as an agenda item. Since then serious attention has been given to the development of approaches and tools for the assessment of change with increasing pressure from the Department of Health to provide quality health care. As a result, a whole growth industry has evolved around the concept of "quality", including quality assurance, quality assessment, quality control, and total quality management. And while considerable controversy surrounds the meaning of such terms, the general consensus is that the health service needs to focus on improving the quality of its health care to patients. There is less agreement on how this might be achieved. Nevertheless, quality health care together with total quality management (TQM) has emerged as a watchword for health care in the 1990s. This chapter discusses the relevance of total quality management, as it pertains to the health service.

One early attempt to improve the quality of care was made in 1986 with the publication of *Better management, better health* by the NHS Training Authority (NHSTA). The report identified three major concerns:

- concern for the consumer
- concern for the quality of care
- concern for the quality of management.

The report provides a framework for judging the quality of all three concerns, each of which forms an integrated, organic process affecting both of the other concerns equally. For example, a concern for the consumer cannot be considered without regard to consideration of the quality of the care. And to provide quality care one must have an effective management system.

DEVELOPMENT OF TOTAL QUALITY MANAGEMENT

The beginnings of the TQM movement can generally be traced to four key figures: W. Edwards Deming, J. M. Juran, P. B. Crosby, and A. V. Feigenbaum, each of whom contributed something unique to its development.

Deming (1982) is recognized as the father of the quality movement and is most closely associated with the post-war Japanese management reconstruction period where his views on quality were enthusiastically embraced by Japanese managers.

Deming maintained that quality does not cost extra and that it should be built in "up stream" at the beginning of the quality process. He proposed the Deming cycle of "Plan-Do-Check-Act" (PDCA) to enable companies to improve their problem-solving processes. If these steps are followed they should result in the Deming chain reaction, which is shown in Figure 20.1. Deming maintained that when quality is improved by improving process (not increasing inspection) the result is improved productivity. Improved productivity leads to decreased costs and the

FIGURE 20.1 The Deming Chain Reaction.

potential for lower prices. Improved quality and lower prices lead to increased market share and the ability to stay in business and provide more jobs. The net result is a greater return on investment (ROI).

Juran (1964) worked closely with Deming during the post-war period but later developed some of his own principles. Juran's major contribution to TQM lies in the distinction he made between control/inspection and prevention. He also exerted considerable influence with what he calls the "managerial breakthrough". He maintained that, since the 1950s, management control systems have accounted for at least 85% of all organizational failures, while worker failure accounts for fewer than 15% of the major problems. Juran argued, therefore, that since management caused the problems, management had to take the responsibility and initiative for improving organizational performance.

The key to achieving the managerial breakthrough, Juran believed, lies in changing managerial attitudes. For example, traditional managerial assumptions, he claimed, rested on the belief that an organization's present level of performance is at least adequate or is incapable of being improved. The goal then becomes one of maintaining performance at the present level by means of the control function and by eliminating any deviations from the norm. While few managers argued against "the breakthrough" concept in principle, most claimed they lacked the time to change from their old system of control and crisis prevention.

Crosby (1979), while espousing many of the principles advocated by Deming and Juran, recognized the importance of the role people play in TQM. He pointed out that TQM is not simply a technical system, but rather depends heavily on the people involved in running the programme. He emphasized that to make it work, it should therefore build on the awareness, understanding, motivation, and commitment of employees at all levels. Crosby devised a quality management maturity grid as a means of measuring the degree to which an organization has begun to implement and integrate TQM into its management system based on what he called the "four absolutes" of quality management:

- Conformity to requirements—If management wants people to do it right first time then they have to make sure they know what "it" is and have everything they need to achieve "it".

- Prevention—To guarantee that quality is achieved means preventing things from going wrong in the first place. Inspecting for mistakes costs extra money and leads to a "fix-it" approach, alleviating the symptoms without tackling the cause.

- Error-free standard of performance—Employees must understand that quality means conformance to requirements every time. However 80% of the time when things are not done right it is likely to be management's fault because the necessary equipment, training or procedures have not been provided.

■ *Quality needs to be measured in money terms*—Quality is measured by the cost of doing things wrong. Once the true cost of poor quality has been calculated, it can be used to identify areas where corrective action is needed and to track the overall improvement.

Feigenbaum's (1983) major contribution to the subject of cost of quality was the recognition that quality costs must be categorized if they are to be managed. Total quality costs is the sum of three major categories: appraisal costs, prevention costs, and failure costs. The goal of Feigenbaum's quality improvement programme is to reduce the total cost of quality to as low a percentage of the cost of operations as possible. An integral part of the programme is developing cost of quality data and tracking them on an ongoing basis. Management must commit itself to:

■ strengthening the quality improvement process itself

■ making sure that quality improvement becomes a habit

■ managing quality and cost as complementary objectives.

The fundamental message to emerge from the work of Deming, Juran, Crosby, and Feigenbaum is that it is managers who should share the primary responsibility for achieving Total Quality Management. To do this, a vast restructuring of fundamental attitudes and assumptions is necessary at all levels of the organization. Only in this way can the necessary "managerial breakthrough" into quality be achieved.

QUALITY DEFINED

The *Oxford English Dictionary* defines quality as "relative nature or kind of character" and "degree of excellence". Crosby (1979) defined it as "conformance to specifications", and Juran (1964) defined it as "fitness for purpose". The British Standards Institute's (BSI) definition is:

> *The totality of feature and characteristics of a product or service that bear on its ability to satisfy stated or implied needs.*

Additionally, the BSI recommends that any usage of the term should involve:

> *a degree of excellence; reflect on measurement of a product in terms of departure from an ideal; and demonstrate fitness for purpose relating to the ability to meet stated needs.*

In the health field, Maxwell (1984) identified six dimensions of quality health care as:

- Access to services
- Relevance to need (for the whole community)
- Effectiveness (for individual patients)
- Equity (fairness)
- Social acceptability
- Efficiency and economy.

Maxwell provided examples of how these dimensions might be operationalized; that is, access can be evaluated in terms of ambulance response rates and waiting time in a casualty department. Relevance could be rated in terms of the various roles played by the accident department and how well they fulfilled their roles. Equity might be assessed in terms of patients' perceptions on how fairly they were treated, while social acceptability could include the conditions, such as privacy and acceptable standards of practice, under which the care was given. Efficiency and economy relate to workload and unit comparisons with other similar units.

Donabedian (1980) identified three components of quality health care as:

Technical care—the application of the science and technology of medicine to the management of a personal health care problem.

Interpersonal relationships—the social and psychological interaction between client and practitioner.

Amenities—décor, temperature, equipment, food, etc.

He implies that quality health care requires a blend of sound technical training and skills provided for service users within a culture which understands and responds to consumers' needs. This wholistic approach to the definition of quality ties in well with the "better management, better health" model described earlier.

While there are minor variations in the definition of quality, depending on whether it is health care or some other product or service being offered, most adopt Juran's and the BSI's definition of "fitness for purpose". This definition at least has the merit of removing the idea of quality being a luxury to something more easily quantifiable, accessible, and tangible. Thus, some of the mystery is removed if we think of quality as representing conformity to some standard against which we can measure it in advance. For example, even if a manager is hindered by lack of resources he or she may still be able to meet certain standards.

TOTAL QUALITY MANAGEMENT DEFINED

Having attempted to define quality one may then attempt to define total quality management (TQM). Collard, Sivyer, and Deloitte (1990) provided a good working definition:

> *A cost-effective system for integrating the continuous quality improvement efforts of people at all levels in an organization to deliver products and services which ensure customer satisfaction.*

This definition implies that TQM is a total and continuous process. Holpp (1989) stated that "total quality means redesigning the organization itself to keep it responsive to those needs as the product goes from one department to another". All advocates of TQM perceive it as being a fundamental cultural shift away from organizing services and products based on error detection and correction to one of error prevention with an emphasis on satisfying customer needs, getting it right every time and on continuous improvement and innovation, or as a recent Incomes Data Service (IDS) Study survey (1980) put it perhaps more succinctly:

> *TQM, in its most advanced form, seeks to create a culture whereby all employees are continually examining and improving the organization of their work with a view to constantly satisfying changing customer requirements.*

ELEMENTS OF TOTAL QUALITY MANAGEMENT

As the name implies, TQM focuses on quality as a key to managerial excellence. The so-called Joiner triangle neatly captures the essential elements of TQM (Figure 20.2). Joiner (1985) identified three areas:

1. The customer as the defining factor in determining quality.
2. Teamwork as a means of unifying goals.
3. A scientific approach to decision making based on data collection and analysis.

At the apex of the quality triangle is a focus on service to *customers*. TQM also uses the *team* approach and endeavours to include everyone in the organization in an effort to break down barriers and drive out fear so everyone can work for the company. The *scientific approach* focuses on data

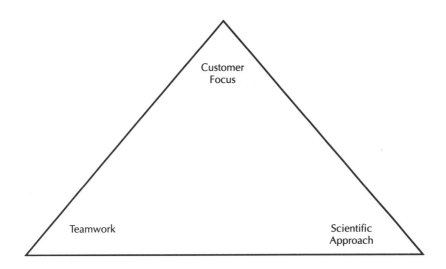

FIGURE 20.2 The 'Joiner Triangle'.
Source: Joiner, B.L., & Scholtes, P.R. (1985). *Total Quality Leadership vs Management by Control,* Joiner and Associates.

collection and study to improve the organizational processes and to improve continuously the product or service. Let's examine these areas in more detail.

Customer Focus

The Griffiths Report (NHS Management Inquiry, 1983) identified a lack of customer focus, including little concern for the views of health care users, as a major health service problem. Since then there has been increasing emphasis on "consumerism" in the NHS. By defining quality as "fitness for purpose" these issues can at least begin to be addressed since this implies that meeting customer requirements is a necessary first step. One of the main aims of TQM, therefore, is customer satisfaction, and on exceeding customer expectations and on getting things right every time. As Drucker (1974) said: "there is only one valid definition of business purpose: *to create a customer.*"

TQM also recognizes that customers can be both external and internal. External customers are the people for whom the product or service is ultimately destined. But for most employees the customer is more likely to be "internal", that is, the worker next involved in the production process. For example, Keyser (1989) noted that:

If the ward is not properly cleaned and the patient suffers, a reprimand to the cleaner may not be the answer. The internal customer–supplier chain may involve: cleaning supervisors, nursing staff, medical records, maintenance staff, recruitment and training, pay scales, the purchasing function right back to suppliers of cleaning materials, or even the beds or the architects and flooring contractors. The customer–supplier transaction needs to examine not only the product service itself but also the relationship and its integrity, the nature of the delivery and the value for money.

Keyser suggests that the questions the supplier needs to ask are:

■ What do you need from me?
■ What do you do with what I give you?
■ Are there any gaps between what I give you and what you need?

Only by answering these questions can the internal customer–client relationship be clarified and an understanding reached of where the work fits into the larger system (see Figure 20.3).

Teamwork (Commitment and Involvement)

In its most developed form, TQM seeks to create a climate or culture in which everyone is continuously examining and improving their work quality with a view to satisfying changing consumer demands. This means getting everyone to work as part of a problem-solving team.

Problem-solving teams are usually of two types: permanent and temporary. "Kaizen" or "focus" teams are usually temporary and are created to deal with specific problems. The success of many of these team approaches in Japan has caused them to be adopted by Western industries. Perhaps the best known is the quality circle approach.

Quality circles (QCs) are employee participation groups that identify

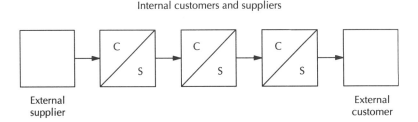

Internal customers and suppliers

External supplier   External customer

FIGURE 20.3 The Customer/Supplier Chain.

ways of improving an organization's services, products, and processes. QCs were adopted enthusiastically in the 1970s and 1980s. However, while most managers attest to their team-building effectiveness, they are less enthusiastic about their effectiveness in resolving quality concerns. This lack of effectiveness is generally attributed to the insufficient support given by top management or to the lack of a shared quality culture. These problems would be eliminated under a full TQM system (Ishikawa, 1985).

Other more permanent group problem-solving methods include brainstorming, Pareto analysis, and force field analysis.

Brainstorming is a familiar and often-used method of generating ideas. It can be used to identify possible causes as well as solutions to a problem. There are two stages to the procedure. The first stage entails listing as many ideas as possible without evaluating them: quantity rather than quality of ideas is the goal. The second phase involves evaluating the feasibility of the ideas.

Pareto analysis is a means of evaluating a list of possible causes. It is named after a famous 19th century sociologist, Wilfred Pareto, who argued that more often than not 80% of the costs are attributable to only 20% of the problems. The so-called 80/20 rule is an attempt to separate "the vital few from the trivial many". The results of the analysis can often be depicted graphically in the form of ogives or histograms.

Force field analysis identifies all forces and pressures in favour of a particular change and those against it in an organization. Force field analysis is discussed by La Monica in Chapter 10.

Scientific Approach

The scientific approach refers to the adoption of problem-solving methods and the use of data, usually by providing statistical feedback and assurance that incremental improvements can be made to the processes. The goal of this is perfection, a never ending process. The Deming approach referred to at the beginning of this chapter is one such method. The Deming PDCA approach may be viewed as a common sense approach to problem solving that has universal application. The major advantage to following Deming's steps is that they prevent premature solutions being adopted and ensure proper follow-through to implementation once a decision has been made. The four steps in the PDCA process are as follows:

1. *Plan* the approach to the problem. Prepare for a trial first and ensure that the appropriate customers are identified and that all personnel involved in the production or service are in attendance.

2. *Do* the experiment. This involves trying out the proposed change and collecting data.

3. *Check* the results. Do this on a group basis and analyse the results. Do the data collected justify the action taken? Where are the delays?

4. *Act* to incorporate the new method and the knowledge gained into the everyday work patterns. Pass on the experience to others and implement the change in line with the results of the trial, setting responsibilities, timing, and specific levels of development (see Figure 20.4).

THE QUALITY CHAIN

Every organizational system consists of a chain of suppliers and customers spread throughout the organization (see Figure 20.3). Everyone in the system is, therefore, at once a customer and a supplier of the person before and after him or her in the chain. This chain, often referred to as the

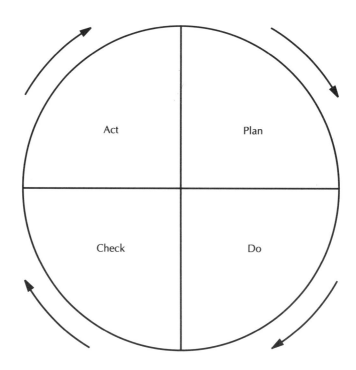

FIGURE 20.4 The Deming Cycle.

"quality chain", may be broken at any point if the links are weak, such as if one person or piece of equipment fails to meet requirements. Failures usually manifest themselves at the interface between the organization and the external customer, for example between the sales assistant and the customer who has brought back faulty goods, but the failures can also occur internally, as when someone in the organization fails to do his or her work properly before passing it on to the next person in the process.

To ensure that there are no weaknesses in the quality chain, quality has to be managed. This means that everyone in the process has to be involved throughout the entire organization. Failure to meet requirements in any part of the chain has a way of multiplying and creating problems elsewhere. The price of quality is the continual examination of the requirements and the ability to meet them. To do this TQM must be driven; it must be the responsibility of senior management and ownership must reside at the top. It is not a short-term programme nor a cost-cutting exercise. Total quality impacts on everyone in the organization. The process for improvement never ends. It is the means through which greater customer satisfaction and an enhanced reputation for the organization are achieved.

Most progressive organizations are now working towards TQM and most TQM programmes proceed in four discrete states: inspection, quality control, quality assurance, and total quality management.

1. *Inspection.* A simple inspection-based system is usually an after-the-fact screening process whereby one or more characteristics of a product are examined and compared with specified requirements to assess its conformity. Such inspection-based systems are usually entirely in-house.

2. *Quality control.* Quality control involves operational techniques and activities aimed at monitoring a process and eliminating causes of unsatisfactory performance at relevant stages of the quality loop (quality spiral) to result in economic effectiveness (ISO 8402 1986). This essentially involves a monitoring activity but also includes finding and eliminating causes of quality problems so that requirements of customers are continually met. Quality control systems are measures leading to lower incidence of non-conformance by greater process control.

3. *Quality assurance.* Quality assurance contains all those planned and systematic actions required to provide adequate confidence that a product or service will satisfy given requirements for quality (ISO 8402 1986). This includes the creation and maintenance of the overall quality system, assessment of its adequacy, the audit of the system's

operation, and review of the system itself. There is a shift in emphasis from detection toward prevention of non-conformance, so one would expect a more comprehensive quality manual, use of statistical process control, and audit of quality systems. A quality assurance system does not necessarily encourage a continual improvement approach to quality; it may only mean that an organization has procedures in place.

4. *Total quality management.* TQM involves the application of quality management principles to all aspects of the business per ISO 8402 1986, the "aspect of the overall management function that determines and implements the quality policy, and as such, is the responsibility of top management". TQM requires that the principles of quality management should be applied in every branch and at every level of the organization, accompanied by greater sophistication in the application of quality management techniques. Advancement towards TQM necessitates a change in behaviour and attitudes throughout the organization.

STAGES OF QUALITY MANAGEMENT

To assess where an organization stands from a quality standpoint, in the public or private sector, Crosby (1979) developed the quality management grid. The grid identifies five stages through which organizations generally pass in developing TQM. These five stages, arranged from least to most desirable, are *uncertainty, awakening, enlightenment, wisdom,* and *certainty.*

> *Uncertainty.* Characterized by management having no knowledge of quality as a positive management tool. Problems are dealt with as they occur. No one is able to identify why there are problems.
>
> *Awakening.* Management begins to recognize that quality management is useful but is still unwilling to commit resources to its implementation. Management begins to ask why it does not have quality and realizes that quality management can help.
>
> *Enlightenment.* Management decides to implement a formal quality programme. A corrective action system and meaningful communications are established. Management becomes committed to quality.
>
> *Wisdom.* Management and the organization reach the stage where permanent changes can be made. Problems are identi-

fied early in their development, and employees actively participate in the quality improvement process. Defect prevention becomes routine.

Certainty. Management and organization reach agreement where permanent changes can be made. The prevention system ensures that few significant problems occur. Quality improvement is a normal activity.

It has been argued that the majority of public services are in the "awakening" stage. That is, they recognize that TQM may be of value but they are prepared to invest only a limited amount of time and money, and tend to fight problems on an *ad hoc* basis, rather than having a total quality perspective. Public services can change this by having a clear quality policy that everyone can understand and by educating all employees in the concepts that form the basis for quality improvement. To improve quality throughout the organization, everyone needs to understand their work in the same way so that they can communicate with their internal customers and suppliers. It is necessary to design the right quality process in order to achieve these quality improvements.

IMPLEMENTING TOTAL QUALITY MANAGEMENT

Any organization seriously committed to improving the quality of patient care and in developing staff potential might do well to consider implementing a TQM programme. Every organization is unique and there is no one TQM programme that is "right" for all organizations. Nevertheless, it is widely recognized by companies that have successfully implemented TQM that such a programme should include the following elements (IDS, 1980):

Training—Training is necessary to enable all employees at all levels to make the maximum contribution to the organization. Part of this training should include identifying who the customers are—both external and internal—and should include the problem-solving skills outlined earlier.

Teamwork—To solve problems, individuals must be able to work in teams either on a permanent or temporary basis.

Quality structure—The quality improvement process must be guided by a structure supported from the top extending down through the organization.

Statistical control and measure of quality—A set of common statistical methods is applied across the organization, e.g. to identify Pareto's "vital few" problems and to measure results.

If TQM is to be implemented successfully it is important to include these elements in the programme.

Additionally, because of the dynamic nature of the health care profession, quality care must be considered as a moving target, constantly changing as the needs of the population change. For this reason, quality should be thought of as being a journey rather than as having a final destination or end point. The health service must, therefore, continually strive to meet the needs of the changing population which it services. It can only do this through continuous improvement achieved through feedback and evaluation of outcomes to employees at all levels. TQM is, therefore, not simply a 'one-off' event, but rather is a continuous, ongoing process to improve an organization's self-renewing capabilities. As such it must be successfully managed. This means that it has to be focused on specific key areas: customers, employees, and processes.

SUMMARY

In summary, the introduction of TQM assumes that in organizations everyone will continually strive for improvement by removing the need for error detection; striving to get it right first time, every time; being better able to define priorities for action by providing agreed care at the lowest cost; by identifying and removing customer dissatisfactions; by increasing customer satisfaction; by improving processes and outcome; by increasing productivity. TQM is a management philosophy that requires total commitment from all levels in the company. Its main aims are:

- A strong customer focus (both external and internal).
- A scientific approach.
- Continuous process improvement.
- Total participation at all levels.

REFERENCES

British Standards, *BS5750*. British Standards Institute.
Collard, R., Sivyer, G., & Deloitte, L. (1990). Total quality. *Personnel Management*, 29, May.
Crosby, P. B. (1979). *Quality is free*. New York: New American Library, McGraw-Hill.
Deming, W. E. (1982). *Out of crisis*. Boston: Massachusetts Institute of Technology.
Donabedian, A. (1980). *The definition of quality and approaches to its assessment*, Vol. 1. Ann Arbor, MI: Health Administration Press.

Drucker, P. (1974). *Management: tasks, responsibilities and practices.* New York: Harper & Row.

Feigenbaum, A. V. (1983). *Total quality control.* New York: McGraw-Hill.

Holpp, L. (1989). Health care: is total quality relevant? *Total quality management,* February, 110–115.

IDS Study (1990). *Total quality management.* IDS Study, No. 457, May. London: Incomes Data Services Ltd.

Ishikawa, A. (1985). Principles of QC circle activities and their effects on productivity in Japan: a corporate analysis. *Management International Review,* 25(3), 33–40.

Joiner, B. L., & Scholtes, P. R. (1985). *Total quality leadership vs. management by control.* Joiner and Associates, Sydney, Australia.

Juran, J. M. (1964). *Managerial breakthrough.* New York: McGraw-Hill.

Keyser, W. (1989). Health care: is total quality relevant? *Total Quality Management,* February.

Maxwell, R. J. (1984). Quality assessment in health. *Journal of the British Medical Association, 288,* 12 May.

National Health Service (1986). *Better management, better health.* Bristol: NHSTA.

NHS Management Inquiry (1983). *Letter to the Secretary of State and Recommendations for Action* (The Griffiths Report). London: DHSS.

Part III

Management Skills: Experiential Exercises

EXERCISE 1 Communication—Are You Good at Following Directions?

Purposes   1. To diagnose reading comprehension.

2. To find out how well one follows directions.

Facility   A classroom large enough to accommodate participants.

Materials   Worksheet A: Following Directions.
Pencil or pen.

Time Required   Thirty minutes.

Group Size   Unlimited.

Design   1. Instruct group members to proceed to Worksheet A and follow the directions.

2. State that members who complete the worksheet should sit quietly until the entire class is finished.

3. When the entire group is done, discuss the experience in the large group. The following questions may form the basis of discussion: Are members good at following directions? Can members scan written messages and still comprehend? If not, why not and can comprehension be learned? If yes, why and how?

(*continued*)

EXERCISE 1 *(continued)*
WORKSHEET A: Following Directions

The following test is designed to find out how well you read and how well you can follow directions. It has been used by a California teacher with junior high school students. It should not take longer than three minutes to complete if you concentrate.

1. Read everything before you do anything.
2. Put your name in the upper right-hand corner of this paper.
3. Circle the word *name* in Step 2.
4. Draw five small squares in the upper left-hand corner of this paper.
5. Put an *x* in each square.
6. Put a circle around each square.
7. Sign your name under the title.
8. After the title write *yes, yes, yes.*
9. Put an *x* in the lower left-hand corner of this paper.
10. Put a circle around each word in Step 7.
11. Draw a triangle around the *x* in Step 9.
12. On the reverse side of this paper, multiply 703 by 1805.
13. Draw a rectangle around the word *paper* in Step 4.
14. Call out your first name when you get to this point in the test.
15. If you think you have followed directions up to this point, call out "I have".
16. On the reverse side of this paper, add 8950 and 9850.
17. Put a circle around your answer. Put a square around the circle.
18. Count out loud in your normal speaking voice backward from ten to one.
19. Now that you have finished reading carefully, do only Steps 1 and 2.

Source: This material was received at the School of Nursing, University of Massachusetts, 1972. Author unknown.

EXERCISE 2   Communication—Observation

Purposes
1. To sharpen observational skills.

2. To increase perception of nonverbal behaviour.

Facility
A classroom large enough to accommodate participants.

Materials
None

Time Required
Twenty minutes.

Group Size
Unlimited pairs.

Design
1. Members should form pairs.

2. Pairs should sit facing one another for two minutes, each person observing everything about his/her partner. If necessary, it can be suggested that certain items be noted, such as: posture, eye contact, placement of hands and feet, facial expressions, dress, jewelry, and so forth.

3. Then members of each pair should turn back-to-back with the agreed-upon partner changing five things about herself or himself.

4. When changes have been accomplished, members should once again face each other. The observing partner should verbalize the noticed changes.

5. Roles are reversed.

6. Discuss the experience.

(*continued*)

Source: Reprinted by permission from La Monica, Elaine L., *The Nursing Process: A Humanistic Approach*, p. 294. Copyright © 1979 by Addison-Wesley Publishing Company, Inc., Menlo Park, Calif. The idea for this exercise came from Kenneth Blanchard, School of Education, University of Massachusetts, 1973.

EXERCISE 2 *(continued)*

Variation

The exercise can be lengthened by using the same pairs and requesting members to change five more things about themselves. This occasionally poses a problem and people often do not know what to change further. During discussion, ask participants if they thought of asking for help from another close member of a pair who was also searching for changes. If they did, how did they feel about needing help on a seemingly simple task? If they did not request assistance, why not?

EXERCISE 3 Communication—Interpreting Nonverbal Behaviour

Purposes
1. To increase awareness of how emotions can be expressed nonverbally.
2. To interpret perceptions of nonverbally expressed emotions.
3. To validate perceptions of nonverbal behaviours.

Facility
Large enough room to accommodate participants sitting around table or on the floor in a circle.

Materials
Small pieces of paper. Two hats or baskets.

Time Required
Thirty minutes or more, depending on group size.

Group Size
Twelve to 15 is ideal; two or more groups may be formed if the group is large.

Design
1. In a large group, ask participants to verbalize emotions/feelings. Write one each on a slip of paper, fold the paper and place in a hat.
2. Repeat Step 1, except this time ask that participants verbalize parts of the body that can be used to express emotions/feelings.
3. A person from the group should then distribute or have participants pick a slip of paper from each hat.
4. Request each participant who has picked an emotion and body part to role play the emotion nonverbally, primarily using the designated body part.

(continued)

Source: Adapted by permission from La Monica, Elaine L., *The Nursing Process: A Humanistic Approach*, p. 295. Copyright © 1979 by Addison-Wesley Publishing Company, Inc., Menlo Park, Calif.

EXERCISE 3 *(continued)*

5. Group participants should then try to guess what feeling is being expressed.

6. Discussion follows.

7. Role players should place papers back in each respective hat, and Steps 3 through 6 should be repeated. This should be done so that all members have a chance to role play.

Variation

If two or more groups of 12 are possible, equalize the number of emotions and body parts for both groups and time how long it takes for groups to carry out the task. Then have groups work against one another; all role plays should result in the group accurately diagnosing the emotion and body part used in expression. Only then may they proceed to the next role play. The group finishing first has the sharpest observational skills, given those present.

EXERCISE 4   Communication—Perceiving

Purposes

1. To increase awareness of the variety of perceptions that can be elicited from a given situation.

2. To raise self-awareness regarding individual perceptual fields.

Facility

Room to accommodate the class size in groups of six.

Materials

Worksheet A: Scenarios.
Paper and pencils.

Time Required

One hour.

Group Size

Unlimited groups of six.

Design

1. Have participants individually read Scenario 1 and write down their perceptions and reactions concerning what happened, their feelings in the situation, and what conclusions they reach.

2. Ask that participants share these notations with their small group.

3. Observe and discuss perceptual differences, possible reasons for such, and rationale for conclusions. Dichotomous differences between members should be studied more fully.

4. Repeat the design with Scenario 2.

Variation

Participants can develop their own scenarios based on actual or hypothetical experiences. They can then share them with their small group and follow the design for as many scenarios as time permits.

(continued)

Source: Adapted by permission from La Monica, Elaine L., *The Nursing Process: A Humanistic Approach*, pp. 296–297. Copyright © 1979 by Addison-Wesley Publishing Company, Inc., Menlo Park, Calif.

EXERCISE 4   (*continued*)
WORKSHEET A: Scenarios

Scenario 1: It is 11:15 A.M. Ms Blue, a supervisor, is making rounds on a surgical unit. She observes a patient with traction of the right leg, a basin of water on the bedside table, the bed stripped, a gown placed over the patient's chest, and the patient, Ms Green, reading a book. As the supervisor enters the room, the patient explains that the student nurse assigned to assist her with a bath had struck his head against the crossbar of the traction frame at 10:30 A.M. The nursing instructor had taken him to the emergency room. On the way to the nurse's staff room, the supervisor notices several nursing personnel, including the ward sister, drinking coffee in the utility room. As she begins calling the Nursing School office to report that a nursing student and instructor had left a patient unattended, the ward sister comes in to tell her about the accident.

Scenario 2*: The setting is a general hospital unit in an urban city. Three people are involved: Ms King, the new head nurse of the medical unit; Ms James, the director of Nursing Services; and Ms Carmichael, the day supervisor of the building. Ms King gives the patients' nursing care file a last-minute check to be sure all patients' activities, treatments, medications, and so forth, are taken care of or are in process. Then she checks the patients, going from room to room. "It's going pretty well," she thinks—she is particularly satisfied with the way Ms Garcia is responding to the care plan now. She has spent a great deal of time working with Ms Garcia. Certainly, Ms King thinks, Ms James can find nothing wrong here; the patients are all receiving excellent care. Ms King has heard a lot about these "spontaneous rounds" by Ms James. Shortly thereafter, Ms James and Ms Carmichael arrive on the unit by the backstairs, so it is some time before Ms King even knows they are there.

During the "rounds" with Ms James and Ms Carmichael, Ms King makes several attempts to comment on certain patients and their progress. Ms James ignores the attempts and starts to jot down notes on her clipboard. Ms James and Ms Carmichael maintain a general conversation about the unit while they finish the rounds. No attempt is made to draw Ms King into the conversation. After rounds

---

*Source: This scenario was received at the College of Nursing, University of Florida, 1966. Author unknown.

are completed on the unit, Ms King asks if there is any additional information they need. Ms James says, "No, however there are a few small items I would like to call to your attention, Ms King. The shelves in the medicine cupboard are rather dusty, and the utility room is very cluttered. Will you please see that these things are taken care of?" With that Ms James and Ms Carmichael leave the unit.

On the way to the next unit Ms James remarks to Ms Carmichael, "On the whole, I think Ms King is doing a good job with her unit. She should make a fine head nurse."

EXERCISE 5   **Communication—Leader/Follower Interactions**

Purposes

1. To focus on verbal and nonverbal messages that may be emitted in the interactions between a manager and a follower.

2. To validate messages received with messages sent.

Facility

Large enough room to accommodate group members seated around tables or in circles on the floor.

Materials

None.

Time Required

One hour or more, depending on group size and number of volunteers.

Group Size

Unlimited groups of 12.

Design

1. Paired volunteers should be given a couple of minutes to develop a hypothetical leader/follower interaction. They should decide which of them is to be the leader and which is to be the follower. A hypothetical leader/follower interaction is a made-up interchange in which the leader is functioning in one of the four leader behaviour styles: (1) high structure, low consideration—telling; (2) high structure, high consideration—selling; (3) high consideration, low structure—participating; and (4) low structure, low consideration—delegating.

2. The pair should then role play the situation with direction being given to the leader that he or she should decide whether to be effective or ineffective in the role. Only the leader should be aware of what is decided.

3. Following the role play, players and the group members should give feedback on their reactions and perceptions of what was nonverbally and verbally communicated. Players should

reveal their intent after group members give feedback.

4. Discuss the experience.

Variations

1. The instructor can prepare the scenes to be role played prior to class.

2. Learners may be given a homework assignment to prepare a scene prior to the class in which the exercise will take place.

EXERCISE 6   Communication—Verbal Directions

Purposes   1. To practise giving verbal directions.

                    2. To validate messages received with messages
                       sent.

Facility   A classroom large enough to accommodate
                    participants.

Materials   Plain paper or construction paper.
                    Pencils, crayons, or magic markers.

Time Required   Thirty to 45 minutes.

Group Size   Unlimited pairs.

Design   1. Members should form into pairs and sit
                       back-to-back.

                    2. One member of each pair should take paper
                       and a pencil/crayon and draw a geometric
                       design. An example of a design is as follows:

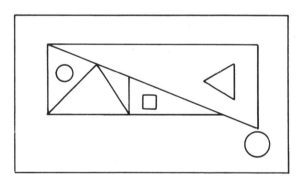

                    3. Provide partner with paper and pencil. Partners
                       should not be able to see each other's work.
                       The member who has drawn a design should
                       verbally describe to the partner, step-by-step,

Source: This exercise is an adaptation of one developed by Hewitt, F. (1981). Introduction to communication. *Nursing Times*, 77, centre pages.

what was drawn. Each step should be one clear statement (for example, put a circle on the top corner of the triangle). Descriptions should not be expressed again or revised. No questions should be asked or answered.

4. The member receiving directions should draw the geometric design as perceived.

5. Upon completion, compare the design that was verbally directed with the original. How good were the directions?

Variation

The design can be repeated with the same partners, only two-way communication is allowed—the receiver can ask the sender questions and receive answers. Discuss the differences between one-way and two-way communication in this experience.

EXERCISE 7 Change—Force Field Analysis for Self-Directed Growth*

Purposes	1. To learn the process of force field analysis.
	2. To develop an awareness of one's needs.
	3. To analyse the need area using a force field approach.
	4. To develop a strategy for meeting one's need.
Facility	None—this exercise is a self-study homework assignment.
Materials	Worksheet A: Problem Areas.
	Worksheet B: Force Field.
	Worksheet C: The Strategy.
	Pen or pencil.
Time Required	One hour.
Group Size	Unlimited—homework assignment.
Design	Explain to participants the purpose of the exercise and then the design of the exercise. Participants can be instructed to do the exercise individually as a home assignment.

1. Using Worksheet A, have participants jot down 10 problems in personal and/or professional aspects of self. Then rank order them from one (low priority) to ten (top priority).

2. Choose the top-priority problem and identify the actual and the optimal situation. Write the resulting problem area statement in the space provided on the top of Worksheet B. Fill in the optimal and actual statement on Worksheet B also. Continue to use Worksheet B for Steps 3 through 6.

---

*Every aspect of this book is directed toward changing people. When a manager leads, it is for the purpose of changing others—moving them from actual to optimal.

3. List the forces that are pushing or driving to solve, eliminate, or overcome the problem.

4. List the forces that are blocking, impeding, or restraining the change.

5. Weigh each of the driving and restraining forces from one (low-energy force) to ten (high-energy force). How does the situation look? Are driving and restraining forces equal?

6. Examine both sets of forces. Can any restraining forces be reduced or eliminated? Can any driving forces be amplified or increased?

7. Focus on the three driving and the three restraining forces that have the highest energy. Develop a step-by-step strategy for increasing each driving force and decreasing each restraining force. Use Worksheet C.

Variation This exercise can be done in class and shared in small groups at the end of Steps 4, 6, and/or 7. The amount of time to do the exercises, of course, increases with group involvement.

(*continued*)

EXERCISE 7   (continued)
WORKSHEET A: Problem Areas

Rank
Order

Problems:

_____   _____
_____   _____
_____   _____
_____   _____
_____   _____
_____   _____
_____   _____
_____   _____
_____   _____
_____   _____
_____   _____
_____   _____
_____   _____
_____   _____
_____   _____
_____   _____

Top priority problem: _____
_____
_____

Actual situation: _____
_____
_____
_____
_____

Optimal situation: _____
_____
_____
_____
_____

EXERCISE 7
WORKSHEET B: Force Field

Problem: _____

Actual situation: _____

Optimal situation: _____

Driving Forces (+)	Weight	Restraining Forces (−)	Weight
_____	____	_____	____
_____	____	_____	____
_____	____	_____	____
_____	____	_____	____
_____	____	_____	____
_____	____	_____	____
_____	____	_____	____
_____	____	_____	____
_____	____	_____	____
_____	____	_____	____
_____	____	_____	____
_____	____	_____	____
_____	____	_____	____
_____	____	_____	____
_____	____	_____	____
_____	____	_____	____

(*continued*)

EXERCISE 7 *(continued)*
WORKSHEET C: The Strategy

Force (+ or −)	Action
1.	A.
	B.
	C.
	D.
	E.
2.	A.
	B.
	C.
	D.
	E.
3.	A.
	B.
	C.
	D.
	E.

Force (+ or −)	Action
4.	A.
	B.
	C.
	D.
	E.
5.	A.
	B.
	C.
	D.
	E.
6.	A.
	B.
	C.
	D.
	E.

EXERCISE 8   Power—The New Car Dilemma

Purposes	1. To further develop group decision-making abilities.
	2. To experience potential and actual power struggles.
	3. To practise the roles of supervisor, follower, or process observer.
Facility	A classroom large enough to accommodate unlimited groups of six.
Materials	Magic markers for name tags.
	For each participant—a name tag for the name of the character to be played. Process observers are called "pros". Worksheet A: General Instructions.
	For each character player—Worksheet B containing further information only on the role to be played. (These descriptions should be individually typed on separate sheets of paper and distributed after members have selected their roles.) *Information from Worksheet B should not be common knowledge to all participants.*
	For each process observer—Worksheet C: Processing the New Car Dilemma.
Time Required	One hour for the exercise and 30 minutes for processing.
Group Size	Unlimited groups of six.

Source: This simulation was adapted into health care from a business exercise. The original material is presented by Maier, N.R., Solem, A.R., & Maier, A.A. (1957). The new truck dilemma. *Supervisory and Executive Development: A Manual for Role Playing.* New York: John Wiley, pp. 20–37.

Design

1. Pairs of teams will work together. One team of six will be players sitting in an inside circle and the other team will be process observers sitting around the players in an outside circle.

2. The team of players should choose the characters to be role played by each player. If the role-play team only contains five players, discard the role of Eileen.

3. After the roles have been selected, players should fill out their name tags and then should receive only the part of Worksheet B that describes their particular character. Instruct players not to discuss roles with anyone else and not to read about other roles. Players should not receive Worksheet B prior to role selection because its contents should not be known by everyone.

4. Process observers should not communicate verbally with the role players. They should use Worksheet C to assist them in observing the players' group dynamics.

5. When all members are ready, the instructor should signal for the role plays to begin. All groups should start role playing at the same time. The role play should last 45 minutes.

6. At the end of the role play, the process observers should report their observations to the group they observed. Group members should also join in the process observations. Were they satisfied with the decision? They should be able to provide rationale for their satisfaction and/or dissatisfaction. A general class discussion should conclude the experience—who received the new car in each group and why? Processes used by groups to make decisions may be shared.

(*continued*)

EXERCISE 8 (continued)
WORKSHEET A: General Instructions

You work for a state supported community care service that investigates reports of child abuse. One of you will be the director, and the others will be members of the professional interdisciplinary team. Each team member has a case load; responsibilities include making home visits, collaborating with professionals in hospitals, meeting doctors in their offices, visiting teachers in schools, and participating in various nonprofit health organizations. The director is usually a promoted staff member, which is true in this case. She has a small case load in comparison with others, spending a great deal of time at the main office in administrative detail and writing grant reports and proposals. She accompanies other team members on various cases as needed; on the average this amounts to two days' time out of five. Of course, this time is spread out over the entire week. Each team member works alone and ordinarily is involved in several cases or assignments in a day.

The team members drive to various locations in the district to do their work. The care service is located in a large town, but cases are referred in from a 50-mile radius of the city. Members drive compact cars that are assigned to them for as long as they work for the care service. The car is used only during working hours. Members drive their personal cars to and from the main office in the morning and in the evening. Members seem to take pride in keeping their business cars looking good; they have a possessive feeling about their cars since other people seldom if ever drive them. Maintenance is requested by the individual team members and is carried out when the members have a block of work to accomplish in the home office.

Here are some facts about the team members and their cars:

EILEEN JONES, BS, RN, a psychiatric nurse, has been with the agency for 17 years and has a 2-year-old Ford.

BILL SMITH, PhD, a state licensed psychologist, has been with the agency for 11 years and has a 5-year-old Dodge.

JOHN ALLEN, MS, a psychiatric social worker, has been with the agency for 10 years and has a 4-year-old Ford.

CHARLIE GOLD, MSN, RN, a psychiatric and paediatric nurse specialist, has been with the agency for 5 years and has a 3-year-old Ford.

Dr MARY HERTZ, a child psychiatrist, has been with the agency for 3 years and has a 5-year-old Chevrolet.

JANICE MARSHALL, PhD, the director, has been with the agency 8 years and has no car assigned to her. She is a psychiatric nurse with a doctorate in psychology. Generally, she rides places with others.

Most of the team members do all of their driving in the town; John and Charlie cover most of the cases in the suburbs.

In role playing your part, accept the facts as given, as well as assuming the attitude supplied in your specific role. From this point on, let your feelings develop in accordance with the events that transpire in the role-playing process. When facts or events arise that are not covered by the roles, make up things that are consistent with the way it might be in a real-life situation.

(continued)

EXERCISE 8   *(continued)*
WORKSHEET B: Character Information

EILEEN JONES: When a new Chevrolet becomes available, you think you should get it because you have seniority, and you do not like your present car. Your own car is a Chevrolet, and you prefer a Chevrolet for business, too. You had one assigned to you before you got the Ford.

BILL SMITH: You feel you deserve a new car. Since the more senior team member has a fairly new car, you feel you should get the next one. You have taken excellent care of your present Dodge and have kept it looking like new. A man deserves to be rewarded if he treats a company car like his own.

JOHN ALLEN: You have to do more driving then most of the other team members because you work in the suburbs. You have a fairly old car and feel you should have a new one because you do so much driving.

CHARLIE GOLD: The heater in your present car is inadequate. Furthermore, since Mary backed into the door of your car, it has never been repaired to fit right. You attribute your frequent colds to the cold air that the door lets in. You want a warm car since you have a good deal of driving to do. As long as it has good tires, brakes, and is comfortable, you do not care about its make.

MARY HERTZ: You have the poorest car in the crew. It is five years old, had been in a bad wreck before you got it, and has never been mechanically sound. You have put up with it for three years and feel the next new car should be yours. You have a good safety record. The only accident you have had was when you sprung the door of Charlie's car when he opened it as you backed out of the garage. You hope the new car is a Ford since you prefer to drive that make.

JANICE MARSHALL: You are the director of the team, each of whom drives a compact car to and from various case assignments. Every so often you get a new car to exchange for an old one, and you have the problem of deciding which of the team members should receive the new car. There are often hard feelings because each member seems to feel he or she is entitled to the new car. You have a tough time being fair—as a matter of fact, most people usually disagree with whatever you decide. You now have to face the issue again because a new car has just been allocated to you for assignment. The new car is a Chevrolet.

In order to handle this problem, you have decided to put the decision up to the team members themselves. You will tell them about the car and pose the problem in terms of what would be the fairest way to assign the car. Do not take a position yourself, because you want to do what the members think is most fair. Your leadership style will be high consideration and low task.

(*continued*)

EXERCISE 8 *(continued)*
WORKSHEET C: Processing the New Car Dilemma

The following items are furnished as a guide for observing what the leader did and how the team reacted:

1. How did the director present the problem?

   A. In presenting the problem, did the director's attitude convey asking for help?

   B. Was the director's presentation of the problem brief and to the point?

   C. Did the director scrupulously avoid suggesting a solution?

2. What occurred in the discussion?

   A. Did all group members participate?

   B. Was there free exchange of feelings between/among group members?

   C. Did the group use social pressure to influence any of its members?

   D. On which member(s) of the team was social pressure used?

   E. Was the director permissive?

   F. Did the director avoid taking sides or favouring any person?

   G. What were the points of disagreement in the group?

3. What did the director do to facilitate problem solving?

   A. Did the director ask questions to help the group explore ideas?

   B. Did the leader and others accept all ideas equally?

   C. Did the director avoid hurrying the group to develop a solution?

D. Did the director avoid favouring any solution?

E. Who supplied the final solution?

F. What, if anything, did the director do to get unanimous agreement on the final solution?

G. What were the bases of the final solution (for example, seniority)?

H. How effective was the leader?

EXERCISE 9   Teaching—A Beginning

Purposes

1. To begin the experience of teaching.

2. To gain experience in using different instructional modes and media to teach a content area.

3. To experience a variety of teaching strategies.

Facility

Large room to accommodate class.

Materials

Specified by the students in their teaching module.

Time Required

Ten minutes per member.

Group Size

Under 25.

Design

1. As a homework assignment, ask learners to think of anything (skill, philosophy, belief, and so on) that they know or do well.

2. Then have them prepare a five- to seven-minute teaching module on the area chosen. The module should include objectives and teaching modes and media.

3. Request that preparation be made for a class presentation.

4. At a subsequent class, have students teach the module to small groups of peers.

5. Encourage group discussion of the experience, focusing on the teacher's experience as well as that of the learner.

Variation

Management or nursing skills or competencies as well as theory can be substituted for the content in the original design.

Source: Adapted by permission from La Monica, Elaine L., *The Nursing Process: A Humanistic Approach*, p. 302. Copyright © 1979 by Addison-Wesley Publishing Company, Inc., Menlo Park, Calif.

EXERCISE 10   Teaching—Applying the Process

Purposes	1. To apply the teaching process.

Purposes

1. To apply the teaching process.

2. To broaden experience in diagnosing the teaching needs of clients and colleagues in a health environment.

3. To increase awareness of the teaching diagnoses that others perceive in the same situation.

4. To identify appropriate objectives and the most effective teaching strategies to accomplish them.

5. To evaluate a teaching intervention.

Facility

Large room to accommodate participants seated in groups of six.

Materials

Worksheet A: Scenarios.

Worksheet B: Instructional Analysis.

Paper and pencils.

Time Required

One to two hours.

Group Size

Unlimited groups of six.

Design

1. Participants should consider themselves as ward sisters. Using all or any combination of the scenarios, ask participants to individually respond to the following in each situation:
   A. Is there a teaching need? If the answer is *yes*, use Worksheet B to complete Step 1. (Worksheet B may have to be duplicated.)
   B. If there is a teaching need, what needs to be taught and to whom? Give rationale for response.

(*continued*)

Source: Adapted by permission from La Monica, Elaine L., *The Nursing Process: A Humanistic Approach*, p. 302. Copyright © 1979 by Addison-Wesley Publishing Company, Inc., Menlo Park, Calif.

EXERCISE 10   *(continued)*

    C. Identify objective(s) for teaching.

    D. Specify teaching strategy: mode(s) and medium (media).

    E. Delineate how the accomplishment of objectives would be evaluated.

2. In groups of six, participants should share and discuss their responses. Different perceptions between/among learners should receive particular attention.

Variations

1. Step 1 may be done as a homework assignment.

2. Individuals or small groups can develop and actually carry out the teaching strategy with their peers, as in Exercise 9.

3. The students' actual clinical placement can be the scene for identifying a learning need and carrying out the process, even to the point of teaching the staff and having them evaluate the programme.

EXERCISE 10
WORKSHEET A: Scenarios

1. Three times in the past two days you've found that elderly patients who have been gotten out of bed rather early in the morning have stayed up sitting in chairs for the rest of the morning. In each case when you noted this, the patient's respiration was either laboured or rapid. The pulse was rapid, and the patient appeared tired and said that he or she was tired.

2. A patient on your unit has been on a Stryker frame for two weeks. You have been told that tomorrow a newly employed graduate nurse and two senior nursing students will be with you for the first time.

3. A patient on your unit has been on a Stryker frame for two weeks. Today when you go in to help turn her, two beginning second year nursing students ask if they may come with you to see what you are doing.

4. During afternoon conference, a patient was mentioned who had just returned from the operating room following "repair of a fractured hip". A nurse said, "We'll have to be careful of his back since he'll have to stay on it for some time."

5. When making rounds on your unit after lunch, you notice that although many patients are in their beds, most of the beds are elevated, and in many cases the linen is rumpled. A TV set is audible through most of the area, and three of your staff members are talking rather loudly in the corridor.

6. On Monday, Mr Smith tells you that his doctor told him he might be going home in a couple of days. Mr Smith has congestive heart failure, has been on digitalis and a diuretic, still has some peripheral oedema, and is on a low-sodium diet. He lives alone.

7. Ms Jones has asked for and received a prescribed narcotic for pain for several days prior to and following her surgery. The nurse assigned to give medications and the one assigned to care for her yesterday both questioned "if she really needed it". The doctor was told of this and gave permission for a PRN placebo. Today it is discussed by others on the team. Ms Jones responded well the first time the placebo was given but then seemed to "want the other medicine" (she recognized that a different injection had been given). The medicine nurse today said she felt Ms Jones had no real need for the narcotic, but another nurse said he thought Ms Jones acted as if she really had pain.

(continued)

EXERCISE 10
WORKSHEET A: *(continued)*

8. When an aide attempting to change a patient's position was experiencing evident difficulty, a graduate nurse came over to the aide, assisted, and then explained the procedure to the aide and patient.

9. You observe a patient walking down the corridor in a coat and hat, carrying a suitcase—an aide is walking beside the patient. A graduate nurse leaves the nurse's station, greets the patient, takes the suitcase, and hands it to the aide. The nurse discusses the patient's plans for discharge as they walk down the hall. The situation was discussed with the aide after the aide returned from taking the patient to the hospital lobby.

10. A team leader asked an aide to do a sugar and acetone test for a patient and reminded the aide not to obtain the urine for testing from the patient's tube (indwelling Foley catheter). The aide took a sample from the drainage bottle and reported the test to the team leader, who then recorded the results.

11. A patient is shaking the side rails and is stating in a loud voice that he wants to go to the bathroom. The aide and practical nurse remove the side rails, explaining to the patient why side rails are necessary. (He had slipped getting out of bed yesterday.) The practical nurse escorts the patient to the bathroom and waits to escort him back to bed.

12. A graduate nurse wheels a patient into the solarium, places the wheelchair close to another patient, and introduces them to each other. The nurse then asks each patient to demonstrate active and passive exercises of their arms. As the nurse leaves the room, the patients continue the exercises and discuss each other's progress.

Source: Scenarios were received by this author at the College of Nursing, University of Florida, 1966. Author unknown.

EXERCISE 10
WORKSHEET B: Instructional Analysis

Scenario No. _____

What needs to be taught and to whom?

Programme objectives:

(*continued*)

EXERCISE 10
WORKSHEET B   (*continued*)

Teaching strategy—mode(s) and medium (media):

Evaluation procedure:

EXERCISE 11 Teaching—Course Evaluations

Purpose   To provide feedback to the course planner/ instructor.

Facility   Regular classroom setting.

Materials   Evaluations A, B, and/or C.

Time Required   Approximately 10 minutes.

Group Size   Unlimited.

Design   The course evaluations may be used when the instructor desires feedback from the learners. Each can be administered in class or taken home for completion.

1. Evaluation A: Usable at any point during the semester in which the class is given. It provides a means for evaluating the needs of students midway through the semester in order for adjustments to be made as indicated by the responses. Instructors must list in the left-hand column the broad content areas covered to date of the evaluation.

2. Evaluation B: This is a short, end-of-course evaluation.

3. Evaluation C: A more descriptive end-of-course report. All evaluations can be either anonymous or identified with the students. They can be openly discussed or not, with relevant participants or the entire group.

(*continued*)

Source: The procedure and Evaluations A and C are reprinted by permission; Evaluation B is adapted by permission. Source: La Monica, Elaine L., *The Nursing Process: A Humanistic Approach*, p. 342–347. Copyright © 1979 by Addison-Wesley Publishing Company, Inc., Menlo Park, Calif.

EXERCISE 11 (continued)
EVALUATION A: Course Content Evaluation

Circle the number that best describes each content area.

Course Content Areas	Too Little 1	Just Right 2	Too Much 3
	1	2	3
	1	2	3
	1	2	3
	1	2	3
	1	2	3
	1	2	3
	1	2	3
	1	2	3
	1	2	3
	1	2	3
	1	2	3
	1	2	3
	1	2	3
	1	2	3
	1	2	3
	1	2	3
	1	2	3
	1	2	3
	1	2	3
	1	2	3
	1	2	3

EXERCISE 11
EVALUATION B: End-of-Course Evaluation

For each item, circle the number that best represents your evaluation.

	Poor			*Average*			*Excellent*		
A. Subject content									
Interesting in terms of new knowledge	1	2	3	4	5	6	7	8	9
Valuable in terms of daily activities	1	2	3	4	5	6	7	8	9
Up-to-date in terms of current trends, issues, and problems	1	2	3	4	5	6	7	8	9
B. Programme leader									
Attitude toward participants	1	2	3	4	5	6	7	8	9
Command of subject matter	1	2	3	4	5	6	7	8	9
Ability to hold participants' interest	1	2	3	4	5	6	7	8	9
Organized presentation of material	1	2	3	4	5	6	7	8	9
Coverage of material	1	2	3	4	5	6	7	8	9
Use of handouts	1	2	3	4	5	6	7	8	9
C. Overall evaluation of programme	1	2	3	4	5	6	7	8	9

D. Programme comments

1. What was of most value to you in the course/programme? ___

_____

_____

_____

2. What was of least value? _____

_____

_____

_____

3. Do you have any specific suggestions about how to improve this course/programme? _____

_____

_____

_____

(*continued*)

EXERCISE 11   *(continued)*
EVALUATION C: End-of-Course Evaluation

Course number and title:

Professor:

Date:

Using the scale provided, rate each item on its overall idea rather than on specific parts.

	Strongly disagree	Moderately disagree	Slightly disagree	Slightly agree	Moderately agree	Strongly agree

CONTENT:

1. The objectives are appropriate for the course content.   1 2 3 4 5 6

2. The objectives were met through class seminars, clinical practicum, and course design.   1 2 3 4 5 6

3. The course has provided me with extensive knowledge in the content area and is applicable in my professional practice.   1 2 3 4 5 6

4. Course requirements cover essential aspects of the course and have learning value.   1 2 3 4 5 6

5. This course has increased my learning, given me new viewpoints and appreciation, and increased my capacity to think and to formulate questions.   1 2 3 4 5 6

6. Contrasting viewpoints, current developments, and related theory were integrated into class topics.   1 2 3 4 5 6

PROCESS:

1. The instructor is clear, states objectives, summarizes major points, presents material in an organized manner, and has extensive knowledge of subject.   1 2 3 4 5 6

2. The instructor is sensitive to the response of the class, encourages student participation, and facilitates questions and discussion.   1 2 3 4 5 6

3. The instructor is available to students, conveys a genuine interest in students, and recognizes their individuality in learning.   1 2 3 4 5 6

4. The instructor enjoys teaching, is enthusiastic, and makes the course content stimulating and alive.   1 2 3 4 5 6

5. The instructor has provided a class environment that increases my motivation to do my best and acquire knowledge independently.   1 2 3 4 5 6

6. This course, as taught by this instructor, is one that I would recommend. On the whole, the course was excellent.   1 2 3 4 5 6

What was of most value in the course?

What was of least value in the course?

Other suggestions/comments.

Source: Adapted from a faculty evaluation form used at the University of Massachusetts, 1975.

EXERCISE 12   Teaching—Self-Diagnosis of Learning Needs

Purposes

1. To diagnose one's own strengths and weaknesses in leading and managing.

2. To diagnose one's own learning needs in relation to management skills.

3. To develop strategies for meeting one's own learning needs.

Facility

Large room to accommodate groups of six to eight.

Materials

Worksheet A: Self-Diagnosis Form.

Pen or pencil.

Time Required

One and one-half hours.

Group Size

Unlimited groups of six to eight.

Design

1. Request that individual learners respond to the Self-Diagnosis Form in class.

2. Request that learners share with the group their learning needs along with strategies for meeting them. Peers should offer alternative strategies to each other.

Variations

1. Step 1 can be done as a homework assignment.

2. This exercise can be used midway through the course to identify learning needs of the majority of the class. Strategies for filling these needs can be developed, and content for meeting the needs can become part of the course substance.

3. The self-diagnosis can be used by in-service and human resource educators to pinpoint areas requiring staff development programmes.

4. The self-diagnosis can form the basis for teacher/learner evaluation conferences.

EXERCISE 12
WORKSHEET A: Self-Diagnosis Form

DIRECTIONS: Select the three areas in which you feel you perform the best. Then select the three areas in which you perform the poorest. This is an evaluation of your comparative strengths and weaknesses, not one comparing you with others. Put comments regarding your choices in the right-hand column. Also comment on as many other areas as are important to you.

Area of Competency	Best	Poorest	Comment
Problem-Solving Method:			
Problem identification			
Problem definition			
Problem analysis			
Diagnosing self			
Diagnosing the system			
Diagnosing the task			
Determining leader behaviour			
Developing alternative solutions			
Choosing an action			
Management Skills:			
Communication			
Change			
Power			
Teaching			
Interviewing			
Assertiveness			
Group dynamics			

(*continued*)

EXERCISE 12
WORKSHEET A: *(continued)*

Conflict resolution   _____   _____   _____

Time management   _____   _____   _____

Performance
  evaluation   _____   _____   _____

Ethics   _____   _____   _____

Other comments/goals

_____

_____

_____

_____

_____

_____

_____

_____

_____

_____

_____

_____

_____

_____

Learning Needs	Strategies for Meeting Them
1.	
2.	
3.	
4.	
5.	

EXERCISE 13   Interviewing—Role Plays

Purposes

1. To develop personal interview formats based on one's individual philosophy of practice.

2. To experience using these formats in role plays with peers.

Facility

A large room where participants can form dyads and interview one another.

Materials

Paper and other writing materials.

Time Required

One hour or more

Group Size

Unlimited dyads

Design

1. As a homework assignment, have participants read Chapters 13 and 18, and other related articles and written materials on the topic.

2. With the information, request each learner to bring to class a structured script for one of the following interview purposes:
   Hiring
   Promotion
   Planning individualized nursing care
   Describing an event.

3. Request that members form into dyads and use their scripts on each other. The student being interviewed should then provide feedback on the process, if requested by the interviewer. Roles should reverse.

4. Personal reactions of the interviewer and interviewee may be shared.

5. Interview formats can then be re-evaluated and changed by the interviewer, based on the results of this experience.

6. Reform into a total group and discuss the experience.

Variations

1. This exercise may be done completely as a homework assignment.

2. Participants may repeat the experience using different purposes for the interview and/or different types of interviews such as the semi-structured and unstructured interview.

EXERCISE 14 Assertiveness—The Compassion Trap

Purpose	To gauge the extent to which one is the Compassion Trap: existing to serve others and providing tenderness and compassion to all at all times.
Facility	A classroom large enough to accommodate participants.
Materials	Worksheet A: The Compassion Trap Quiz.
	Worksheet B: Scoring Key.
	Pen or pencil.
Time Required	Thirty minutes.
Group Size	Unlimited
Design	1. Instruct members to respond individually to the items in Worksheet A, following directions on the instrument.
	2. After completing Step 1, go to Worksheet B to score responses and to read interpretations.
	3. Discuss findings in small groups.
Variation	This can be a self-study assignment.

EXERCISE 14
WORKSHEET A: The Compassion Trap Quiz

DIRECTIONS: Gauge the extent to which you are in the Compassion Trap by taking the quiz below. Answer each question honestly. If you have not personally experienced some situations, choose the response that most closely approximates the way you think you would respond. After you have finished, go to Worksheet B and add up your score according to the key. The interpretation of your score will tell you how "trapped" you really are.

1. You have been seeing this man socially for several weeks, but you are beginning to feel bored and uninterested in continuing the relationship. He likes you very much and would like to see you more often. Do you:
   A. Tell him you'd prefer not to see him, feeling you've been honest with yourself?
   B. Feel a sudden attack of the Hong-Kong flu coming on?
   C. Continue to be the object of his affections, because leaving would really hurt his ego?
   D. Tell him that he bores you to tears, and that even if you were both marooned on a desert island, you would camp out on the opposite shore?
2. You invited a friend of yours who lives out of the state to spend her/his two-week vacation with you at your home. It is now one month later, and your friend shows no intention of leaving, or reimbursing you for food and telephone bills. You would like your friend to leave. Do you:
   A. Not mention anything about your expenses or feelings, because you don't want to damage the friendship?
   B. Leave a note saying that you're terribly sorry, but your mother has decided to live with you, and you'll need the room?
   C. Tell your friend that you really value your friendship, and that her/his extended visit is putting a strain on it. You ask that your friend make plans to leave?
   D. Put all of your friend's belongings out on the doorstep with a note: "Don't call me; I'll call you"?
3. You are enjoying one of your rare visits to San Francisco, and you are staying with your brother and sister-in-law. One of your favourite things to do in San Francisco is to sample the fine restaurants. Your brother and sister-in-law are terrible cooks, but they

(continued)

EXERCISE 14
WORKSHEET A: *(continued)*

insist on "treating" you by cooking for you themselves. You would much prefer going out to eat. Do you:

A. Decide to have dinner at your brother and sister-in-law's home because you don't want to disappoint them by refusing their offer?

B. Tell them that you appreciate their thoughtfulness, and explain that one of the reasons you come to San Francisco is to enjoy the restaurants? You suggest that all of you go out to eat instead.

C. Loudly tell them that you're not there for their food?

D. Call and claim that you are unavoidably detained, tell them not to wait dinner for you, and then sneak out and eat by yourself?

4. You are working on a project that is very important to you. Some friends drop by unexpectedly. You'd really like to continue working on your project. Do you:

A. Shelve your project, prepare hors d'oeuvres, and apologize for your cluttered living room?

B. Loudly berate your friends for not having called first?

C. Explain that you're in the middle of an important project and arrange to see them at a mutually convenient time?

D. Ignore your friends and continue working on your project while they are there, hoping they'll get the message?

5. Your 10-year-old daughter customarily walks to school, but today she wants you to drive her. You have driven her on rainy days, but it is not raining today. She continues to ask you to drive her, adding, "Besides, everyone else's mother drives them". Do you:

A. Tell your daughter she can walk to school today, as usual?

B. Begin by telling your daughter that you won't drive her to school but after a short time you give in and drive her, feeling guilty that you hesitated?

C. Reply "Oh, okay, I'll drive you", thinking of all the other children whose mothers faithfully drive them? You will feel like a neglectful mother if you don't drive your daughter to school.

D. Threaten to call the truant officer and report on your daughter if she doesn't leave for school immediately?

EXERCISE 14
WORKSHEET B: Scoring Key

1. A.	An assertive choice	(3)
B.	Honesty is the best policy here.	(0)
C.	Don't forget *your* feelings.	(0)
D.	Don't forget *his* feelings.	(0)
2. A.	You'll feel resentful later. You're trapped.	(0)
B.	This may get her/him out, but how do you feel about trapping yourself with *that* one?	(1)
C.	Right. This will also get her/him out, and leave you with your self-respect.	(3)
D.	This will get your friend out of your life, also.	(0)
3. A.	This Compassion Trap will result in your disappointment and indigestion.	(0)
B.	The assertive thing to do.	(3)
C.	Better look for a hotel room—your brother and sister-in-law won't want to have you as a guest for some time.	(0)
D.	You'll soon run out of excuses. Then what?	(0)
4. A.	The Compassion Trap.	(0)
B.	Only if you *never* want to see them again.	(0)
C.	Ain't it the truth?	(3)
D.	You're wasting time; it may take hours for them to get the hint!	(0)
5. A.	You've got it!	(3)
B.	A good start—but you're in the Compassion Trap here.	(1)
C.	Are you really neglectful? The Compassion Trap again.	(0)
D.	You avoided the Compassion Trap, but stepped into the Aggression Trap!	(0)

Add up your total points and gauge the extent of *your* Compassion Trap.

14+: We couldn't ask for more. You can choose what to do without being trapped. Be on the lookout, though, for other situations that may trap you.

9—13: You can avoid the Compassion Trap most of the time, and you're moving in the right direction. Give some extra attention to the people/situations that continue to trap you, and attempt more assertive ways of handling them.

(*continued*)

EXERCISE 14
WORKSHEET B: *(continued)*

2—8: Consider the price you are paying when you do things at the expense of your own happiness. With some practice, you can leave the Compassion Trap and enjoy what you choose to do. Be an assertive person and be loved for it.

EXERCISE 15   Assertiveness—Self-Assessment

Purposes	1. To evaluate the frequency of one's assertions.
	2. To identify areas of communication that require further assertiveness training.
Facility	A classroom large enough to accommodate participants.
Materials	Worksheet A: Assertion Self-Assessment Table
	Worksheet B: Problem Areas
	Pen or pencil, blackboard, and chalk or newsprint and magic markers.
Time Required	One to one and one-half hours
Group Size	Unlimited
Design	1. Individuals working alone should read Worksheet A and use the following question with each row and column heading: "Do I (behaviours) to/from/of/with (persons) when it is appropriate?" For instance, beginning with the upper left-hand cell, form the following question: Do I give compliments to friends of the same sex when it is appropriate?
	2. In answering the question for each cell, participants should write in the word that best describes how often they engage in the behaviour in that situation. Choose *usually, sometimes*, or *seldom*. For example, if one seldom gives compliments to friends of the same sex when appropriate, one would write the word *seldom* in the upper left-hand cell of the table.

(*continued*)

Source: From *Assert Yourself: How to Be Your Own Person*, by J. Galassi and M. Galassi. Copyright © 1977 by Human Sciences Press, New York. Reprinted by permission.

EXERCISE 15   (*continued*)

3. Complete each cell in the table in the manner described in Steps 1 and 2.

4. After completing the table, members should find the places where they answered with *seldom* and *sometimes.* Are there one or more behaviours (for example, making requests) for which one has given a number of *seldom* or *sometimes* answers? If there are, the behaviours should be listed on Worksheet B under the individual problem areas for behaviours.

5. Participants should again look at the places where the words *seldom* and *sometimes* are written. Are there one or more persons (for example, spouses, boyfriends, girlfriends) for whom one has given a number of *seldom* or *sometimes* answers? If there are, list those persons on Worksheet B under the individual problem areas for persons.

6. Inform participants that answers of *seldom* and *sometimes* occasionally do not group into any particular behaviour or persons. This is not uncommon since people often have difficulty expressing only certain feelings with only certain people.

7. Have participants form into groups of six to eight. Request that they share and discuss their problem areas with each other and specify three problem areas each in "behaviours" and "persons" that are shared by the greatest number of people in the group—the group modes. Jot these in the appropriate area on Worksheet B.

8. Reassemble as a total class and record the problem areas for each group on the blackboard. Modal problem areas for the class can be identified and special attention can be given these areas in assertiveness training. Individual problem areas can be worked on in the small-group activities that usually occur in assertiveness training programmes and classes.

Variations

1. Steps 1 through 6 can be done as a homework assignment.

2. Galassi and Galassi (1986) also presented a design for evaluating the presence of anxiety, areas of aggression, knowledge of appropriate behaviour, and knowledge of personal rights, all using the same table. Details can be found in the original source and in a chapter by Galassi, J. and Galassi, M. (1986). Assessment procedures for assertive behaviours. In R. Alberti (Ed.). *Assertiveness: Innovations, applications, issues.* San Luis Obispo, CA: Impact.

(continued)

EXERCISE 15 *(continued)*
WORKSHEET A: Assertion Self-Assessment Table

Persons

Behaviours	Friends of the same sex	Friends of the opposite sex	Intimate relations (spouse, boyfriend, girlfriend)	Parents, in-laws and other family members	Children	Authority figures (bosses, professors, doctors)	Business contacts (sales-persons, waiters)	Co-workers, colleagues, and subordinates
Expression of positive feelings								
Give compliments								
Receive compliments								
Make requests (ask for favours, help)								

Express liking, love, and affection

Initiate and maintain conversations

Self-Affirmation

Stand up for your legitimate rights

Refuse requests

Express personal opinions including disagreement

(continued)

EXERCISE 15
WORKSHEET A: *(continued)*

Persons

Behaviours	Friends of the same sex	Friends of the opposite sex	Intimate relations (spouse, boyfriend, girlfriend)	Parents, in-laws and other family members	Children	Authority figures (bosses, professors, doctors)	Business contacts (sales-persons, waiters)	Co-workers, colleagues, and subordinates
Expression of negative feelings								
Express justified annoyance and displeasure								
Express justified anger								

EXERCISE 15
WORKSHEET B: Problem Areas

INDIVIDUAL PROBLEM AREAS:

Behaviours   Persons

_____   _____

_____   _____

_____   _____

_____   _____

_____   _____

_____   _____

_____   _____

_____   _____

_____   _____

_____   _____

_____   _____

_____   _____

_____   _____

GROUP PROBLEM AREAS:

Behaviours   Persons

_____   _____

_____   _____

_____   _____

_____   _____

_____   _____

_____   _____

_____   _____

_____   _____

_____   _____

_____   _____

EXERCISE 16   Assertiveness—Situations to Role Play

Purposes

1. To role play assertiveness in common situations.

2. To receive feedback on one's own assertiveness.

3. To recognize assertiveness in others.

4. To give feedback to others on their assertiveness.

Facility

A classroom large enough to accommodate the class in groups of six to eight.

Materials

Worksheet A: Situations.

Worksheet B: Responses.

Worksheet C: Practice Situations.

Pencil or pen.

Time Required

One to one and one-half hours.

Group Size

Unlimited groups of six to eight.

Design

1. Lecture or discussion on assertion theory should precede this exercise.

2. Have participants individually respond to the situations in Worksheet A, using the space provided following each situation.

3. After completing Step 1, ask participants to form into groups of six to eight and practise role playing the five situations in pairs. Participants not involved in the immediate role play should give feedback to the players on their assertiveness.

4. After group members have completed Steps 2 and 3, hand out Worksheet B and have them compare their responses with the examples of responses provided. Discuss these results.

5. Worksheet C, Practice Situations, can be used as small groups wish to role play assertiveness techniques in various situations, according to individual and group needs. The process noted in Step 3 can be applied.

(*continued*)

EXERCISE 16   *(continued)*
WORKSHEET A: Situations

1. You and Jessica are associates on a patient care unit. Jessica asks you to give her a ride home every afternoon from now on. You don't want to do it. You say:

_____

_____

_____

_____

_____

2. It is your lunch hour. You're waiting for a friend. She breezes in a half-hour late and, without any reference to her lateness, asks, "How are you?" You answer:

_____

_____

_____

_____

_____

3. Just as you're about to leave for the hospital, your cousin George calls you on the telephone. He starts to tell you about a problem he's been having with his parents. You're anxious to get off the phone. You say:

_____

_____

_____

_____

_____

4. You're standing in line in a restaurant waiting to be seated. The hostess says, "Who's next?" It is your turn. The woman next to you says, "I am". You turn to her and:

_____

_____

_____

_____

_____

5. You're at an agencywide directors' meeting. An associate speaks up and urges members not to appropriate extra funds to the nursing budget. He gives inaccurate information in his attempt to persuade people that there is no need for extra positions. You disagree with his ideas and his data. You:

_____

_____

_____

_____

_____

(*continued*)

Source. The situations and responses from Worksheets A and B, Exercise 16, are a slight modification of those presented in *The New Assertive Woman*, by L. Bloom, K. Coburn, and J. Pearlman. Copyright © 1975 by Delacorte Press. Reprinted by permission.

EXERCISE 16 *(continued)*
WORKSHEET B: Responses

Responses to Situation 1:

- ◼ "Well. . . uh. . . I guess I could. . . (pause). . . Uh. . . O.K." (*Nonassertive:* pauses with apparent hesitancy)

- ◼ "I'd love to take you, but sometimes I have to stop at the market on the way home. And sometimes I leave late." (*Nonassertive:* excuses)

- ◼ "What's the matter? Haven't you and Norman gotten around to buying that second car yet?" (*Aggressive:* sarcastic)

- ◼ "You've got nerve! Do you think I have nothing better to do than chauffeur you around?" (*Aggressive:* attempt to make the requester feel guilty)

- ◼ "I know it's a pain to wait around for Norman to pick you up, but I'd rather not be tied down to giving you a ride every day. I'd be happy to do it once a week, though." (*Assertive:* compromise)

- ◼ "I understand that you don't like having to wait for Norman to pick you up every day, but I really don't want to be tied down to having to take you." (*Assertive:* direct refusal)

Responses to Situation 2:

- ◼ "Fine, thanks," said with a smile. (*Nonassertive:* denial of actual feelings)

- ◼ "O.K., I guess," said with a frown on your face. (*Nonassertive:* attempt to communicate the real message, but indirectly)

- ◼ "What do you mean, how am I? How do you think I am, sitting here, waiting for you and staring at the ceiling? Do you ever stop to think of anyone but yourself?" (*Aggressive:* attempt to humiliate the latecomer)

- ◼ "Well, I'd been looking forward to our lunch, but since I've been waiting so long, I've really gotten upset. Now we'll have only a half-hour together." (*Assertive:* a direct statement of feelings)

Responses to Situation 3:

- You listen. . . and listen. . . and listen. . . . (*Nonassertive:* accommodation of the other's needs at the expense of your own)

- "Look, I'm too busy to talk to you now. You've always got some little problem, and I have more important things to do. Good-bye." (*Aggressive:* disregard of the other's wishes and feelings)

- "I'd like to hear more about it later. I was just on my way to work when you called. I'll call you back tonight." (*Assertive:* direct statement of wishes)

Responses to Situation 4:

- Smile. (*Nonassertive:* accommodation of the other's needs at the expense of your own)

- Frown silently. (*Nonassertive:* attempt at indirect communication of your wishes)

- Mutter under your breath, "Some people are so pushy"—but you say nothing directly to anyone. (*Nonassertive:* repression of your own wishes)

- "No you're not. I was here first. You can't take advantage of me, lady." (*Aggressive:* hostile overreaction)

- "I believe I was here before you." (*Assertive:* direct expression of your own wishes)

Responses to Situation 5:

- Say nothing to anyone. (*Nonassertive:* refrain from expressing your own opinion)

- Stand up and say, "I don't know much about this. I'm no expert, but. . . ." (*Nonassertive:* self-demeaning and self-deprecating)

- Whisper to the person sitting next to you about how stupid the speaker is. (*Nonassertive:* indirect, inhibited behaviour)

- Stand up and say, "You're a liar. You don't know what you're talking about." (*Aggressive:* intent to humiliate)

(*continued*)

EXERCISE 16
WORKSHEET B: *(continued)*

- Stand up and say, "I've heard what you have to say, and I disagree with you. I would like you to listen to my point of view." (*Assertive:* stand up for legitimate rights without violating the other's rights)

EXERCISE 16 *(continued)*
WORKSHEET C: Practice Situations

Family Situations

Slumber Party. Your 12-year-old daughter is having a slumber party with five other girls. It is past 2 A.M.; the girls should have settled down to sleep by now, but they're still making a lot of noise.

Alternative Responses:

(a) You toss and turn in bed, wishing your spouse would get up and say something to the girls. You're really angry, but just lie there trying to block out the sounds.

(b) Jumping out of bed, you scold the girls angrily, especially your daughter, for their conduct.

(c) Talking to the girls in a firm tone, so they'll know you mean business, you tell them that you've had enough for tonight. You point out that you need to get up early tomorrow, and that everyone needs to get to sleep.

Late for Dinner. Your wife was supposed to be home for dinner right after work. Instead, she returns hours later explaining she was out with the girls for a few drinks. She is obviously drunk.

Alternative Responses:

(a) You say nothing about how thoughtless she has been, but simply start preparing something for her to eat.

(b) Screaming, yelling, and crying, you tell her that she is a drunken fool, doesn't care about your feelings, is a poor example for the children. You ask about what the neighbours will think. You demand that she get her own dinner.

(c) You calmly and firmly let her know that she should have informed you beforehand that she was going out for few drinks and would likely be late. Telling her that her cold dinner is in the kitchen, you add that you expect to discuss her behaviour further tomorrow.

Visiting Relative. Aunt Margaret, with whom you prefer not to spend much time, is on the telephone. She has just told you of her plans to spend three weeks visiting you, beginning next week.

Alternative Responses:

(a) You think, "Oh, no!" but say, "We'd love to have you come and stay as long as you like!"

(continued)

EXERCISE 16
WORKSHEET C: *(continued)*

(b) You tell her the children have just come down with bad colds, and the spare bed has a broken spring and you'll be going to cousin Bill's weekend after next—none of which is true.

(c) You say, "We'll be glad to have you come for the weekend, but we simply can't invite you for longer. A short visit is happier for everyone, and we'll want to see each other again sooner. We have lots of school and community activities which take up most of our evenings after work."

Past Midnight. Your teenage son has just returned from a school party. It is 3 o'clock in the morning, and you have been frantic, concerned primarily for his well-being, since you had expected him home before midnight.

Alternative Responses:

(a) You turn over and go to sleep.

(b) You shout, "Where the hell have you been? Do you have any idea what time it is? You've kept me up all night! You thoughtless, inconsiderate, selfish, no-good bum—I ought to make you sleep in the street!"

(c) You say, "I've been very worried about you, son. You said you'd be home before midnight, and I've been frantic for hours. Are you all right? I wish you'd call me! Tomorrow we'll discuss your arrangements for staying out late."

Consumer Situations

Haircut. At the barber shop, the barber has just finished cutting your hair and turns the chair toward the mirror so you can inspect. You feel that you would like the sides trimmed more.

Alternative Responses:

(a) You nod your head and say, "That's ok".

(b) Abruptly you demand that he do a more thorough job, adding sarcastically, "You sure didn't take much off the sides, did you?"

(c) You tell the barber you would like to have the sides trimmed more.

Short-changed. As you are leaving a store after a small purchase, you discover that you have been short-changed by three pounds.

Alternative Responses:

(a) Pausing for a moment, you try to decide if £3 is worth the effort. After a few moments, you decide it is not and go on your way.

(b) You hurry back into the store and loudly demand your money, making a derogatory comment about "cashiers who can't add".

(c) Re-entering the store, you catch the attention of the clerk, saying that you were short-changed by three pounds. In the process of explaining, you display the change you received back.

Waiting in Line. You are standing near a cash register waiting to pay for your purchase and have it wrapped. Others, who have come after you, are being waited on first. You are getting tired of waiting.

Alternative Responses:

(a) You give up and decide not to buy the article.

(b) Shouting, "You sure get poor service in this store!" you slam the intended purchase down on the counter and walk out.

(c) In a voice loud enough to be heard, you tell the clerk you were ahead of people who have already been served. You ask to be waited on now.

Phone Blues. You are at home, hoping for a restful day. The phone rings, and you answer to a voice stating your full name and asking if that is you. The call is long distance, so you feel it might be important. Then you hear, "This is Rocky Road Magazine. We are conducting a readership survey. Have you heard of our magazine?"

Alternative Responses:

(a) You are polite, don't interrupt, and answer all of the caller's questions. Soon you hear a "sales pitch" instead of a readership survey. The call lasts ten minutes.

(b) You yell, "You people are a bunch of vultures! Don't you know anything about telephone privacy? Stick it in your ear!" You slam down the phone.

(c) You state firmly, "I am not interested". The caller replies, "I only want to ask you a few questions". You repeat firmly, "I am not interested". You hang up the phone.

Employment Situations

Working Late. You and your partner have an engagement this evening which has been planned for several weeks. You plan to leave immediately after work. During the day, however, your supervisor asks you to stay late this evening to work on a special assignment.

Alternative Responses:

(a) You say nothing about your important plans and simply agree to stay until the work is finished.

(*continued*)

EXERCISE 16
WORKSHEET C: *(continued)*

(b) In a nervous, abrupt voice you say, "No, I will not work late tonight!" Adding a brief criticism of the boss for not planning the work schedule better, you then turn back to your work.

(c) In a firm, pleasant voice, explain your important plans and say you will not be able to stay this evening to work on the special assignment, but perhaps you can help find an alternative solution.

Deniable Passion. One of your co-workers has been making sexual overtures toward you. You are not the least bit interested and have begun to feel harassed.

Alternative Responses:

(a) You begin wearing clothing that is less appealing, change your hair style, and start looking down each time the person approaches.

(b) The next time the person makes an overture you state, "I hate your guts! You are scum! You are so ugly that Frankenstein wouldn't have you."

(c) After a recent incident, you sit and talk quietly with the person. You note that you are feeling pursued and do not wish to be, giving examples of what you mean. Finally you say that if the approaches do not stop, you will file a report with your employer.

Below Par. One of your employees has been doing sub-standard work recently. You decide it is best to deal with the situation before it gets out of control.

Alternative Responses:

(a) "I'm sorry to bring this up, but I know you must have a good reason why your work has seemed to slide a little lately."

(b) "Things between us are not right. You have been making me mad lately by doing a lousy job. If you don't shape up pronto, you will be out of here."

(c) "I am very concerned about your work performance recently. You won't be receiving a pay increase this period. Let's analyze what's been going on and see what improvements you can make for the future."

Job Error. You have made a mistake on the job. Your supervisor discovers it and is letting you know rather harshly that you should not have been so careless.

Alternative Responses:

(a) Overapologizing, you say, "I'm sorry. I was stupid. How silly of me. I'll never let it happen again!"

(b) You bristle up and say, "You have no business whatsoever criticizing my work. Leave me alone, and don't bother me in the future. I'm capable of handling my own job!"

(c) You agree that you made the mistake, saying, "It was my mistake. I will be more careful next time. However, I feel you are being somewhat harsh and I see no need for that."

Late to Work. One of your subordinates has been coming in late consistently for the last three or four days.

Alternative Responses:

(a) You grumble to yourself or to others about the situations, but say nothing to the person, hoping he will start coming in early.

(b) You tell the worker off, indicating that he has no right to take advantage of you and that he had better get to work on time or else you will see that he is fired.

(c) You point out to the worker that you have observed him coming in late recently and wonder, "Is there an explanation I should know about? You'll have to start coming to work on time. You should have come to me and explained the situation, rather than saying nothing at all, and leaving me up in the air."

School and Community Situations

Quiet Prof. In a lecture with 300 students, the professor speaks softly and you know that many others are having trouble hearing him as you are.

Alternative Responses:

(a) You continue to strain to hear, eventually moving closer to the front of the room, but say nothing about his too-soft voice.

(b) You yell out, "Speak up!"

(c) You raise your hand, get the professor's attention, and ask if he would please speak louder.

Clarification. At a Lion's Club meeting, the President is discussing the procedures for the annual high school speech contest. You are puzzled by several of his statements and believe he has incorrectly described the rules.

(continued)

EXERCISE 16
WORKSHEET C: (continued)

Alternative Responses:

(a) You say nothing, but continue to puzzle over the question, looking up your notes from last year's contest later in the day.

(b) You interrupt, telling him he is wrong, pointing out the mistake and correcting him from your own knowledge of the contest. You tone is derisive, and your choice of words obviously makes him ill-at-ease.

(c) You ask the President to further explain the procedures, expressing your confusion and noting the source of your conflicting information.

Morals. You are one of eleven people in a discussion group on human sexuality. The concepts being supported by three or four of the more verbal students are contrary to your personal moral code.

Alternative Responses:

(a) You listen quietly, not disagreeing openly with the other members or describing your own views.

(b) You loudly denounce the views which have been expressed. Your defense of your own beliefs is strong, and you urge others to accept your point of view as the only correct one.

(c) You speak up in support of your own beliefs, identifying yourself with an apparently unpopular position, but not disparaging the beliefs of others in the group.

Know It All. As a member of the community beautification committee, you are dismayed by the continued dominance of group discussion by Ms Brown, an opinionated member who has "the answer" to every question. She has begun another tirade. As usual, no one has said anything about it after several minutes.

Alternative Responses:

(a) Your irritation increases, but you remain silent.

(b) You explode verbally, curse Ms Brown for "not giving anyone else a chance", and declare her ideas out-of-date and worthless.

(c) You interrupt, saying, "Excuse me, Ms Brown". When recognized, you express your personal irritation about Ms Brown's monopoly on the group's time. Speaking directly to her as well as the other group members, you suggest a discussion procedure which will permit all members an opportunity to take part, and will minimize dominance by a single individual.

Social Situations

Breaking the Ice. At a party where you don't know anyone except the host, you want to circulate and get to know others. You walk up to three people talking.

Alternative Responses:

(a) You stand close to them and smile but say nothing, waiting for them to notice you.

(b) You listen to the subject they are talking about, then break in and disagree with someone's viewpoint.

(c) You break into the conversation and introduce yourself.

(d) You wait for a pause in the conversation, then introduce yourself and ask if you may join in.

Making a Date. You'd like to ask out a person you have met and talked with three or four times recently.

Alternative Responses:

(a) You sit around the telephone going over in your mind what you will say and how your friend will respond. Several times you lift the phone and are almost finished dialling, then hang up.

(b) You phone and as soon as your friend answers, you respond by saying, "Hi, baby, we're going out together this weekend!" Seemingly taken aback, your friend asks who is calling.

(c) You call, and when your friend answers, you say who is calling and ask how school (job, etc.) is going. The reply is, "Fine, except I am worried about a test I will be taking soon". Following the lead, you talk for a few minutes about the test. Then you say that you would like to go together to a show on Friday evening.

Smoke Gets in Your Lungs. You are at a public meeting in a large room. A man enters the room and sits down next to you, puffing enthusiastically on a large cigar. The smoke is very offensive to you.

Alternative Responses:

(a) You suffer the offensive smoke in silence, deciding it is the right of the other person to smoke if he wishes.

(b) You become very angry, demand that he move or put out the cigar and loudly assail the evils and health hazards of the smoking habit.

(c) You firmly but politely ask him to refrain from smoking because it is offensive to you.

(d) You ask him to sit in another seat if he prefers to continue smoking, since you were there first.

(continued)

EXERCISE 16
WORKSHEET C: (continued)

Family Situations

Holy Terror. Your son's pre-school teacher tells you he is hitting the other children. At home he "runs the show", staying up late, roughing up the pets, not eating properly. In the past you have thought his behaviour "cute".

Alternative Responses:

(a) You talk gently to your son about not hitting the other children. He says the other kids are mean, but that he is sorry. He jumps in your lap and you say, "You are such a sweet boy, I love you".

(b) You grab your son roughly and say that if he hits anyone else that you will beat his bottom till it is raw.

(c) After discussing the issue with the teacher and ruling out any physical causes, you sign up the entire family for counselling.

Plastic Money. Finances are tight. When you receive the credit card bill for the month, you are shocked. Your spouse has charges that seem excessive and unnecessary.

Alternative Responses:

(a) You go to the bank and cash a check for an equal amount of money. After spending it, you feel that you have gained your revenge. You don't mention the credit card.

(b) You realize that you also have over-spent before. You still feel upset, but decide to be understanding this time.

(c) You arrange an appropriate time to discuss the finances, and tell your partner that when you opened the statement, you were shocked at the charges. Asking your spouse for an explanation, you also express your wish to establish agreeable guidelines for the use of the credit card.

Source: From *Your Perfect Right: A Guide to Assertive Living,* 5th ed., © 1986, by Robert E. Alberti and Michael L. Emmons. Reproduced for Springer Publishing Company, Inc., by permission of Impact Publishers, Inc., P.O. Box 1094, San Luis Obispo, CA 93406. Further reproduction prohibited.

EXERCISE 17   Group Process—Observation Sheets

Purposes	1. To gain experience in studying small-group processes.
	2. To gain experience in communicating with group members on process observations (giving and receiving feedback).
	3. To provide feedback on group functioning in relation to task accomplishment.
	4. To foster team building.
Facility	Room large enough to accommodate group members seated around tables or in circles on the floor.
Materials	Worksheet A, B, or C: Evaluation of Group Effectiveness.
Time Required	Ten to 30 minutes for each worksheet.
Group Size	Unlimited small groups of six to eight members.
Design	These worksheets are to be used following any of the exercises in this book when the members of the group wish to study their group process in relation to accomplishment of their group task (how they functioned as a group).
	1. At the conclusion of group work, reserve ten minutes or more for group processing. Request members to individually respond to the items in Worksheet A, B, or C.

(*continued*)

Source: Adapted by permission from La Monica, Elaine L., *The Nursing Process: A Humanistic Approach*, p. 307–310. Copyright © 1979 by Addison-Wesley Publishing Company, Inc., Menlo Park, Calif.

EXERCISE 17   *(continued)*

2. Instruct the total group to share their responses with one another, amplifying their rationale for choices. Differences in point allocation should be discussed since they point out various group members' perceptions.

Note: Worksheet A is the least complicated instrument, while Worksheet C is the most complicated. The worksheets should be used progressively from A to C as groups move toward above-average maturity in group-processing activities.

EXERCISE 17
WORKSHEET A: Evaluation of Group Effectiveness

Rate the group on each statement below, with 4 representing your greatest agreement and 1 representing your least agreement with the statement. Circle the number that best approximates your rating of the behaviour exhibited by the group.

	Disagree		*Agree*	
1. Group members understood the problem under discussion.	1	2	3	4
2. Group members stayed on the topic.	1	2	3	4
3. Group members avoided premature closure on discussion.	1	2	3	4
4. Group members contributed equally to the discussion.	1	2	3	4
5. Group members agreed with group consensus and/or discussions.	1	2	3	4
6. Group members discussed their opinions openly without hiding personal feelings.	1	2	3	4
7. Group members were able to resolve conflict or discontent.	1	2	3	4
8. Group members displayed commitment to the group tasks.	1	2	3	4
9. Group members indicated satisfaction with the group process.	1	2	3	4
10. Group members indicated satisfaction with the group outcomes.	1	2	3	4

(continued)

Source: This instrument was obtained by this author at the School of Education, University of Massachusetts, 1974. Author unknown.

EXERCISE 17 (continued)
WORKSHEET B: Evaluation of Group Effectiveness

The following five items will be used to critique work-group activity: climate, conflict, communications, decision making, commitment to objectives.

- *Individual evaluation.* Each person will evaluate the activity of the work group, distributing 100 points among the alternatives for each item.

- *Work group evaluation.* The group will discuss the point allocation for every item in order to reach consensus on a single distribution that represents member understanding of how work-group activity took place. Any approach that assures that the thinking of each member on each item is heard and considered may be used. Averaging of individual answers to get a single work-group rating is to be avoided. The purpose is to probe for differences in points of view.

CLIMATE:

1. _____ One or more people tried to take over and control the decisions; it was a competitive, tense, win–lose conflict.

2. _____ The discussion was penetrating and challenging—a very rewarding session to which we all were committed.

3. _____ The discussion was polite, easygoing, and pleasant—a very friendly session.

4. _____ The discussion was rather flat and lifeless; comments slid from point to point with little evidence of commitment.

CONFLICT:

1. _____ There was considerable unnecessary and unprofitable disagreement; competitiveness resulted in win–lose conflict.

2. _____ Disagreements were explored to help the group produce the best possible decisions; conflict was confronted and resolved.

3. _____ We were quite polite and pleasant; we took care to avoid conflict.

4. _____ There was very little open disagreement or conflict.

COMMUNICATION:

1. _____ Ideas and opinions were expressed to "win one's own point"; few members listened to conflicting points of view.

2. _____ Ideas and opinions were expressed openly and with candour; close attention was paid to both majority and minority opinions so that we could fully understand all points of view.

3. _____ Ideas and opinions were expressed politely; we listened to all contributions attentively; no feelings were hurt.

4. _____ Ideas and opinions were expressed with little conviction, and people listened with little evidence of concern.

DECISION MAKING:

1. _____ To complete the task, decisions were "railroaded" by one or a few.

2. _____ Once each member understood all points of view, the work group reached a decision to which all were committed.

3. _____ Decisions were made in a way that gave maximum consideration to all people; we did not want to "rock the boat".

4. _____ Compromise was the key to decision making; the traditional decisions resulted from majority rule.

COMMITMENT TO OBJECTIVES:

1. _____ We attempted to stay directly with the problem, and we solved it as quickly and efficiently as possible.

2. _____ There was an attempt to look at the problem as broadly and deeply as possible. Involvement and creativity characterized the discussion.

3. _____ We often seemed to be more interested in harmony than in getting the job done.

4. _____ There was little consistent focus on the problem; we solved the problem as rapidly as possible based on precedents.

(continued)

Source: This instrument was obtained by this author at the School of Education, University of Massachusetts, 1974. Author unknown.

EXERCISE 17 (*continued*)
WORKSHEET C: Evaluation of Group Effectiveness

DIRECTIONS: Insert group members' names, including your own, in the diagonal lettered spaces. Place check marks in the column corresponding to the roles played by each group member, again including yourself. Briefly jot down the context in which the roles were played.

Names of Members / Task Roles	A	B	C	D	E	F	G	H	I	J	K	L
1. Initiator												
2. Information seeker												
3. Evaluator												
4. Coordinator												
5. Procedural technician												
6. Recorder												
Maintenance Roles												
1. Encourager												
2. Harmonizer												
3. Compromiser												
4. Standard setter												
5. Gatekeeper												
Self-Oriented Roles												
1. Aggressor												
2. Blocker												
3. Recognition seeker												
4. Playboy												
5. Dominator												
6. Help seeker												

Source: This instrument was obtained by this author at the School of Education, University of Massachusetts, 1974. Author unknown.

EXERCISE 18   Group Process—Self-Diagnosis

Purposes	1. To raise consciousness of one's own behaviour in groups.
	2. To self-diagnose learning needs regarding small-group functioning.
Facility	None—homework assignment.
Materials	Worksheet A: Self-Diagnosis of Small Group Behaviour.
Time Required	Fifteen to 30 minutes.
Group Size	Unlimited—individual homework assignment.
Design	1. Using Worksheet A, have class members respond to the items in terms of the categories represented.
	2. Ask that they consider the following: A. Why do they take certain functions most often? B. Why are certain functions never or rarely carried out? C. How can they experience functions they would like to practise? What assistance, if any, is needed?
Variation	Self-diagnosis can be discussed within small groups; familiar members can offer feedback on their perceptions.

(*continued*)

Source: Reprinted by permission from La Monica, Elaine L., *The Nursing Process: A Humanistic Approach*, pp. 311–313. Copyright © 1979 by Addison-Wesley Publishing Company, Inc., Menlo Park, Calif.

EXERCISE 18 *(continued)*
WORKSHEET A: Self-Diagnosis of Small-Group Behaviour

Listed below are functions that are performed by members of discussion groups. Considering each category, check the columns that apply to you.

Frequency of Behaviour(s)

	I perceive myself to use most often	I seldom use	I never use	I would like to practise
Task Roles				
1. Initiator				
2. Information seeker				
3. Evaluator				
4. Coordinator				
5. Procedural technician				
6. Recorder				
Maintenance Roles				
1. Encourager				
2. Harmonizer				
3. Compromiser				
4. Standard setter				
5. Gatekeeper				

Frequency of Behaviour(s)

Self-Oriented Roles	I perceive myself to use most often	I seldom use	I never use	I would like to practise
1. Aggressor				
2. Blocker				
3. Recognition seeker				
4. Playboy				
5. Dominator				
6. Help seeker				

(continued)

EXERCISE 18
WORKSHEET A: *(continued)*

Respond to each question explicitly. Use extra paper if necessary.

A. Why do I use certain roles most often?

B. Why are certain roles never or rarely carried out?

C. How can I experience roles that I would like to practise? What assistance, if any, do I need?

EXERCISE 19 Conflict Resolution—Saturn's First Hospital Station

Purposes   1. To develop group collaboration and planning.

2. To experience conflict resolution.

3. To foster group team building.

4. To facilitate setting group goals.

Facility   A classroom large enough to accommodate participants.

Materials   Paper and pencil or pen.

Blackboard and chalk.

Time Required   One and one-half to two hours.

Group Size   No more than five groups of six to eight participants.

Design   1. Explain the following to the group: The entire class has been carefully selected to set up the first space hospital station on the planet Saturn. The class will be transported tomorrow on Columbia 6. Members will spend the rest of their lives on Saturn. The shuttle that transports people and equipment will visit Uranus and Mars after stopping at Saturn and then return to Earth. The next visit to Saturn for transporting equipment and personnel is unknown, but it will not be before ten Earth years have passed. The class must decide what is needed to survive and what is needed to equip the hospital. Due to constraints of space on Columbia 6, each person can bring only five

(*continued*)

Source: The idea for this exercise came from one entitled "Noah's Ark" at the School of Education, University of Massachusetts, 1973.

EXERCISE 19 (*continued*)

specific items on board; these items include personal and hospital needs. Air concentration that is needed to sustain human life is guaranteed as is water. Nothing else is promised.

2. Have members individually write down the five items that they wish to bring. (5 minutes)

3. After completing Step 2, notify the class that you have received word that extra fuel is required on board as a result of a meteor storm that is expected between Saturn and Uranus. The space allocated to the hospital crew has been cut. Class members should therefore form into pairs (have triads if there is an odd number in the group) and select five things out of their combined list of ten items to bring to Saturn. (10 minutes)

4. After Step 3 has been completed, a spacegram is received with the following message: "President orders that the intergalactic missile tracking station be housed on Saturn." The effect of this message on the hospital crew is elation. However, all materials for the missile tracking station must be transported in tomorrow's voyage. Space is again decreased and each group of six to eight can only bring five items on board the shuttle to Saturn. After grouping into six to eight members, have each group decide what five items to bring. Pairs (triads) formed in Step 3 should be in the same group. (15 minutes)

5. When groups have selected their five items, announce the following: There is a massive surplus in the country's budget—enough for a sister hospital station in Uranus. The president has selected the crew for Uranus; both crews will be transported together. *Each crew* will bring only five items due to the shortage of space on the ship. Each group should be instructed to choose a negotiator and plan a strategy for selling other groups on the im-

portance of taking their items (15 minutes). Negotiators from each group will then meet around a table at the head of the class to select the five items that will be brought to Saturn. Negotiations will take place in three rounds within the following time limits: Round 1— meeting of negotiators (15 minutes); Round 2 —negotiators consult with their groups (15 minutes); Round 3—meeting of negotiators (15 minutes). The decision on the five items must be made by the end of Round 3. Only the negotiators can talk during Rounds 1 and 3; groups must be quiet.

6. After the five items have been selected, list them on a blackboard and discuss the experience with the class as a whole. Questions that can be asked and areas that usually engender discussion are:
   A. What did the items chosen by individuals represent in comparison with those chosen by groups?
   B. Was their movement from counting on self to counting on others and the interactions between and among others?
   C. Were the resources of the group studied? Could people build things, grow things, and so forth?
   D. Did the final items represent any particular area of Maslow's hierarchy? Explain.
   E. How was the negotiator chosen? Were needed attributes of the negotiator specified?
   F. Was creative problem solving evident as the experience developed?
   G. What was learned from the experience that applies in the present?

EXERCISE 20   Conflict Resolution—Contingency Contracting

Purposes
1. To apply types of contingency contracting to real or hypothetical situations.

2. To role play one type of contingency contract.

3. To receive feedback from peers on the role play.

Facility
A classroom to accommodate participants working in pairs with space between dyads.

Materials
Worksheets A, B, C, D, and E—Types of Contingency Contracts.

Pencil or pen.

Time Required
Forty-five minutes.

Group Size
Unlimited pairs.

Design
1. Instruct participants to individually choose one of the five worksheets and jot down an experienced or hypothetical example that requires the particular contingency contract. If necessary, refer to Chapter 16 for the definitions and examples of each type of contract.

2. Participants should form into pairs and role play the examples. The writer of the example should be the leader first; the other member should be the follower. Members of pairs should provide feedback to each other. If time permits, roles should switch using the same two situations.

3. After dyads have completed Step 2, have two or three dyads volunteer and share their experiences with the group.

EXERCISE 20
WORKSHEET A: Leader-Control Contingency Contract

Example:

_____

_____

_____

_____

_____

_____

_____

_____

_____

_____

_____

_____

_____

_____

_____

_____

_____

_____

_____

_____

_____

_____

_____

_____

_____

_____

(_continued_)

EXERCISE 20   *(continued)*
WORKSHEET B: Partial-Control-by-Follower
                       Contingency Contract

Example:

_____

_____

_____

_____

_____

_____

_____

_____

_____

_____

_____

_____

_____

_____

_____

_____

_____

_____

_____

_____

_____

_____

_____

_____

_____

EXERCISE 20
WORKSHEET C: Equal-Control-by-Leader-and-Follower
                      Contingency Contract

Example:

_____

_____

_____

_____

_____

_____

_____

_____

_____

_____

_____

_____

_____

_____

_____

_____

_____

_____

_____

_____

_____

_____

_____

(continued)

EXERCISE 20 *(continued)*
WORKSHEET D: Partial-Control-by-Leader Contingency Contract

Example:

_____

_____

_____

_____

_____

_____

_____

_____

_____

_____

_____

_____

_____

_____

_____

_____

_____

_____

_____

_____

_____

_____

_____

_____

_____

EXERCISE 20
WORKSHEET E: Follower-Control Contingency Contract

Example:

_____

_____

_____

_____

_____

_____

_____

_____

_____

_____

_____

_____

_____

_____

_____

_____

_____

_____

_____

_____

_____

_____

_____

_____

_____

EXERCISE 21:   Time Management—Time Analysis Sheets

Purposes

1. To facilitate identification of time wasters.

2. To analyse time wasters.

3. To use time more effectively.

Facility

None—this exercise is a self-study homework assignment.

Materials

Worksheet A: Time Analysis Worksheet.
Worksheet B: Biggest Time Wasters.
Worksheet C: Time Log.
Pen or pencil.

Time Required

Variable.

Group Size

Unlimited—homework assignment.

Design

Three worksheets are provided for use in individual analysis for professional and/or personal aspects of one's life. It is suggested that they be used in order—Worksheet A through Worksheet C—for the first time. Then they can be reused over and over as one wishes to be in more and more control of time.

Worksheets A and B require simply filling in the blanks.

Worksheet C requires specifying daily goals and keeping a log of activities for the day. The log can then be analysed using Worksheets A and/or B with new goals set for the next day. Progress can be traced by reviewing these sheets.

Variation

Group members can be encouraged to share analyses with peers. Class time can be allotted for small- and large-group discussion.

EXERCISE 21
WORKSHEET A: Time Analysis Worksheet

What items am I spending too much time on?	What am I doing that does not need to be done at all?
What items am I spending too little time on?	What am I doing that could be done better (or more economically, more effectively) by others?
Items in which I can make my most important savings.	Ways by which I can avoid overusing the time of others.
Other ways in which I can make effective savings.	Other suggestions.

(*continued*)

Source: Brown, D., *The use of time: A looking-into-leadership monograph.* Fairfax, VA: Leadership Resources, 1980, p. 9. Reproduced by permission.

EXERCISE 21 *(continued)*
WORKSHEET B: Biggest Time Wasters

Specifically, my biggest time wasters are:

1. _____

2. _____

3. _____

4. _____

5. _____

6. _____

7. _____

8. _____

	Imposed by	Cause	Solution
1.	_____	_____	_____
			_____
2.	_____	_____	_____
			_____
3.	_____	_____	_____
			_____
4.	_____	_____	_____
			_____
5.	_____	_____	_____
			_____
6.	_____	_____	_____
			_____
7.	_____	_____	_____
			_____
8.	_____	_____	_____
			_____

Source: Graf P. 1979. *Time management.* Unpublished material.

EXERCISE 21
WORKSHEET C: Time Log

Date _____

Day of the week _____

Goals: 1. _____   4. _____

       2. _____   5. _____

       3. _____   6. _____

Time	Activity	Priority Rating A, B, or C	Comments
8:00 8:30			
9:00 9:30			
10:00 10:30			
11:00 11:30			
12:00 12:30			
1:00 1:30			
2:00 2:30			

(continued)

EXERCISE 21
WORKSHEET C: (continued)

Time	Activity	Priority Rating A, B, or C	Comments
3:00 3:30			
4:00 4:30			
5:00 5:30			
6:00 6:30			
7:00 7:30			
8:00 8:30			
Evening			

Source: Graf P. 1979. *Time management*. Unpublished material. Reprinted by permission of the author.

EXERCISE 22 Performance Appraisal—Rating Scale for Clinical Staff Nursing

Purposes
1. To appraise the clinical performance of a staff nurse.

2. To practise using a Likert-type rating scale for appraising performance.

3. To develop strategies for meeting the clinical learning needs of a staff nurse.

Facility
None. This is a clinical assignment.

Materials
Worksheet A: Clinical Nurse Performance Appraisal Form.

Pen or pencil.

Time Required
One hour or more.

Group Size
Unlimited dyads.

Design
1. As a homework assignment, have participants read Chapter 18, plus other related articles and written materials on the topic.

2. Ask that participants form into comfortable pairs—teaming with a peer who is seen as nonthreatening and/or is a friend. Using Worksheet A, ask that each pair member observe the other's clinical practice for a period of one to two shifts, trying particularly to assess the areas noted in the performance appraisal form.

3. Using Worksheet A, each pair member should appraise their partner's performance in writing. Following the written appraisal, the pair should meet and role play discussion of the performance appraisals. Each pair member should have the opportunity to be the appraiser and the person being appraised. Together, they should develop an action plan for the next month.

(*continued*)

EXERCISE 22 *(continued)*

Variation

The pair member being appraised may complete Worksheet A as a self-report prior to the role-play discussion. Then both appraisals can be discussed with reference to the appraisee's performance. Also, the period being appraised can be longer than one to two shifts, depending on the available time.

EXERCISE 22
WORKSHEET A: Clinical Nurse Performance Appraisal Form

Name of Appraisee _____

Name of Appraiser _____

Date of Appraisal _____

	Unacceptable	Acceptable	Distinguished	Not Observed	Not Applicable
Clinical Skills					
Data Collection					
Taking Nursing Histories					
Interviewing					
Interpreting Clinical Data					
Consulting with Colleagues					
Talking with Families					
Conducting Physical Assessments					
Nursing Diagnosis					
Processing Data					
Determining Diagnoses					
Setting Priorities					
Nursing Orders					
Writing Nursing Orders					
Maintaining Individualized Care					
Providing Care					
Giving Direct Care					
Effectively Using Interpersonal Processes					
Quality of Technical Skills					
Quality of Teaching Methods					

(continued)

EXERCISE 22
WORKSHEET A: *(continued)*

	Unacceptable	Acceptable	Distinguished	Not Observed	Not Applicable
Advocating for the Client/Family					
Making Appropriate Referrals					
Coordinating Care					
Delegating Care Appropriately					
Supervising Other Nursing Personnel					
Evaluating Outcome					

Goals for Next Appraisal Period   *Date for Next Appraisal* _____

1. _____

_____

_____

_____

2. _____

_____

_____

_____

3. _____

_____

_____

_____

4. _____

_____

_____

_____

5. _____

_____

_____

_____

Part IV

MANAGEMENT STRUCTURE AND PROCESSES

The purpose of Part IV is to discuss some important structural and process aspects of managing health care organizations that managers need to understand in order to manage and work more effectively within the macro system of the NHS.

"Structure" refers to aspects of the organization's design; while "process", as used here, refers to certain dynamic aspects of an organization's wider context (e.g., the external environment and the internal organizational culture). The main theme of this section is how environment, structure and culture interact with one another. Thus, Chapter 21 provides a historical perspective by discussing how the NHS has evolved to its present form and how it has changed its management structure as new demands have been placed upon it. Chapter 22 discusses the demands and constraints imposed by both the external and internal environments in which a "typical" NHS organization operates. Chaper 23 discusses formal design characteristics, together with ways in which a manager can structure an organization to meet effectively the challenge of the environmental demands and constraints. Chapter 24 discusses the kinds of cultures which develop within organizations, together with the effect they have on employee performance.

How these management structures and processes affect overall organizational performance is also covered.

CHAPTER 21

Development of the National Health Service

by Philip I. Morgan, PhD

To lead and manage any organizational system successfully requires an understanding of its history and management structure. This chapter, therefore, provides a brief overview of the changing role of the management and organizational structure of the National Health Service (NHS) since its inception in 1948. Also highlighted are some of the major pieces of NHS legislation implemented in Britain since that time.

THE NATIONAL HEALTH SERVICE 1948–1972

The origins of the establishment of the British National Health Service can be traced back to a series of reports made by the Ministry of Health as early as the 1920s. For example, the Dawson Report (1920) recommended the provision of a comprehensive scheme of hospitals and primary health care. Reports from the National Health Insurance (1926) and the British Medical Association (1930, 1938) all pointed to the shortcomings of the existing pattern of services and made various recommendations for change. However, it was not until 1946 and the publication of the National Health Service Bill by the Labour Party Minister of Health, Aneurin Bevin, that the NHS became a viable entity. The Bill which was to make the NHS a reality was fully enacted in 1948 after some initial objections, most notably from the British Medical Association (BMA). However, these were overcome through negotiations. The Act set out the Health Minister's responsibility to develop "the establishment . . . of a comprehensive health service designed to secure improvements in physical and mental health . . . and the prevention, diagnosis and treatment of illness". Under the NHS Act the Health Minister was directly responsible to Parliament for providing all hospital and specialist services (see Figure 21.1). Additionally, the Central Health Council and its Standing Advisory Committees were established. Under the new structure the council's purpose was to review developments in the NHS and to advise and make recommendations to the Minister. The resulting structure of the NHS represented a political compromise between the government and the various provider groups.

Under the Health Minister, the Permanent Secretary, and the Central Services Council the structure was divided laterally into three groups:

1. Executive Councils, which were responsible for the administration of GPs, dentists, opticians, and pharmacists. These councils were appointed partly by local professionals and partly by the Ministry of Health (MoH), which also provided their funding.

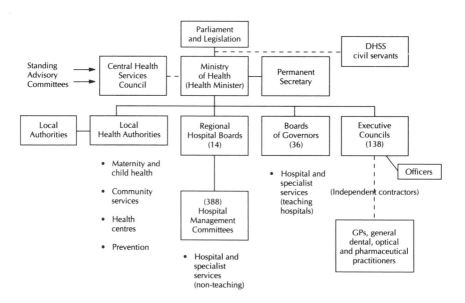

FIGURE 21.1 Structure of 1948 NHS.

Source: Riserborough, P.A., & Walter, M. (1988). *Management in health care*. London: Wright.

2. Local Authorities, which were responsible for a variety of environmental and personal health services, including maternity, health visitors, midwives, health education, and ambulance services.

3. Regional Hospital Boards (RHBs), Hospital Management Committees (HMCs), and Boards of Governors. Teaching hospitals were organized under boards of governors, directly under the MoH, while most other hospitals were administered under Regional Hospital Boards.

Originally, 14 Regional Hospital Boards (RHBs) were set up in England and Wales, individually centred around a university medical school. Later, this number was increased to 15 RHBs with the addition of Wessex. They were seen as mainly planning agencies rather than as an additional management tier (which they later became). Teaching hospitals were administered separately by a Board of Governors.

The NHS was thus founded on existing hospitals owned by local authorities and charitable organizations. The major changes were that the hospitals were no longer controlled by local authorities, and municipal and voluntary hospitals were amalgamated to form hospital groups, each of which was managed by a Hospital Management Committee. Many other services, however, such as home nursing and care of the mentally handicapped did remain under the aegis of local authorities.

An important feature of the newly established NHS was the state support for financing and planning medical care in order to bring it within the reach of the whole population. By nationalizing the hospitals, the government in principle made a commitment "to provide medical care without charge to the user at the time of consumption" (Brown, 1973).

Leavitt and Wall (1984) noted, however, that the 1948 Act did little to eliminate much of the inequalities of service between regions, arguing that:

> Because the administrative structure, with its bias towards hospital matters, had the strongest influence on policy-making in the central department, there was inadequate local liaison between hospital and community staff, with the result that services for the acutely ill tended to improve more rapidly while the needs of the chronically ill and disabled were comparatively neglected.

The structure imposed certain constraints on the NHS. For example, the division of responsibility between the executive councils, local health authorities, and the hospital service made effective coordination between them difficult. An ineffective administrative control system allowed the objectives of local bodies to be achieved rather than the implementation of the national policy. Thus, in the hospital service there was a lack of direction and general uncertainty about responsibilities. A poor quality of care was provided to patient groups and consequently a less than optimum use of resources (Haywood, 1974). Resources varied at regional and local levels which resulted in the demand for more resources of better hospitals, better facilities, more supporting staff, and better pay.

Because the NHS was divided into three areas (hospital, family practitioner services, and other health services delivered by local authorities) this created a problem of unified management. Consequently, during the late 1950s to early 1970s, various proposals were made to combine these three divisions under one unified area board. Most of these proposals met with only limited success. However, in 1962, the Porritt Committee Report recommended that the health services should be consolidated under the control of area boards to be administered by local government. The proposed reorganization by the Porritt Committee had three major objectives: (1) to unify health services—previously under the RHBs, HMCs, board of governors, executive councils, and local health authorities—under one authority; (2) to improve coordination between health authorities and related government services; and (3) to introduce better management. These objectives were largely accomplished and as a result of the reorganization, Regional Health Authorities (RHAs) replaced Regional Hospital Boards and were given greater responsibilities. In England, 90 Area Health Authorities (AHAs) were organized under the RHAs.

Also, in the 1960s, a major plan was developed for acute hospitals. District General Hospitals (DGHs) were built with modern medical specialities, each serving a defined population. In addition, each region had its own medical school. Hitherto, teaching hospitals were concentrated mainly in London and Scotland, leaving large sections of the country isolated from most modern medical advances.

In the 1970s, attention was given to the linkage between the various parts of the NHS. Regions were subdivided into "districts" and a further geographical division was created between regions and districts which matched local authority boundaries. Once established these so-called "areas" could then begin to coordinate the various NHS activities. As a direct result, many working parties were set up in England and Wales to devise new ways of allocating funding from Whitehall to regions and to districts. One of the best known was the Resource Allocation Working Party (RAWP) which developed a formula for assessing regional needs by means of mortality and population. As a result, a major redistribution of resources based on actual need rather than precedent was implemented.

"CONSENSUS" AND "DIPLOMATIC" MANAGEMENT 1972–1982

In 1972, a DHSS document known as the "Grey Book" was published (DHSS, 1972). It was heavily influenced by recommendations made by Brunel University's Health Services Organization Research Unit and McKinsey & Co., a management consultant group. The Grey Book set out the definitive philosophy for the management arrangements for the 1974 NHS reorganization. It advocated that management should be based on teams of equals, who should manage and make decisions by consensus. "Consensus management" meant no one person or group retained power; instead, decisions had to be made collectively after discussion of alternatives. The Grey Book proposed that team management should be implemented at three levels: district, area and region.

The advantage of team management was that it fostered multidisciplinary cooperation; the disadvantage was that it took time to manage and could cause considerable delays. Since the powers of veto are left in the hands of only one or two members of the team, difficult decisions may never be resolved. Moreover, under this new structure, district chief officers were not subordinate to area officers, since there was no line management accountability between them. The district management team (DMT) was directly accountable to the AHA, there being no authority at district level. Riserborough and Walter (1988) note that area officers were the AHA's principal advisors with planning responsibilities; although they monitored the work of districts and reported to the AHA, they had no control over district officers. Many problems arose from this confusing structure.

An attempt to remedy the problem was made in 1973 by the National Health Reorganization Act by unifying hospitals and various specialist services previously run by executive councils and local authorities. Only the occupational health services, environmental health services, and personal social services remained separate. The additional management tier created by the 90 AHAs generally had identical boundaries to metropolitan counties and non-metropolitan districts.

The 1974 Reorganization

In 1974, the NHS was reorganized along more modern businesslike lines and given a new corporate structure (see Figure 21.2). The chief management innovations were an emphasis on management training, together with a general streamlining of some of the inconsistencies of the administrative structure. This made it possible to develop coherent local plans in keeping with a national health service. Additionally, health councils and area health authorities (AHAs) were developed. This improved local

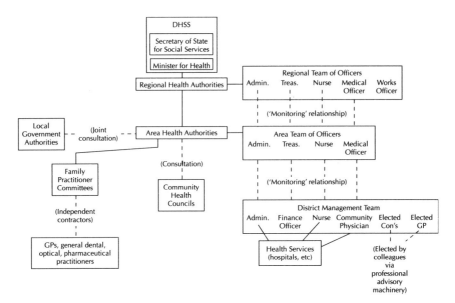

FIGURE 21.2 Structure of the 1974 NHS (England and Wales).

representation by ensuring that their input would be considered in the planning process.

Regions and districts were to be managed by distinct management teams; however, there was no general manager to oversee the process. Hence, there was no central chain of command—a fundamental prerequisite for all large business. Instead, management by consensus held sway whereby management was conducted by groups of "equal" fellow professionals, each representing a particular occupational group's interests. Each district was represented by a district management team (DMT).

The 1976 Royal Commission

In 1976, a NHS Royal Commission was set up to consider the best use of management of the NHS's financial and manpower resources. The Commission criticized the new reorganization as creating an unnecessary extra management level, resulting in unnecessary paperwork and delays in decision making. Their report, published in 1979, criticized the NHS as having: "too many tiers; too many administrators, in all disciplines; failure to take quick decisions; money wasted" (DHSS, 1979). To remedy these problems, the Commission recommended the abolition of the area tier and proposed that Family Practitioner Committees' (FPCs) functions should be merged with those of health authorities. The preferred solution to the problem was to dismantle the AHAs; however, others thought that the regional level should be abolished.

However, a Conservative government rejected the Royal Commission proposal to merge the functions of the FPCs with those of health authorities. They also rejected the idea of delegating accountability of regions. In December 1979, the Secretary of State published *Patients first*, dealing with the structure and management of the NHS. It made four major recommendations:

1. Strengthening management at local level, with greater delegation of responsibility to those at unit level or in community service.

2. Simplifying the organizational structure by removing the AHA level and replacing it with the District Health Authority (DHA) at district (or local) level. These were to be based on the district general hospital and its catchment area being re-established as the basis for organizing health care.

3. Simplifying the professional advisory machinery.

4. Streamlining and simplifying the planning system.

These recommendations were largely endorsed by April 1982 and the AHAs were abolished and the DHAs installed in their place. Decision making therefore became more local and less remote (see Figure 21.2).

The reorganization of the NHS in 1974 placed emphasis on the structure and abolished HMCs and the addition of a new health authority. This was to make comprehensive planning possible so as to allow centralized policies to be issued down the hierarchy.

The 1974 reorganization was intended to achieve the following results:

- Integration of the tripartite functional organization into a new unified organization where "a fully integrated. . . service in which every aspect of health care can be provided by members of the health care professions. . ." (DHSS, 1972).

- Better coordination and decentralization of the administration between health authorities and related local government services. The First Green Paper (1968) suggested that health and local government could be jointly administered. The Second Green Paper (1970) favoured the separate administration of health services within the same boundaries of local authorities. The boundaries of AHAs were made the same size as those of local authorities with strategic planning of resources for primary care.

- Better management. This was prompted by various reports prior to the reorganization: the Farquharson Lang Report

(1962) on the administrative practices of hospital authorities, the Salmon Report (1966) on nursing staff structure, and the Cogwheel Report (1967) on the organization of medical staff. The reorganization based the administration on the concepts of "maximum responsibility delegated downwards" linked by "clear lines of accountability upwards", which would be exercised by sound management structures at each level (DHSS, 1972).

- Increased participation and democrative representation of medical professionals at all levels. Thus, clinicians became members of DMTs, RHAs and AHAs.

One of the major changes of the reorganization of the NHS in 1982 was that of structural integration to district level with the removal of AHAs. It was now the responsibility of each new DHA to determine its own management arrangements, and to decide on the numbers and types of functional manager it required. At district level, management teams, DMTs based on consensus decision making, were to remain. Below district level, hospitals and community services became management units. Each unit was to be managed by a unit administrator, a senior doctor and a senior nurse. All functional managers would report to the unit administrator. The new structure is shown in Figure 21.3.

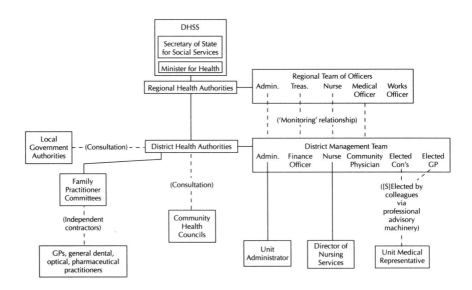

FIGURE 21.3 Structure of the 1982 NHS (England and Wales).

RHAs continued to be responsible for the allocation of capital and revenue to districts with each RHA chairman accountable to the Secretary of State for developments in the region. It followed that district chairmen would be accountable to regional chairmen.

THE GRIFFITHS REPORT 1983—"GENERAL MANAGEMENT"

Following the reorganization of 1982, the Health Service Minister, Norman Fowler, announced the need for an inquiry into the effective use of manpower and resources in the NHS, citing the apparent inability of the NHS to achieve improvements in cost and management effectiveness. The result was the publication of the Griffiths Report (named after its Chairman, Sir Roy Griffiths, Managing Director of Sainsbury, PLC).

The Griffiths Report was perhaps one of the most significant and far-reaching reorganizations of the structure of the NHS. The report recommended the adoption of the concept of "general management" to replace functional or consensus management. To comprehend the rationale for the recommended changes it is necessary to have some understanding of the problems inherent in the system prior to the report.

Pre-1982 management was characterized by smoothing over real differences and attempting to reconcile conflicts between various groups within the NHS (Harrison, 1988). As noted earlier, the managers ran the organization based on consensus and were often reduced to playing a diplomatic role in working with multidisciplinary groups. For this reason, pre-1982, pre-Griffiths management style is often described as "diplomatic management".

Harrison (1988) summarized much of the research findings prior to the publication of the Griffiths Report under four major headings: pluralism, reactiveness, incrementalism, and introversion (see Table 21.1).

1. *Pluralism:* Harrison reported that managers were not the most influential actors in the NHS. Instead, he found that the medical profession exerted the most influence on re- source decisions in the NHS. Also, he found that decisions were made with reference to the lowest common denom- inator. No single person was in charge; hence, there was no accountability.

2. *Reactiveness:* Harrison argued that managers were problem- driven and lacked any concern for how the decision was to be implemented. Rather than being proactive, problems tended to be dealt with on an *ad hoc* basis. The manager's

TABLE 21.1 Correspondence of Research Findings and the Griffiths Analysis

Academic Research	Griffiths "Diagnosis"	Griffiths Prescriptions
Pluralism	Lowest common denominator decisions No one in charge	General management in place of consensus
Reactiveness	Lack of concern with implementation for managers	Extension of review process Incentives
Incrementalism	Lack of performance orientation	Extension of review process Cost-improvement programmes Management budgets
Introversion	Lack of attention to consumers	More concern with consumer market research

Source: Harrison, S. (1988). *Managing the national health service: shifting the frontier?* London: Chapman & Hall, p. 70.

main consideration was in trying to deal with complaints, without creating further dissatisfactions elsewhere.

3. *Incrementalism:* Managers were reluctant to question the value of existing patterns of service or to propose major changes to them. The practice among managers was to seek more resources rather than try to find ways of using current resources more wisely.

4. *Introversion:* Managers behaved "as if" other groups of employees, rather than the public, were the clients of the NHS. The tendency was to focus on serving health service staff rather than the general public (Schulz and Harrison, 1983; Harrison, Hagwood, & Fussell 1984).

The Griffiths Report paralleled Harrison, Hagwood, and Fussell's findings and concluded that there were five major areas of weakness in the health service management structure:

1. Lack of strategic central direction.

2. Lack of individual managerial responsibility leading to "lowest common denominator" decisions.

3. Lack of objectives to guide action and a lack of motivation to implement plans and policies.

4. Lack of orientation towards performance, including disinclination to conduct financial evaluation, to collect the right kinds of data or to be concerned with productivity.

5. Lack of customer focus, including little concern to collect information about the views of health service users.

To remedy these problems the Griffiths Report recommended a management reorganization through the establishment of a Management Board reporting to an NHS Supervisory Board. It also recommended that general managers were to be introduced at all levels who would be responsible for making final decisions. The general manager's duties were as follows:

■ to achieve objectives;
■ to break down inappropriate professional boundaries;
■ to involve doctors more closely in management;
■ to improve the measurement of health outcomes;
■ to ensure devolution to unit level;
■ to improve sensitivity of service to the views of the consumer.

The core of the 1984 reorganization was the assertion of central managerial control over all health service workers. The new management system was based on the following principles:

■ systematic monitoring
■ a single chain of command
■ an integrated structure
■ the rule of generalists not specialists
■ greater devolution as well as greater central control
■ flexible staff and flexible structures
■ hybrid staff members who would know something of everyone's job.

The new structure was to allow a smooth flow of precise information to the centre with every individual within the organization taking on a greater personal responsibility. Radical devolution coupled with modern information systems and regular reviews gave potential scope for a new, more strategic role for senior management.

In short, the Griffiths reforms put general managers in charge of the NHS and made them accountable at all three levels: regional, district, and unit (see Figure 21.4).

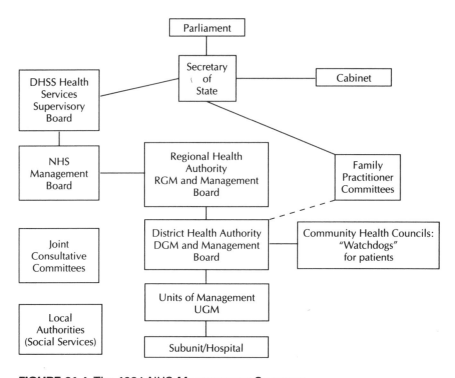

FIGURE 21.4 The 1984 NHS Management Structure.

Source: Riserborough, P.A., & Walter, M. (1988). *Management in health care.* London: Wright.

However, Pollit *et al.* (1991) argued that the new managerialism was founded on distrust. Based on a three-year study of the impact of general management in the NHS, the researchers concluded that the Griffiths model demands proof of performance reviews of RHAs and DHAs. Individuals and authorities are called to answer if they do not produce according to plan. The Griffiths Report fails to offer a convincing analysis of the relationship between the business of running the NHS and the workings of the political system in which the service is set.

Also, Strong and Robinson (1990) argued that:

> Griffiths. . . for all its radicalism, was only a partial break with the past. There was now a chain of command which reached from the top to the bottom of the organization. There was a new headquarters staff with a potential flexibility to match the exigencies of local need and form. But the service was still trapped, for general managers at least, within a national straightjacket. Local initiative was frustrated by ministers, by civil servants, by supervisory management tiers and by powerful professional bodies. Doctors still gave orders, nanny still knew best.

CONSUMERISM—1989 AND BEYOND

With the publication of two White Papers in 1989 (DHSS, 1989), *Working for patients* and *Caring for people*, a new era of NHS management was born. The main characteristics of this new era can be summarized as an increasing emphasis on consumerism and value for money, together with a further professionalization of standards by means of clinical audits and an emphasis on income generation and entrepreneurialism. For example, *Working for patients* contained seven key proposals:

1. *More delegation of responsibility to local level:* Responsibilities were to be delegated from regions to districts and from districts to hospitals to make the service more responsive to patients' needs.

2. *Self-governing hospitals:* To encourage a better service to patients, hospitals were able to apply for a new self-governing status within the NHS as NHS Hospital Trusts.

3. *New funding arrangements:* To enable hospitals which best meet patients' needs to get the money to do so, the money required to treat patients was to be able to cross administrative boundaries.

4. *Additional consultants:* To reduce waiting times and improve the quality of service, over 100 new permanent consultant posts were to be created by 1992.

5. *GP practice budgets:* To help family doctors improve their service to patients, large GP practices were enabled to apply for their own NHS budgets and to obtain a defined range of services direct from hospitals.

6. *Reformed management bodies:* To improve the effectiveness of NHS management, regional, district, and family practitioner management bodies were to be reduced in size and reformed along business lines.

7. *Better audit arrangements:* To ensure that all who deliver patient services make the best use of resources, quality of service and value for money would be more rigorously audited.

Working for patients had the objective of facilitating and providing better quality and greater choice of services for patients. Its intent was to create a market in which hospitals, as the providers of health care, compete with one another to win contracts from district health authorities. The contracts will enable districts to increase their control over the amount and quality of the health care they purchase, while competition will encourage hospitals to provide services which are of low cost but sufficient quality.

Several issues have since emerged. First, the main reforms are to be achieved through incentives, rather than through structural reorganization where control is through trust. Second, there must be a balance between freedom to compete and manage one's affairs and regulation to provide comprehensive and accessible services (Nichol, 1989). Managers are required to monitor closely the cost and quality of their services, while doctors are expected to play a key role in management and budgeting. Competition is to be used as a stimulus to create greater incentives for efficiency. The most important quality needed is the ability to manage change. One of the key roles will be for all managers to give leadership in the creation of a positive climate. Managers will need to look at the skills needed and arrange for the necessary training to be given.

However, Strong and Robinson (1990) argued that "NHS PLC" may expect a few problems of its very own making. These include:

1. The change of emphasis in the nature of health services means that there is a focus on the integration of the trades within the service, on flexible forms of local administrative structure, and on the systematic monitoring of individual performance. This could prove difficult, especially with regard to internecine rivalries within the health service.

2. The start-up costs for entry into hospital markets are high with real competition between hospitals and will involve a huge increase in the distances which patients have to travel in order to receive care.

3. Achieving quality care is a third major problem. How can the regulatory structure work if there are few indicators of quality? The benefits of competition are premised on the assumption that purchasers possess serious information about the product. However, this is particularly difficult to accomplish in the health service since most consumers operate on the basis of partial or complete ignorance of the quality of care they might expect to receive.

As can be seen from the foregoing, the 1989 White Papers have pointed the way to increasing decentralization and autonomy in the health service. The creation of self-governing hospital trusts whereby hospitals who meet certain criteria have been able to "opt out" and assume responsibility for managing their own budgets and making many of their own decisions regarding patient care is obviously a step in this direction. Also, GPs are now able to manage their practices like small businesses.

SUMMARY

In summary, from 1948 until 1982 the NHS was increasingly preoccupied with a series of organizational and management changes. Since it began in 1948, the NHS hospitals were run by hospital management committees to provide the needs of effective management. The 1960s and 1970s were characterized by a general belief in the efficacy of changing the organizational structure and on management training as a means of improving the service. The 1974 and 1982 reorganizations were introduced to improve the administration of the NHS. However, criticism grew that those in charge of the NHS too often lacked management expertise and vision, and that those in authority had insufficient power to discharge their responsibilities effectively. The 1983 Griffiths Report made recommendations to remedy these perceived deficiencies.

Moreover, in the 1980s, a Conservative government initiated several other related reforms aimed at further decentralizing the service. All of this has had the effect of dismantling much of the bureaucratic structure of the NHS with the intent of making the service more self-supporting and cost-effective.

These new initiatives are bold experiments; however, as of this writing much remains to be resolved and it is difficult to see just how far reform can be taken in this direction and just what the results of these new measures will be.

REFERENCES

Brown, R.G.S. (1973). *The changing National Health Service.* UK: Routledge and Kegan Paul.

Cogwheel Report (1967). *First report of the Joint Working Party on the Organisation of Medical Work in Hospitals* (Chairman, Sir G. Godber). London: HMSO.

Department of Health and Social Security (1989). *Caring for people.* London: DoH.

Department of Health and Social Security (1972). *Management arrangements for the reorganized National Health Service (The Grey Book).* London: HMSO.

Department of Health and Social Security (1989). *Working for patients: the health service; caring for the 1990s.* London: DoH. (Cm 555).

DHSS and Welsh Office (1979). *Patients first: consultative paper on the structure and management of the National Health Service in England and Wales.* London: HMSO.

Farquharson Lang Report (1966). *Administrative Practice of hospital boards in Scotland.* Edinburgh: HMSO.

First Green Paper (1968). *The administrative structure of medical and related services in England and Wales.* London: HMSO.

Griffiths, R. (1983). *National Health Service management inquiry.* Letter to the Secretary of State and recommendations for action. London: DHSS.

Ham, C. (1982). *Health policy in Britain.* UK: Macmillan Press Ltd.

Harrison, S. (1988). *Managing the National Health Service: shifting the frontier?* London: Chapman & Hall.

Harrison, S., Hagwood, S., & Fussell, C. (1984). Problems and solutions: the perception of NHS managers. *Hospital and Health Services Review, 80*(4), July. UK: Longman Group.

Haywood, S. (1974). *Managing the Health Service.* London: Allen & Unwin Ltd.

Leavitt, R., & Wall, A. (1984). *The reorganised National Health Service* (3rd ed.). London: Croom Helm.

NHS Management Inquiry (1983). *Letter to the Secretary of State and recommendations for action* (The Griffiths Report). London: DHSS.

Nichol, D. (1989). Working for patients, the role of managers in implementing the White Paper. *Health Service Management, 85*(3), 107–109.

Pollit, C., Harrison, S., Hunter, D. J., & Marnoch, G. (1991). General management in the National Health Service: The Initial Impact 1983–1988. *Public Administration, 69*, Spring, 61–83.

Riserborough, P.A., & Walter, M. (1988). *Management in health care.* London: Wright.

Salmon Report (1966). *Report of the Committee on Senior Nursing Staff Structure* (Chairman, B. Salmon). London: HMSO.

Schulz, R. I., & Harrison, S. (1983). *Teams and top managers in the NHS: a survey and a strategy.* London: King's Fund Project Paper No. 41.

Second Green Paper (1970). *The future structure of the National Health Service.* London: HMSO.

Strong, P., & Robinson, J. (1990). *The NHS under new management.* Milton Keynes: Open University Press.

The National Health Service Act, 1946 (1946). London: HMSO.

CHAPTER 22

The Environment

by Philip I. Morgan, PhD

In order to provide a basic understanding of the various concepts discussed so far it may be useful at this juncture to discuss the managerial processes in terms of a larger contextual framework. For convenience we can call this wider framework the "environment".

An organization's environment consists of the forces and conditions that surround and pervade it (Hodgetts & Altman, 1979). Since an organization's success or failure is wholly dependent on how effectively it copes with the competing demands of its environment, one useful way of understanding the essential components of that environment is to describe two simple models. The models should enable us to conceptualize the processes common to any managerial endeavour and help us to begin to pull together the various elements around which this book has been organized. This chapter provides a short description of the models and identifies relevant chapters in the book pertaining to parts of the models.

For example, if we examine a typical general hospital, we can identify two environmental components: one *external* and the other *internal*. The external environment can be further subdivided into two: (1) the general, and (2) the task environment (see Figure 22.1).

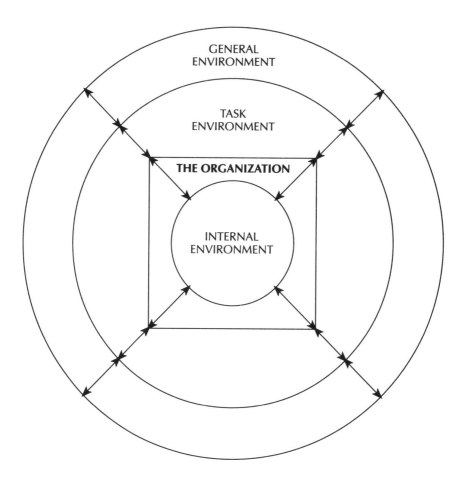

FIGURE 22.1 The Organization and its Environment.

THE EXTERNAL ENVIRONMENT

The General Environment

The *general* environment consists of all the nonspecific dimensions in the organization's surroundings that might affect its activities and which pose a threat or an opportunity to it. The dimensions in the general environment consist of the following (see Figure 22.2):

> *Political–legal dimension*—which refers to the type of political system and laws governing the behaviour of the organization. For example, much of the change in the NHS has been gener-

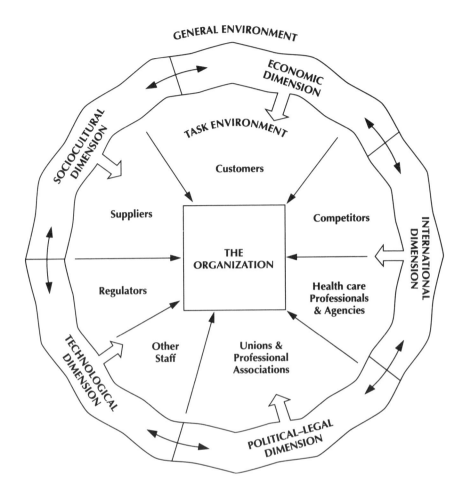

FIGURE 22.2 The General and Task Environments.

ated by the government in terms of the many White Paper reforms, related legislation, and parliamentary acts passed. This dimension has always been one of the main driving forces for change in the NHS.

Economic dimension—which refers to the government's monetary and fiscal policies regarding employment and economic cycles. These policies have a direct effect on the provision of health care. In times of economic scarcity, health care managers have to make adjustments to expenditure and the allocation of resources. At the same time they have to try to ensure equity of treatment for all patients.

Sociocultural dimension—which refers to the customs, mores, values and ideologies that characterize the society in which the organization operates. For example, changing expectations and increased standards of education mean that the general public now expect hospital waiting times to be reduced and to be kept better informed about any treatment they may receive. Consumers have also grown to expect value for money in health care and are more willing to challenge the conventional wisdom of their GP regarding their treatment.

Technological dimension—which refers to new scientific and technological developments which improve the service. In addition to medical technological breakthroughs, information technology is now indispensable to management and budgetary control.

International dimension—which refers to those areas of an organization's activities extending beyond the boundaries of a single country. For example, the World Health Organization (WHO) has established objectives and standards of health care that have to be met by all developed countries within a specified timeframe. These factors mean that managers have to adopt an increasingly global perspective to the delivery of health care.

The Task Environment

The task environment includes those external groups and forces with which the organization has direct contact and transactions (Duncan, 1972). These various groups are sometimes referred to as "stakeholders" and include (see Figure 22.2):

Competitors: other service organizations in the same marketplace that compete with the focal organization for customers and resources. Increasingly, competition will play a key role in the new market-driven economies in which hospitals operate.

Suppliers: other organizations that provide resources for the focal organization in the form of material and services. Peters (1989) argued that establishing what he calls "value-added" relationships with suppliers who share one's values can be advantageous. Doing so often means that in times of scarcity they will give the hospital preferential treatment.

Regulators: groups that have the potential to actively control, regulate and/or influence an organization's policies and practices. These include central government politicians who regulate, and provide funding to, the NHS.

Customers: people or organizations that receive products and services (usually in exchange for money). These may be direct customers, such as patients or clients, but may also include "gatekeeping" consumers in the form of GPs and community representatives serving patients. Other NHS customers include the purchasers of health care, represented by District Health Authorities (DHAs), GP fundholders, local authorities and social services.

Health care professionals and agencies: people or organizations with whom the organization has contractual obligations. These include various clinicians (usually supported by Royal Colleges), paramedical groups (e.g. speech therapists) and nurses.

Unions and professional associations: organized groups who negotiate with management and regulators over conditions of work, salaries, benefits, etc. These include the BMA, the RCN, the National Union of Public Employees (NUPE), and the Confederation of Health Service Employees (COHSE).

Other staff groups: generally non-medical personnel, especially support staff, including medical records, catering, receptionists, etc.

All of these elements in the task environment may be either a source of strength or weakness to a particular organization.

THE INTERNAL ENVIRONMENT

A third environment is the *internal* environment of the organization itself. A way of conceptualizing this internal organizational process is by means of a model adapted from the work of Nadler and Tushman (1977; see Figure 22.3). The model conceives of the organization as an open system which is influenced by the demands of the task environment. The internal organizational components, in their turn, attempt to respond to the demands of the environment. Thus, a continuous set of transactions is set in motion.

The primary components of the internal environment consist of the self, the tasks, the processes and skills, the formal organizational design, the organizational culture, the individual employees or people system, together with the leadership function and shared vision of the organization.

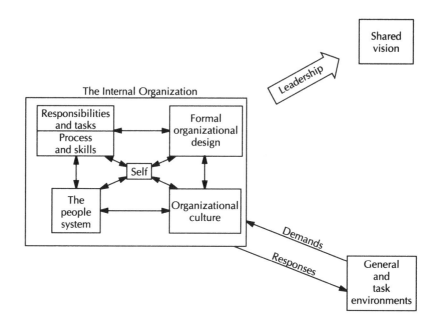

FIGURE 22.3 The Internal Organization, based on Nadler & Tushman's Model.

The *self* consists of the thoughts, feelings, values, motivations, behaviours, and experiences from the point of view of the individual manager working within the system (see Chapter 3).

The *task* responsibilities consist of the work that has to be done, its nature, and the quantity and quality of the service provided (see especially Chapters 6, 7 and 20).

The *processes* and *skills* refer to the actions necessary to perform the tasks, including communicating, interviewing, and managing change and power conflicts, time, stress, and performance evaluation, etc. (see Chapters 9–19).

The *formal structure* consists of the organizational hierarchy, the lines of authority and accountability, information and control systems, job descriptions, reward mechanisms, policies, and procedures. These characteristics have to operate in a way that supports the primary task and at the same time enables it to remain responsive to the external environment (see Chapter 23).

The *organizational culture* is rather more intangible and consists of the attitudes, values, rites and rituals, power bases, allegiances, tribalism, beliefs, norms, informal sanctions, and rewards operating in an organization (see Chapter 24). It also includes the shared vision or future description of the organization and provides a focus for the organization's energy, and serves to unify staff in pursuit of common goals.

The *people system* consists of the different personalities that constitute the organization together with their individual skills, knowledge, aptitudes, motivation, experience, and behaviours. Management's task is to match up the individuals and their needs to the organization's requirements so that tasks can be accomplished efficiently and effectively (see Chapter 4).

Two other parts of the model are the *leadership* and the shared *vision* the leader has for the organization. Leadership is the process of directing, motivating, and educating individuals to accomplish organizational goals (see Chapter 5).

SUMMARY

The models presented provide a means of analysing the three environments and a focus for discussing each characteristic as well as how they fit together. Thus, both the internal organizational elements and the external environments are in a constant dynamic state of equilibrium with each other. Changing one of the elements automatically affects all others. Corresponding adjustments, therefore, have to be made to accommodate and/or compensate for the change.

By analysing the forces in the general environment and determining the interactive effects these have on the task and internal environments, management can develop appropriate strategies and structures to meet these demands.

The model described is useful to the extent that it enables one to conceptualize and analyse the current situation and identify ways in which an organization might change in response to internal and external demands placed upon it.

REFERENCES

Duncan, R. (1972). Characteristics of organizational environments and perceived environmental uncertainty. *Administrative Science Quarterly, 17*, 314.

Hodgetts, R. M., & Altman, S. (1979). *Organizational behavior*. Philadelphia: W. B. Saunders Co.

Nadler, D., & Tushman, M. (1977). *Perspectives in behavior*. New York: McGraw-Hill.

Peters, T. (1989). Tomorrow's companies. *The Economist*, March.

CHAPTER 23

Formal Organization Design
by Philip I. Morgan, PhD

Donabedian (1980) has noted that an organization's structure "is probably the most important means of protecting and promoting the quality of care". In structuring an organization, management must select from among several design options those elements that appear to have the optimum chance of achieving the organization's purpose. In making this selection, management must steer a difficult course between the demands of the environment and the needs of employees. Doing this requires: (1) a clear understanding of the organization's goals, strategy, and people; and (2) a thorough understanding of the various design components available.

The purpose of this chapter is to examine some of the basic tools involved in structuring an organization. It begins with an historical overview of some of the classical approaches to organizational design (Taylor, 1911; Fayol, 1929; Weber, 1978). Secondly, it then reviews how contingency organizational theory has extended and modified these principles (Burns & Stalker, 1961; Lawrence & Lorsch, 1969). Thirdly, it examines some basic design tools, such as job descriptions, formalization, specialization, delegation, span of control, chain of command, centralization versus decentralization, and departmentalization. Finally, it examines some views of the future forms of organizational structure based on the work of Mintzberg (1980), Schol (1967) and futurist writer, Alvin Toffler (1970, 1981, 1985).

Historically speaking, organizational design theory has undergone many revisions and modifications to the earlier principles developed by classical management theorists at the turn of the century. Nevertheless, the classical period contributed much to our understanding of basic design principles as well as describing how people might be expected to behave in them. Most organizations still employ many of these same principles as a starting point from which to develop their own operations and structures. The chapter begins by reviewing some of these design principles as they pertain to the NHS.

CLASSICAL ORGANIZATION DESIGN

Classical theorists (Taylor, 1911; Fayol, 1929; Weber, 1978) were committed to a rational approach to organizational design. They attempted to formulate universal principles which would be appropriate to all circumstances. They maintained that, although no two formal structures are alike, it was possible to develop general principles and basic rules which would serve as guidelines for designing organizations. These components are now generally modified in actual practice to meet the specific requirements of particular organizations.

Among the principles espoused by classical design theorists the following are perhaps the most typical:

1. *Work specialization and division of labour*. The way to produce maximum efficiency is to have one person assigned to one task and one task only.

2. *Authority and responsibility should be equal.* A person must be given the authority as well as the responsibility to get the job done.

3. *Unity of command.* Each employee should have one supervisor and only one supervisor to whom he or she reports.

4. *Unity of management.* One manager should be assigned to one plan for all operations having the same objective.

5. *Optimum span of control.* There should be an optimum number of subordinates over which a supervisor can comfortably supervise.

Max Weber (1864–1920), a German sociologist, devised a highly formalized system based on rational principles which he called the bureaucratic ideal. For Weber, bureaucracy was the "ideal" system because it was rational, orderly, efficient, and the "one best way" of organizing. According to Weber, bureaucracies have the following six basic characteristics:

1. A distinct division of work with each position being filled by an expert.
2. A consistent set of abstract rules and procedures to ensure that tasks are performed uniformly.
3. An established hierarchy of positions, authority, or offices so that a chain of command exists from the top to the bottom of the organization.
4. Rules and procedures which are applied in an impersonal and objective manner so that favouritism is avoided.
5. Employment is based on technical qualifications and the incumbent is protected from arbitrary dismissal.
6. Job security in the form of fixed salaries, tenure, and retirement pensions.

Many would maintain that all of these characteristics perfectly describe today's NHS. The possible exception is item 6, since general managers have only limited tenure (usually three to five years). However, for a creative individual this is probably as long as he or she would be willing to serve in this role.

The main advantage to the ideal bureaucracy is that it is logically and systematically designed. The rules ensure uniformity of standards and impersonality in implementing these rules and standards. The adoption of these rules would, Weber believed, help to avoid nepotism and ensure more equitable treatment for all employees.

The main disadvantage to bureaucracies is that they often produce a degree of standardization that stifles initiative and discourages creativity and risk-taking. The tendency is to produce a kind of "organization man" mentality in which everyone conforms to some average requirements. Nevertheless, a certain degree of bureaucracy is necessary to any organization and many large-scale organizations have adopted many of Weber's bureaucratic principles in some modified form. A major problem facing the NHS today is how to maintain the delicate balance between excessive bureaucratic control to keep down costs and at the same time search for more innovative solutions to provide better health care with the fewer resources now available.

CONTINGENCY THEORY

While classical theory believed that there was "one best way" to structure an organization, more recent research has suggested that it is more reasonable to identify the conditions under which particular designs would be appropriate and to view the organization from a wholistic perspective. This approach is known as contingency theory.

Contingency organizational design operates on some basic "if-then" propositions. For instance:

1. If the organization operates in a highly volatile and competitive environment, then decentralization of authority is appropriate so that swift on-the-spot decisions can be made at a local level.

2. If subordinates are capable and desire more autonomy and responsibility, then the manager should delegate more.

3. If the organization's size increases, the manager should implement rules and policies so as to manage more effectively the larger number of personnel.

Contingency research on organizational structure has generally focused on how environment, size, technology, and strategy affect structure. We shall discuss some relevant research findings related to environment and structure before turning our attention to the "nuts and bolts" of organizing.

Environment and Structure

Burns and Stalker (1961) conducted a highly influential study of 20 UK firms with different markets and growth rates in an attempt to determine how technological change affects the management process, structure, and market environment. They identified two diametrically opposed environments: stable and unstable. Stable environments are relatively unchanging over time; unstable environments are subject to rapid growth and uncertainty. Burns and Stalker found that two quite different organizational designs were necessary for the very different environments; one they labelled mechanistic and the other organic. These structures could be thought of as being arranged along a continuum, as shown in Figure 23.1.

Mechanistically designed companies tended to operate in relatively certain environments where activities are structured in predictable ways with centralized authority, job specialization, and written rules and procedures. This type of structure most closely resembles the bureaucratic model described earlier. For example, the rayon manufacturing industries were found to operate in relatively stable, unchanging environments.

Organic designs are characterized by highly volatile, unstable and unpredictable environments requiring more flexibility, autonomy, and

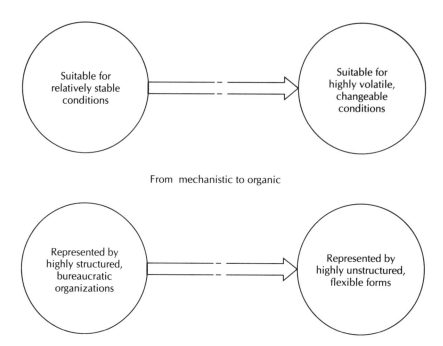

FIGURE 23.1 The Continuum of Organizational Designs: From Mechanistic to Organic.

decentralized authority. The electronics industry, is one such example, where firms have found it necessary to decentralize operations and to keep the organizational design fairly fluid so that managers can respond quickly to market changes.

Burns and Stalker (1961) determined that the requirements of the situation dictate the most appropriate or "ideal" organizational design. As a company's environment becomes more stable, a more mechanistic design should be adopted. Conversely, for a company which is moving into a more dynamic environment, a more organic design is required. They found that the latter is perhaps the most difficult to achieve since, for this to happen, a great deal of change is required throughout the system. Also, highly mechanistic companies may find the transition difficult to make because of their being bound by many rules and procedures.

Lawrence and Lorsch (1969), building on the work of Burns and Stalker, advanced another organizational contingency theory based on their research. They examined managers' behaviour in manufacturing, sales, and research and development in three different kinds of industries (plastics, packaged-goods, and standardized container industries), in terms of the particular organization's goal orientation, time orientation, interpersonal orientation, and structural formality. As a result they identified two basic concepts: *differentiation* and *integration.*

Differentiation refers to the degree to which an organization's activities are highly specialized; integration refers to the degree to which the various departments are integrated within the larger organization.

Their findings revealed that the most successful organizations were those that had hightly differentiated departments but at the same time had various *ad hoc* groups which worked towards integration of the whole system. Each department's structure was highly dependent upon its time pressure, goals, interpersonal needs, and degree of formality in achieving its tasks. For example, research and development department managers usually have much longer time horizons than production department managers whose main concern is normally the immediate one of increasing productivity.

Each sub-environment could vary along three dimensions:

1. Rate of change of conditions over time.
2. Certainty of information about conditions at any particular time.
3. Time span of feedback on results of employee decision.

Lawrence and Lorsch argued that these variables determine the degree of diversity (or uncertainty) in the environment that the organization faces and as a result the amount of differentiation required. Thus, they found that there was greater differentiation among the subsystems and a greater need for achieving integration among the various units.

They also found that the way in which conflicts were resolved was largely dependent upon the degree of successful integration of units. Decision making was much more decentralized and conflict was also resolved much lower down. Also, communication tended to be open and confrontational. There was much more willingness to argue, to work through a problem, rather than attempting to suppress conflict.

Burns and Stalker's, and Lawrence and Lorsch's research enables us to recognize that there is no specific "one best way" to organize a company or a department. Instead, the most effective structure for any organization or department is determined largely by its goals, its tasks, its technology, and its environment.

STRUCTURAL TOOLS

Having examined some of the basic classical systems and contingency theories related to organizational structure, we now turn our attention to the basic structural tools themselves. These consist of: job descriptions, degree of formalization, work specialization, delegation, span of control, chain of command, centralization vs decentralization, and departmentalization.

Job Description

The job description spells out the duties and responsibilities for a given job incumbent and is the basic unit of an organization's structure. An effective job description should define each employee's areas of responsibility, accountability, and authority. Part of the problem in writing job descriptions for NHS members is, of course, that the health service is so diverse and largely uncoordinated. As a result, most job descriptions are ill-defined. An example of an ill-defined job description is the GP's contract which is usually couched in vague generalities. This is largely due to the fact that GPs and consultants tend to band together to protect their clinical freedom from what they see as government interference. The White Paper published in 1989 (DoH, 1989) recommends that fuller job descriptions be provided to NHS employees. Fortunately, this seems to have been accepted by most health authorities and the trend seems likely to continue.

Formalization

In developing a job description, attention must be given to the degree of formalization required by the organization. Formalization refers to the extent to which jobs are standardized and "controlled". Some jobs need to be more formalized than others and those that are tend to be associated with bureaucratic structures. More formalized jobs may be governed by rules and standard operating procedures (SOPs). For example, in cases where accidents or emergencies are likely to occur, certain rules or procedures may be formulated which then become part of an individual's job description. Obviously, the more formalized the jobs, the less discretion permitted to employees. However, by following certain rules and procedures there is less likelihood of an accident occurring or the wrong procedure being followed. Formalization is, therefore, a method of reducing uncertainty in the performance of one's job.

Work Specialization

Work specialization refers to the degree to which jobs and tasks are divided up. Adam Smith, the eighteenth century economist, is credited with being the first to argue that specialization would increase productivity by suggesting that if one man did one task and one task only, he could improve his productivity several-fold. For example, in the production of steel pins, Smith maintained that if one man did one job and only one job, 10 men could produce 48,000 pins per day, whereas each man performing all of the necessary tasks by himself would only produce 20 pins per man per day.

While specialization expedites production, it generally does so at the expense of employee job satisfaction. The major problem is that much of the craft element is taken out of the work, together with much of the sense of accomplishment and achievement. Also, if the job is too specialized, employees often become bored and complain that the job lacks challenge. The resultant monotony and boredom may cause the quality of the work to deteriorate, and absenteeism and turnover to increase. A manager must bear these points in mind when deciding how best to divide tasks up into individual jobs.

Delegation

Delegation is the process of assigning tasks to subordinates together with the establishment of authority patterns between supervisor and staff. For example, a ward sister or other subordinate may be given authority to request certain information, access classified files or requisition supplies, etc. In assigning responsibility an employee must also be granted the necessary authority to get the job done. At the same time, the employee must also be made accountable to his or her manager for accomplishing the work.

Delegation enables managers to get more work done in an effective and efficient manner. Managers who consistently fail to delegate and insist on doing everything themselves are generally ineffective. Firstly, this is generally not the best use of their time and, secondly, by failing to delegate they deny others the opportunity to develop work experience so that they may become more useful and promotable within the organization.

Span of Control

Span of control or span of management refers to the number of subordinates who are supervised by and report to a specific manager. Determining the appropriate span for a particular set of circumstances has preoccupied managers and researchers for years. For example, Graicunas (1947) was one of the first to try to quantify span of control problems. He identified three types of interaction with and between subordinates:

1. *Direct*—the manager's one-on-one contact with each individual subordinate.

2. *Cross*—the relationship among the subordinates themselves.

3. *Group*—the relationships between groups or subordinates.

Based on these definitions, Graicunas devised the formula:

$$I = N \left(\frac{2^N}{2} + N - 1 \right)$$

Here I is the total number of interactions with and among subordinates and N is the number of subordinates. Thus, if a manager has 2 subordinates, 6 potential interactions exist. If the number of subordinates increases to 3, the possible interaction total is 18; with 5 subordinates, there are 180 possible interactions. Graicunas's formula demonstrates that adding additional subordinates produces more overall complexity to the group than the previous one did. However, the formula still does not specify what N should be.

Steiglitz (1966) also identified criteria that may help to determine the appropriate span of control, such as degree of competence, the physical dispersion of staff, the amount of work that must be supervised, required degree of interaction, degree of standardization of the procedures, similarity of task, frequency of new problems, and individual preferences. All of these factors need to be considered in determining an appropriate span of control.

Chain of Command

"Chain of command" is a military term used to refer to the line of executive authority running, in a hierarchical organization, from the apex of the pyramid to the lowest "shop-floor" operative. It is this line down which orders, instructions and requests for information are supposed to travel.

Classical theorists recommended that this line should be as short and direct as possible with, ideally, each person in the organizational hierarchy having one "boss" to whom he or she reports. Line managers have the right to command subordinates because of the authority vested in the position they occupy in the chain of command. Not all organizational members are part of line management, of course. For example, those members who are hired to provide specialist services in an advisory capacity to top management are referred to as "staff" (e.g. accountants, legal advisors, computer experts, etc.). The main difference between line and staff members is that line people "tell" subordinates what to do, whereas staff people "sell" or advise others what to do.

The span of control and the size of an organization determine whether an organization will have a tall or flat structure. Researchers have long debated whether tall or flat structures are more appropriate, and under what circumstances. Classical theorists maintained that narrow spans were preferable to wide (i.e., 3–6 or 5–7 people). However, narrow spans tend to produce very tall organizational structures. For example, in an organization of 63 with a span of control of 2 it would take 6 hierarchical levels, whereas a span of 8 needs only 3 levels for 73 people. Another problem with tall structures is that the more levels there are, the more need there is to provide differential pay rates for each level.

Porter and Lawler (1965) claimed to have found a correlation between organizational size and job satisfaction. They found that in firms with less than 5000 employees, flat structures tended to provide more employee job satisfaction, whereas in larger companies (those with over 5000 employees) tall structures tended to produce greater employee job satisfaction. The researchers also found that top-level managers felt greater job satisfaction in taller structures and lower-level managers tended to be more satisfied in flatter structures. To date, however, there is no clear evidence to demonstrate conclusively that flat is always superior to tall, or vice versa.

Centralization vs Decentralization

Centralization vs decentralization refers to the degree to which decision making is concentrated or devolved in the organization. Under decentralization, decision making may be dispersed down to the lowest department or unit; centralization refers to decision making which is concentrated at a single point at the top in the organizational structure. There are advantages and disadvantages to both centralization and decentralization, as outlined in Table 23.1.

Because of their sheer size and complexity there is a great deal of variety in the way in which various health service organizations are structured. Some are highly decentralized. GPs, for example, usually enjoy a great deal of autonomy and flexibility in the way in which they organize their practices. Others are very highly centralized. For example, since the 1980s various Departments of Health and Regions in Scotland and Wales have generally required more detailed information and accountability from individual authorities. These trends seem likely to continue.

There is also an increasing trend towards decentralization among hospital authorities who are currently being allowed to become "self-governing trusts" (DoH, 1989). On the other hand, the top of the NHS through the creation of the Policy Board chaired by the Secretary of State is still highly centralized. This body defines strategy, objectives, and finances in terms of government policy. This, in essence, creates a clear chain of command extending from districts to regions to the Chief Executive and finally to the Secretary of State. Also, The Griffiths Report

TABLE 23.1 Benefits and Drawbacks of Centralization vs Decentralization

	Centralization	*Decentralization*
Benefits	Assures uniformity of standards and policies among the organization units. Permits the use of outstanding talent in managers by the whole organization rather than a single unit. Ensures uniform decisions. Helps eliminate duplication of effort and activity.	Reduces the total responsibility to more manageable units. Encourages more involvement of the personnel in the decision-making process. Shortens lines of communication. Brings decision making closer to those affected by the decision. Disperses power and authority among many people
Drawbacks	Makes great demands on a few managers instead of spreading responsibility. Forces top managers to possess a broad view, which may be beyond their ability. Gives vast amounts of authority and power to a few people. Reduces a sense of participation for all but a few.	Allows a lack of uniformity of standards and policies among organizational units. Necessitates making of decisions without capable managers, who may be unavailable or unwilling to participate. Can create coordination problems among the various organizational units. Can lead to interunit rivalry, which can interfere with the organization's overall effectiveness. Requires training programs, which can be time-consuming and costly.

Source: Adapted from F. J. Carvell (1975). *Human relations in business* (2nd ed.). New York: Macmillan Publishing Co. Inc., p. 356.

(DHSS, 1983) expressed concern at the delays caused by "consensus management" and recommended that a more centralized management structure should be vested in "one person at each level who would take personal responsibility for securing action" (DHSS, 1984).

In determining the degree of centralization vs decentralization required in an organization, consideration should always be given to which system is more likely to achieve organizational goals more effectively and efficiently. For example, if a hospital needs to respond quickly to a customer need or emergency situation, where immediate action needs to be taken and where delay would jeopardize lives, decentralization would be appropriate. However, if standardization and uniformity of treatment is the goal, then centralization would be more appropriate.

Departmentalization

Departmentalization refers to the process of grouping jobs horizontally into more manageable units. Departmentalization by function is one of the most common forms. (Other common forms are by geographical area, by product, by equipment, by time, and by sequence.) We shall discuss one of the more common forms here, departmentalization by function, together with another common alternative—matrix designs.

Functional Design

Departmentalization by function refers to the practice of dividing up key activities according to specific functional specialities, e.g. pathology, radiography, personnel, etc. For example, Figure 23.2 shows a "typical" Regional Health Authority organized along functional lines. Operations are divided into departments based on their functional speciality, each of whom all report to a functional director.

This traditional way of organizing has several advantages. First, this type of design makes for greater operating efficiency. It also means that the people within each functional area can become specialized and proficient within their own departments. And since a manager need concentrate only on his or her specialist function, training within the department is also simplified. Another advantage to this type of design is that there is usually a high degree of formal control since command and authority pass from the top down through the various functional areas.

The main disadvantages of functional designs are that people may become too specialized within their departments and develop "tunnel vision" making coordination difficult. It also encourages "empire building", in-fighting, and "turf protection" within the functional unit and can lead to an "us versus them" mentality so that organizational conflict between departments becomes inevitable.

It is in this lack of cooperation between the various functional divisions that this type of structure shows its main weaknesses. For example, people tend to get "locked into" a way of thinking which promotes "win–lose" situations. Thus, when budgets are being determined for each department, each director may try to secure the largest share for his or her department to the detriment of the whole organization.

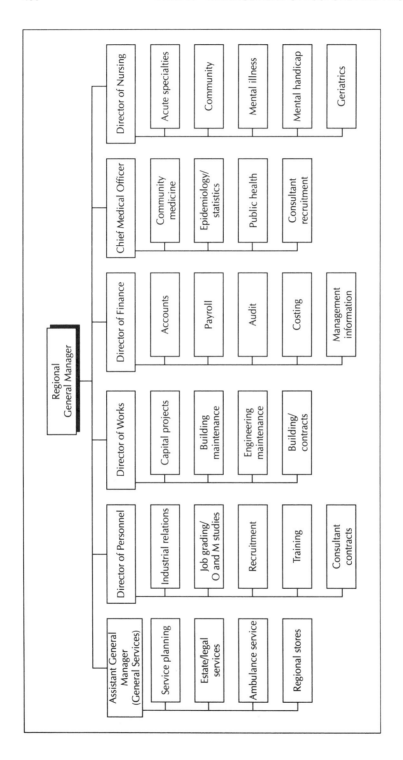

FIGURE 23.2 The Organizational structure of a Regional Health Authority.
Source: *Open University, Managing Health Services, 1991.*

Matrix Design

Matrix designs are sometimes proposed as an alternative and as a way of avoiding the problems just cited. Matrix designs can be extremely effective, especially where project work is the norm and people are required to work together in interdisciplinary teams. The key characteristics of matrix designs are: (1) that two or more chains of command or lines of authority or functional lines of authority are overlaid; (2) authority over employees in each unit of the matrix is shared between the functional manager and the project manager; and (3) employees are responsible to both managers on a continuous basis.

Figure 23.3 is an example of a matrix organizational structure for a Regional Health Authority, Department of Works. In this situation the department runs a variety of projects all requiring different skills at different times. In this case, groups can be formed and disbanded as needed. This has the effect of breaking down the barriers typical of most functional organizational structures and creating an *esprit de corps* among all organizational members.

The main advantages to using a matrix organization design include:

Increased cooperation. Traditional lines authority and responsibility are broken up since employees work as teams within their functional units. They can also serve as links between their unit and the task team. "Empire building" within functional areas is also greatly reduced. Conflict resolution may be generally easier to attain since units tend to be working toward common goals rather than competing with each other.

Increased flexibility. Teams can be created and disbanded according to the needs and demands of the environment. Interaction between project and functional areas generally ensures that groups remain responsive to the changing needs of the environment.

More efficient use of human resources. Matrix designs enable organizations to take full advantage of their highly specialized staff. Since this expertise is shared by several teams, much wastage and duplication of effort is eliminated and synergy can also be more easily attained.

Increased personal development. Team members are given opportunities to develop their skills and knowledge. Since they have to interact with various functional areas, they may begin to appreciate others' viewpoints. Moreover, having their own views challenged by others from different disciplines or functional areas stimulates thinking and causes them to take less for

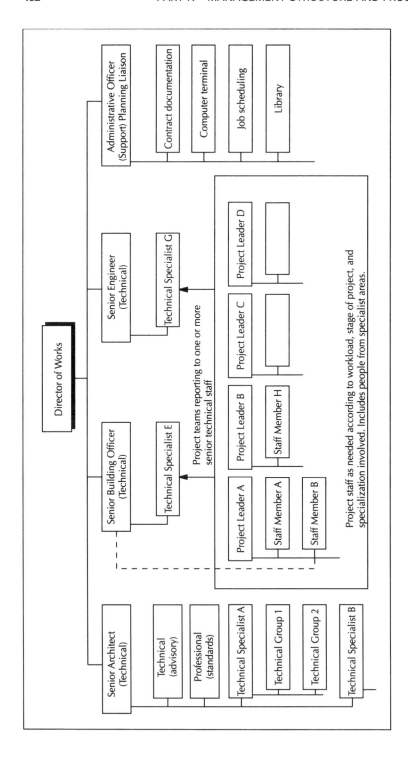

FIGURE 23.3 A matrix structure for a Regional Health Authority Works Department.

Souce: Open University, 1991. *Managing Health Services.*

granted. In the process, they generally gain a more complete picture of the whole organization and its purpose.

The main disadvantages are that:

Power and authority are confused. Because employees have to report to more than one supervisor, they may be unclear as to priorities. If employees are reporting to two or more project managers as well as to a functional manager, there may be conflicting demands placed upon them. Alternatively, some employees may be encouraged to "goof off" in the hopes that in the confusion their lack of input won't be missed.

It is time consuming and costly. Matrix designs are more time consuming because of the added time needed to coordinate activities. Matrix designs also generally necessitate hiring more staff and more managers, thus increasing the operating costs (Griffin, 1984).

Some of these disadvantages can be minimized by clearly specifying areas of responsibility and authority for both superiors and subordinates. Matrix designs do offer a viable alternative to more traditional functional forms. For this reason, they have been adapted by many public and private sector organizations.

FUTURE ORGANIZATIONAL STRUCTURES: "NETWORKS"

As health care organizations increase in size and complexity, and as environments become more uncertain, what will future organizational structures be like? Many writers (Bennis, 1969; Perrow, 1972) have suggested that bureaucracies will tend to die out to be replaced by more flexible organic structures. Katz and Kahn (1978) and other management theorists have also promoted the idea that future structures will have to be extremely adaptable and open to the environment. Where they are decentralized, future structures also need to be more transitory and ad hoc and will need to be flexible at all levels—operational, strategic, and administrative (Mintzberg, 1980).

It has also been predicted that future technology-based companies will consist of central units comprising the financial and technological capital of the company, surrounded by a group of relatively independent constellations of small technology-based satellites (Schol, 1967). These new "network" structures described by Schol, Galbraith (1977) and others appear to offer this necessary flexibility. Under this system, many firms are becoming "shell or core corporations" sitting in the middle of a constellation of supplier and service relations who contract out to other agents such functions as manufacturing, distribution, marketing, or sometimes even financial activities. Benetton is a fairly typical example of this new type of company. Benetton exists as a small central organization which is mainly concerned with financial investments and protection of proprietary technologies on cloth and wool dyeing. Everything else is done on a network system. Each Benetton shop is franchised and most of the manufacturing and production work is contracted out. High technology is a key feature in Benetton's success. For instance, managers rely on computers to design clothes and monitor preferences. Benetton could well serve as a model of what many future organizations may become.

The logical extension of the current purchaser–provider split in the health service would appear to presage this looser network type of organizational structure. These so-called "network" organizational structures have several advantages: they need much less capital investment, have lower overhead expenses, are more suited to entrepreneurial activities, and are more flexible and fast moving by being better able to adapt to a changing environment. Moreover, they can easily use low-cost labour and can better tap into outside expertise and knowledge.

The disadvantages to such structures are that they are vulnerable to competition from suppliers, and companies have less control over services and, as a result, they offer employees much less job security.

Toffler (1985) and Mintzberg (1980) described similar "network organization" structures, which can be characterized in Mintzberg's term as "adhocracies". An adhocracy is characterized by a flexible, adaptive, and fluid type of design of the organic type which avoids specialization, formality, and unity of command. In his book, *The third wave*, Toffler (1981) suggested that industrialization has come full circle and that we have entered a new "information age" where organizations are much less dependent on the infrastructure and much more able to capitalize on more fluid structures. Toffler identified three significant "waves" or periods of industrial development, commencing with the pre-industrial revolution in Britain. The first wave, he asserted, was characterized by "cottage industries" where people worked from their homes; the second wave occurred during the industrial revolution where everyone worked under the factory system; the third wave, according to Toffler, is characterized by a new kind of cottage industry where people may once again work from their own homes, linked by computer terminal to a central mainframe computer. This is generally referred to as "homeworking" or the "electronic cottage". Increasingly, information technology is revolutionizing the way people work, enabling them to become much less dependent on the infrastructure.

How do these changes affect the health service? To begin with, contrary to Bennis's predictions about the demise of bureaucracies, to some extent certain areas of the NHS are becoming more, rather than less, bureaucratized with the increasing emphasis placed on centralized authority and maintenance of the chain of command. Yet in another sense it would appear that "network" organizational structures are becoming popular also. This is especially true with a provider role moving to a purchaser role in the NHS. Also, as "privatization" continues, "management by contract" rather than "management by command" will reinforce the *ad hoc* nature of the health service. It also seems clear that "homeworking" is a definite possibility for some sections of the workforce in the NHS, for example, among clerical and support workers. There is considerable evidence that this trend has already occurred in the private sector. For example, Norwich Union now has a large proportion of its workforce employed at home, linked to a central computer system. The savings to the company in terms of overhead costs have been substantial. It now seems possible for hospital medical records departments to operate successfully in this way. However, employee legislation needs to catch up with this new development since, under this new system, employees may not be legally covered for accidents and other exigencies in the same way that they would if they were working in an office.

SUMMARY

It is probably obvious from the foregoing discussion that our understanding of the factors affecting organizational design is far from complete. While classical theorists contributed much to our understanding of what principles make for an effectively run organization, we are now able to take an altogether more eclectic approach when designing organizations and borrow from a wide variety of alternative structures which have developed since. What is clear is that there is no panacea or "best way" of structuring all organizations. Each design has its advantages and limitations.

The current view is that one should take a contingency or systems approach to organizational design based upon considerations of both internal and external organizational constraints and demands. It all depends on what one wants to accomplish. Perhaps Peter Drucker (1974) best summed the situation up when he said:

> *The simplest organization structure that will do the job is the best one. What makes an organization structure "good" are the problems it does not create. The simpler the structure, the less that can go wrong. Some design principles are more difficult and problematic than others. But none is without difficul-*

ties and problems. None is primarily people-focused rather than task-focused; none is more "creative", "free", or "more democratic". Design principles are tools; and tools are neither good nor bad in themselves. They can be used properly or improperly, and that is all. To obtain the greatest possible simplicity and the greatest "fit", organization design has to start out with a clear focus on key activities needed to produce key results. They have to be structured and positioned in the simplest possible design. Above all, the architect of the organization needs to keep in mind the purpose of the structure he is designing.

REFERENCES

Bennis, W. G. (1969). *Organization development: its nature, origins and prospects.* Reading, MA.: Addison-Wesley.

Burns, T., & Stalker, G. M. (1961). *The management of innovation.* London: Tavistock.

Carvell, F. J. (1975). *Human relations in business* (2nd ed.). New York: Macmillan.

Department of Health and Social Security (1989). *Caring for people.* London: DoH.

Department of Health and Social Security (1984). *Health service management: implementation of the NHS management inquiry report.* London: DHSS.

Department of Health and Social Security (1989). *Working for patients: the health service; caring for the 1990s.* London: DoH (Cm 555).

Donabedian, A. (1980). *The definition of quality and approaches to its assessment,* Vol. 1. Ann Arbor, MI: Health Administration Press.

Drucker, P. (1974). *Management: tasks, responsibilities and practices.* New York: Harper & Row.

Fayol, H. (1929). *Industrial and general administration,* translated by J. A. Coubrough. Geneva: International Management Institute, 19–33.

Galbraith, J. R. (1977). *Organizational design.* Reading, MA: Addison-Wesley.

Graicunas, A. V. (1947). Relationships in organizations. In L. Gulick and L. Urwick (eds.). *Papers on the science of administration.* New York: Columbia University Press, 183–187.

Griffin, R. W. (1984). *Management.* New York: Houghton Mifflin.

Katz, D., & Kahn, R. L. (1966). *The social psychology of organizations.* New York: Wiley.

Katz, D., & Kahn, R. L. (1978). *The social psychology of organizations* (2nd ed.). New York: Wiley.

Lawrence, P. R., & Lorsch, J. W. (1969). Differentiation and integration in complex organizations. *Administrative Science Quarterly, 12* (June), 1–47.

Mintzberg, H. (1980). Structure in 5s: a synthesis of the research on organization design. *Management Science, 226,* 322 ff.

NHS Management Inquiry (1983). *Letter to the Secretary of State and recommendations for action* (The Griffiths Report). London: DHSS.

Perrow, C. (1972). *Complex organizations: a critical essay.* Glenville, IL: Scott, Foresman.

Schol, D. (1967). *Technological change: the new hierarchy.* London: Penguin.

Smith, A. *An inquiry into the nature and causes of the wealth of nations.* (1776; reprinted edition, New York: Modern Library, 1937).

Steiglitz, H. (1966). On concepts of corporate structure. *The Conference Board Record* (Feb.).

Taylor, F. W. (1911). *Principles of scientific management.* New York: Harper.

Toffler, A. (1970). *Future shock.* New York: Random House.

Toffler, A. (1985). *The adaptive corporation.* Aldershot: Gower.
Toffler, A. (1981). *The third wave.* London: Pan.
Weber, M. (1978). *The Protestant ethic and the spirit of capitalism.* New York: Basic
    Books (first edition, London: Allen & Unwin, 1930).

Organizational Culture
by Philip I. Morgan, PhD

The importance of culture in determining an organization's effectiveness has received widespread attention in recent years. While not an entirely new concept—it has been discussed in the literature for over 100 years—it has been given a new impetus by the "excellence writers" exemplified by the work of Ouchi (1981), Peters and Waterman (1982), Deal and Kennedy (1982), and Pascale and Athos (1982). The common theme among these popular, best-selling authors is the emphasis they place on the part played by shared values and beliefs in shaping successful organizations.

Peters and Waterman (1982), for example, maintain that managerial excellence does not consist of the more traditional quantitative approaches of financial planning and computerized control methods, but rather arises from the more qualitative aspects of an organization's culture. This includes staying close to the customer, of having a set of shared values and beliefs, and by sanctioning open communications at all levels.

This chapter examines the concept of culture as a means of understanding and promoting more effective behaviour in organizations. Also examined are ways of classifying organizational cultures according to the dominant patterns they exhibit, together with ways of changing these patterns in order to improve organizational effectiveness. The chapter concludes with an examination of some of the culture trends now emerging in health care organizations.

DEFINITION OF "CULTURE"

Definitions of "culture" vary considerably. Kroeber and Kluckhohn (1952) in a comprehensive review of the literature identified 164 different definitions of the term. Part of the problem is that, within the discipline of social anthropology, culture has been interpreted in two main ways by two different groups of researchers. One group views culture in a very broad sense as part of the general social structure (Levi-Strauss, 1958; Geertz, 1973; etc.). In this sense, culture is seen as enmeshed in and inseparable from the social class and ethnic group, including social behaviour and organizational transactions in which it operates (Malinowski, 1944; Radcliffe-Brown, 1952). (This view of culture is discussed later in the chapter, with reference to the work of Ouchi, 1981.)

A second view conceives of culture as, to some extent, independent of the social context. Here culture is seen as consisting of stories, slogans, legends; icons, organizational logos, or national flags (Lynn Meek, 1988). In this latter definition, values are seen as the cornerstone of the organization's culture that underpins the shared belief systems about what constitutes appropriate behaviour for members in an organization. These symbols convey meanings which can positively motivate people to act in an organization to improve productivity. It is this latter view of culture that is adopted by the so-called "excellence" writers and researchers in the organizational culture field. For example, Deal and Kennedy (1982) viewed culture as:

> a stable collection of values, symbols, heroes, rituals and stories that operate beneath the surface exerting a powerful influence on behaviour in the work place.

Peters and Waterman (1982) also viewed organizational culture as a system of shared values, norms, and routines that manifests itself through "the rich tapestry of anecdote, mythical fairy-tale, all of which serve to communicate and reinforce shared values and beliefs within an organization".

Additionally, both Peters and Waterman (1982), and Deal and Kennedy (1982) perceived culture as a hidden system that influences individual behaviour largely at a subconscious level. Schein (1983) noted the subconscious element in culture and emphasized the underlying assumptions behind the values (Figure 24.1). He defined culture as:

a . . . pattern of basic assumptions which a given group has invented, discerned or developed in learning to cope with its problem of external adaptation and internal integration, which have worked well enough to be considered valid, and therefore . . . (are) . . . taught to new members on the correct way to perceive, think and feel in relation to those problems.

(These assumptions) . . . lie behind the values . . . and . . . determine the behaviour patterns and visible artifacts such as architecture, office layout, dress codes and so on.

FIGURE 24.1 Level of Culture and their Interaction.
Source: Schein, E.H. (1985). *Organization Culture and Leadership*. San Francisco: Josey-Bass, p. 14.

Whatever the minor variations in definition, most writers agree that organizational culture refers to the pattern of shared values (about what is important) together with the beliefs and expectations (about how things function or operate), and that these values, beliefs, and expectations in turn create behavioural norms ("the way we do things around here").

The general consensus among the popular writers is that "strong cultures" (i.e. those organizations with well-developed belief systems and common shared values) tend also to be the best run and most productive organizations (Deal & Kennedy, 1982; Ouchi, 1981; Pascale & Athos, 1981; Peters & Waterman, 1982; Peters & Austin, 1985).

Peters and Waterman (1982) insisted that it is the dominance and cohesiveness of the culture that is an essential feature of the excellent companies they studied. These excellent companies tend to be organized around a core set of values. For example, they cited Hewlett-Packard and IBM's dominant values of customer service which, they state, serve as a means of ensuring that everyone from top management down to the employee on the shop floor is committed to working as a team, and toward a common goal.

FUNCTIONS OF ORGANIZATIONAL CULTURE

Martin and Siehl (1983) identified *four* major functions served by an organization's culture:

1. *A knowledge function.* The myths, legends, and stories that form an organization's general knowledge pool facilitates employees' understanding of an organization's history and general approach, all of which serve as a guide to how one is expected to behave in the organization.

2. *A means of establishing commitment to the corporate philosophy and values.* All organizations have cultures; however, some cultures are more effective than others in promoting excellence. What makes a culture effective according to Peters and Waterman is where it tends to create a climate in which employees feel a sense of involvement and a sense of participation in their work. To do this it is necessary to establish common purposes and goals, to open channels of communication, and to encourage participative decision making and problem solving at the lowest levels. It may also involve centring employee behaviour around certain dominant values.

3. *A control mechanism by which employee behaviour is channelled away from undesirable patterns to desirable patterns.* Where the values, beliefs, and assumptions are widely held there is little need for management to exercise more traditional methods of control over members' behaviour. In this situation, the organizational values have become internalized by the individual members. In this case, employee behaviour can be channelled away from undesirable behaviour to more desirable behaviour patterns by means of the organizational culture.

4. *A means of increasing organizational effectiveness under certain conditions.* For example, Denison (1984) examined 34 companies and found evidence of a high correlation between an organization's culture and its performance. He found that

companies with "participative cultures" and well-organized workplaces generally performed significantly better than companies that did not have these qualities.

FACTORS INFLUENCING THE DEVELOPMENT OF CULTURES

Although many of the excellent companies identified by Peters and Waterman exhibited certain common characteristics, in some cases their cultures are quite different. This has led researchers to look further afield for answers and to ask themselves: Just what are the cultural factors and conditions that give rise to effective organizations? While there is general agreement among researchers that an organization's culture is, among other things, a function of several interrelated factors, including its history, its management processes, its leadership, and so on, some have argued that effective cultures have more to do with the wider spheres of influence in which organizations function such as the social context (Pascal & Athos, 1982) or the racial or national identity of the participants (Hofstede, 1980). The social context theory seems to have gained most acceptance among researchers in the field. Some of the evidence that supports it will now be examined.

The Social Context

As previously noted, some anthropologists have argued that an organizational culture is inseparable from the wider society and that this plays a major role in influencing the organizational culture. For example, the phenomenal success of Japanese companies can largely be attributed to the wider influence of the Japanese society itself. The major differences between Japanese and Western societies and companies have been well documented and these differences cannot be discounted in attempting to explain their success. The main differences between Japanese and US companies have been described by Ouchi (1981), were introduced in Chapter 5 of this work and are summarized in Figure 24.1.

Ouchi argued that Western companies need to take a new direction in order to compete with Japanese companies and so improve their productivity. Ouchi suggested that future organizations should take an eclectic approach and draw on the "best" features of both successful Japanese and US companies and combine them to fit Western culture. He called this hybrid concept Theory Z and proposed that it should comprise:

■ Long-term employment
■ Consensual decision making

- Individual responsibility
- Slow evaluation and promotion
- Implicit information control with explicit formalized measures of performance
- Moderately specialized career paths

Theory Z organizations, Ouchi argued, will combine the more individual-istic approach of Western organizations with the group-oriented cooperative approach to decision making advocated by the Japanese (see Figure 24.2).

**ORGANIZATION TYPE A
(AMERICAN)**

1. Short-term employment
2. Individual decision making
3. Individual responsibility
4. Rapid evaluation and promotion
5. Explicit control mechanisms
6. Specialized career path
7. Segmented concern for employee as an employee

**ORGANIZATION TYPE J
(JAPANESE)**

1. Lifetime employment
2. Collective decision making
3. Collective responsibility
4. Slow evaluation and pro-motion
5. Implicit control mechanism
6. Nonspecialized career path
7. Holistic concern for employee as a person

1. Long-term employment
2. Collective decision making
3. Individual responsibility
4. Slow evaluation and promotion
5. Implicit, informal control with explicit, formalized measures
6. Moderately specialized career paths
7. Holistic concern, including family

**ORGANIZATION TYPE Z
(MODIFIED AMERICAN)**

FIGURE 24.2 Comparison between American, Japanese and Theory Z Organizations.

Source: Ouchi, W.G. (1981). *Theory Z: how American business can meet the Japanese challenge.* Reading, MA: Addison-Wesley.

Criticism

It should be noted that many of the excellence writers have been severely criticized. For example, Sullivan (1983) criticized Ouchi's Theory Z for his lack of real data supporting the idea that Type Z organizations are more productive than traditional organizations. This was later refuted by an experiment conducted by Mead Corporation's CEO who successfully implemented a Theory Z culture within the corporation. Also, Peters and Waterman's work has been criticized on methodological grounds. Carroll (1983) argued that the researchers did not consider the part played by proprietary technology, market dominance, control of critical raw materials, and national policies in contributing to the companies' effectiveness. Other critics have indicated that Peters and Waterman failed to examine the extent to which the excellence characteristics were prevalent in ineffective organizations. Yet despite these criticisms, there is growing support for the notion that an organization's culture plays a considerable role in determining its effectiveness.

CULTURAL TYPES

Harrison (1972) was among the first to develop a basic taxonomy for classifying various cultures according to a predominant set of characteristics. Harrison used the term "organizational ideologies". However, Handy (1985b), who popularized Harrison's ideas, preferred to use the word "cultures" and this term seems to have stuck. According to these writers there are essentially four kinds of cultures: *power, role, task,* and *person.*

The *power culture,* according to Harrison and Handy, depends on a single source of power and on developing trust and empathy for its effectiveness. In this culture, control of the organization's resources is maintained by people who exert real power in the organization. Power resides in the person and rests on her or his ability and willingness to administer rewards and punishments. Handy uses the diagram of a web to symbolize this type of culture whereby the rays of the web emanate from the centre and are connected by functional power rings. Handy noted that the power culture flourishes in small entrepreneurial organizations, among people who are "power-orientated, politically-minded, risk-taking and rate security as a minor element in their psychological contract". Handy noted that this structure tends to become less viable as the organization grows. At best the type of leadership exhibited in this type of culture is based on strength, justice, and paternalistic benevolence. At worst, it tends towards a rule by fear with abuse of power for personal advantage.

A *role culture* was described by Handy as a bureaucracy and is symbolized by a Greek temple. Power is exercised through the pillars of the organization representing the clear lines of authority and chain of command with each employee having a clearly defined role. This type of culture balances the leader's power with a system of bureaucratic structures and procedures. At best, the organization provides security and stability. When operating in a relatively unchanging environment it can be very efficient since much of the routine work can be made subject to impersonal rules and systems of checks and balances. At worst, this type of culture can become hidebound by rules and procedures which may strangle any initiative on the part of its employees. The role organization is best suited to stable environments, such as monopolies, with stable markets, or where the product has a long shelf-life. Employees who have a strong need for security and predictability and who have a low tolerance for ambiguity tend to be best suited to specialist or bureaucratic situations found in most role organizations.

Task cultures are generally goal oriented; the whole focus is on accomplishing the task. Handy represented the task structure as a net, some of the strands of which are thicker and stronger than others. Matrix organizations are typical of task cultures; much of the power and influence is located at the intersections of strands. Tasks are usually accomplished by teams while power is utilized through group consensus. Teams or task forces are quickly formed for specific purposes and disbanded just as quickly. Extreme flexibility of this culture means that it is adaptable and able to respond to the changing nature of the environment.

Task cultures are best suited to competitive markets where speed and reaction time are essential. Employees who enjoy a great deal of autonomy, who can tolerate ambiguity, and are self-motivated find this type of environment most compatible. Power is decentralized and top managers exercise little control. However, where resources are limited or where the organization gets too big to be organized into task groups, the whole culture becomes either a role or power culture.

A *person culture* exists primarily to serve certain individuals within the organization. Handy represented this type of culture as a constellation of stars. Examples of this type are barristers, professors, architectural partnerships and consultancy firms. Since organizations tend to have objectives over and above the goals and objectives of individuals, organizations of this type are rare. Nevertheless, some employees still adhere to the values of a people culture and in organizations of this type power is based on the expertise of the individuals. Handy noted that little control can be exercised by top management in this type of organization.

Naturally, few organizations fit neatly into any one single culture. Most organizations exhibit characteristics of various kinds and demonstrate attributes of more than one type. For example, a surgical unit may be classified as having a person culture while the nursing division may have a role culture even though both divisions belong to the same hospital. Nevertheless, Handy's culture typology is a useful way of classifying organizations according to dominant patterns of behaviour and expectations of participants.

CHANGING THE NHS CULTURE—FROM ROLE TO TASK

It can be argued that the recent proposed changes to the NHS have been attempts to change the organization's culture in the broadest sense, from a role to a task culture. Despite these attempts, the health service is still very much a role culture; it still operates very much as a bureaucracy and it is not quick to change and adapt to a new environment.

One reason that has prevented the health service from becoming more task oriented is because it still does not have clear-cut goals. It cannot decide whether care should be preventative, wholistic, or simply palliative. There is even a lack of clarity about what constitutes "health"— there is considerable debate among authorities in the field over just this issue.

A second reason preventing the NHS adopting a task orientation might be attributed to what is referred to in NHS circles as "tribalism". That is, the NHS is composed of various "tribes"—midwives, nurses, doctors, and other professionals, represented by various professional bodies (the RCM, RCN, BMA, etc.)—all of whom have slightly different goals and perceptions of what constitutes effective care, and all of whom are pulling in somewhat different directions. General managers have found it difficult to bring these groups together in order to make them work as a team. For this reason, the 1989 White Papers gave general managers greater powers for making, appointing, and rewarding NHS members.

OCCUPATIONAL CULTURES

Occupations also develop cultures and as such may become subcultures within the larger organizational culture. Again, occupational cultures develop in the same way as organizational cultures, i.e. groups with common interests and beliefs band together to give meaning to their work.

Any occupational culture interested in preserving its identity must somehow differentiate itself from other groups. It does this through a simultaneous process of identifying the characteristics of the "in-group" (the profession) and the "out-group" (anyone who does not belong to the profession) and by protecting and preserving its own expertise. This is accomplished through a dress code, language, professional qualifications, and the "tools of the trade" (Van Maanen & Barley, 1984). For example, nurses wear uniforms which identify them and distinguish them from other health service groups. Doctors wear white coats and carry stethoscopes. The language used by both groups is rather specialized and esoteric. Doctors use a lot of Latinized names to diagnose and treat illnesses. Additionally, the shared sense of stress and danger associated with health care serves further to tie these occupational groups together while the legends and heroes that develop in the culture foster an 'us vs them" attitude to any groups outside the profession.

All of this distinguishes them from other occupational classes and increases the profession's control over its members. Moreover, attempts made to regulate the profession by external groups, according to Van Maanen and Barley (1984), are strongly condemned as interference from people who simply do not understand the problems. (Witness the BMA's reaction to the many governmental reforms since 1948.) Perceived external threats to the rights of professionals to regulate themselves and ways to avoid them become part of the rituals at national conferences held by professionals.

Similarly, the public's perception of the integrity and expertise of the profession must be maintained whatever the costs. Any perceived threats to undermine the public's trust in them is immediately dealt with most severely. In most cases, degradation rites are invoked, i.e. scapegoats are identified (usually high-status people within the profession) followed by an investigative ritual to ascertain guilt followed by a removal from office.

Occupational cultures represent a major problem for NHS managers, and may be one of the greatest challenges facing them in the near future as occupational groups become increasingly "tribalized" as they become more specialized.

CHANGING THE ORGANIZATIONAL CULTURE

There is considerable debate among researchers as to whether an organizational culture can be changed or only "managed" once it is in place. For example, Nord (1985) believed that managers can change anything they do not like in the culture. Deal and Kennedy (1982) also believed that what they call the "symbolic manager" can change an organization by using culture as a mechanism to shape and develop it.

Most of these writers believe that any behaviour that is learned can be unlearned. However, it isn't usually quite this simple. First, simply changing behaviour alone will not change the culture; a change in values, beliefs, and attitudes must also occur (Nordstrom & Allen, 1987). Secondly, organizational cultures take on a life of their own and become self-perpetuating and self-reinforcing. Once developed they provide a degree of certainty and become a source of stability for members. People feel comfortable within them since they know what behaviour is expected of them. There is, therefore, an in-built resistance to change the present culture. For instance, an organization's culture may perpetuate the norm of not challenging the leader's authority or questioning his or her decisions. This type of culture may simply produce corporate "yes-men" and the organization may become stale through a rigidly controlled managerial style. This could be altered by deliberately changing the reward system so that employees might be systematically allowed to take risks and by adopting the norm of challenging the leader's decisions. (For a more detailed discussion see Chapter 10.)

According to Schein (1983) there are *five* major areas which managers may concentrate on in order successfully to manage an organization's culture. These include:

1. *What managers pay attention to, measure, and control.* When behaviour is acknowledged and either rewarded or punished this sends a strong message throughout the organization to employees as to what behaviour is expected of them.

2. *Reactions to critical incidents and crises.* Depending upon the way in which crises or critical incidents are handled by management they may either reinforce the existing culture or trigger a new system of values to emerge that may become part of the new culture.

3. *Role modelling, teaching, and coaching.* Leaders are in a position to reinforce effective organizational behaviours. Employees look to others for leads and setting a good example is one way of reinforcing this. Above all, it is important for a manager to maintain consistency between what is said and what is done. For example, if a manager preaches one set of rules yet fails to live up to these rules, his or her credibility and leadership will be jeopardised.

4. *Criteria for allocating rewards and status.* People learn what is appropriate and acceptable behaviour in organizations not only through their own experiences but through observing what happens to others. Where organizations sometimes go wrong is in failing to be consistent in their administration of these rewards or punishments. Thus, if someone is "goofing off" and nothing happens to him or her, this will signal to others that it is acceptable to do likewise. Similarly, a failure to reward desirable behaviours will cause these behaviours to be extinguished.

5. *Criteria for recruitment, selection, promotion, and removal.* Recruitment and selection is obviously one area in which the organizational culture is perpetuated. In selection, for exam-

ple, it is a well-known fact that interviewers tend to select interviewees who are most like them in terms of values, tastes, and outlook. Schein notes also that the criteria used to fire or promote people in the organization will quickly become known throughout the organization and will tend to strengthen the existing culture.

With reference to point **3** above, heroes or role models are important, particularly the stories and myths that surround them. The current spate of biographies on private sector entrepreneurs tends to foster this belief in the manager as hero. The story of how Hewlett and Packard started their enterprise in a garage and then went on to develop the immensely successful computer firm serves to further bolster the belief that anyone can be successful if they work hard at it. Such stories inspire employees and spur them to greater effort. Unfortunately, there are fewer heroes in the public sector. However, Florence Nightingale may serve as both an inspiration and role model for many nurses entering the profession.

IMPLEMENTING A CULTURE CHANGE PROGRAMME

To implement successful culture change first of all requires clear leadership and commitment from top management. Leaders should provide a clear vision of what the organization can become. Nordstrom and Allen (1987) noted that corporate culture is heavily influenced by corporate leaders. A leader's well-formulated vision should be broad enough to encompass all of the organization's activities while still allowing for change, yet be specific enough for employees to be able to relate their own personal organizational contribution to that vision.

Culture change is also facilitated by an analysis of the current culture together with a re-examination of the current value system and assumptions under which it is operating. Nordstrom and Allen observed that a health care culture should be understood before it can be changed. It is highly recommended that the commitment of the people involved be gained through ensuring early involvement in the process. This also helps to overcome resistance to change.

Although research on changing organizational cultures is inconclusive, the following steps are recommended, adapted from Huse and Cummings (1985) and based on the work of researchers in the field (Schwartz & Davis, 1981; Sathe, 1983; Utall, 1983).

1. *Develop a clear strategic vision.* A clear vision of what the organization can become, coupled with effective skills in communicating this vision to others, provides purpose and

direction for the cultural change. A good way of beginning to develop this mission and strategy is to identify the basic values the organization considers important.

2. *Gain the commitment of top management.* To be successful, culture change must be managed from the top. Without this commitment and pressure to change, nothing will be accomplished. Top managers may serve as role models to others who must demonstrate by their actions their clear commitment to the new culture programme.

3. *Use symbolic leadership.* Deal and Kennedy suggest that a symbolic leader, using organizational culture as a tool, can shape and change it. Symbolic leadership involves using behaviours to symbolize the values and behaviours desired. It is suggested that, to be effective, such leaders need to develop a kind of missionary zeal with regard to the new value system espoused.

4. *Support organizational change.* Effective culture change should be supported through modifications in the structure, management style, information, and control and reward systems. These changes will strengthen and reinforce the switchover to the new culture.

5. *Select and socialize newcomers.* Pascale (1985) defines socialization with reference to organizational culture as the systematic process by which new employees are inducted into the organization's culture. What the excellence writers suggest is that, although organizations are set up for specific purposes and in order to achieve certain goals, the organization through its membership serves a specific adaptive social function and thereby develops a unique corporate identity of its own with its own set of values, assumptions, and myths. This process in turn serves to integrate new organizational members and comes to have a greater significance over and above that for which it was originally designed. What sometimes happens, therefore, is that inductees are socialized informally by organization members in ways that are detrimental to overall organizational effectiveness.

Many organizations lose a valuable opportunity to induct successfully a new recruit into the organization. To do this, a training programme for inductees may be formalized to the extent that the company's corporate philosophy, value system, and expected behaviour and mission are fully explained. In addition, the formal reward system should reinforce the behaviours the organization considers necessary and desirable.

FUTURE ORGANIZATIONAL CULTURES

Handy (1985a) perceived a growing conflict in the past few years between the organizational imperatives of increased size, conformity and control and the individual's growing need for greater opportunities, freedom and drives towards personal expression and autonomy in tackling their work. Handy claimed organizations cannot succeed if they continue to increase their size and attempt virtually to control employees' behaviour. Instead, Handy claimed that the organizational cultures of the future will be hybrids and will include "federalism", i.e. high autonomy for each section of the organization, each part of which will be small and autonomous. The new federal structures should provide:

1. A sense of "community" and personal involvement for employees. The anonymity and impersonality of the organization will be much reduced producing a semi-autonomous "village" within the organization.
2. Highly expert professional care with a flat collegial structure.
3. Many workers employed on a short-term contractual basis. The division between management and workers will be obliterated.
4. A greatly reduced middle management.

Handy believed that information technology combined with the flexibility of more contractual relationships and obligations will permit organizational structures to become more of a network than a pyramidal structure.

Handy cited the hospital as an example of this new "federal" type of organization. And there is some evidence to suggest that this is accurate as hospitals increasingly continue to contract out many ancillary services. However, Handy's thesis has been criticized on at least two counts. First, there is little evidence that middle management is decreasing. If anything, since *The Griffiths Report*, managers seem to be growing in influence. Increasingly also, managers are being recruited who do not have a health service background. Secondly, Handy's predictions assume full employment and steady growth. In a recession as resources become scarcer there is less likelihood that the new federalism will spread. Instead, as has been shown, when resources are scarce, people are willing to accept authoritarian leadership and will usually forego many of the desirable characteristics of federalism (*Managing Health Services*, 1990).

SUMMARY

Ouchi, Peters and Waterman, Deal and Kennedy, and Pascale and Athos have all emphasized the importance played by an organization's culture in determining its effectiveness. Although definitions differ, most writers agree that organizational culture refers to the pattern of shared values (what is important), beliefs (about how things work), and expectations about how to behave (the way we do things around here). It also includes myths, rituals, and ceremonies.

Peters and Waterman maintained that "strong cultures" that emphasize cohesiveness are a feature of excellent companies, ensuring as they do that everyone from the top down works as a member of a team. Harrison and Handy classified organizations as *power, role, task,* and *person* cultures. Each culture develops unique patterns of behaviours and expectations.

Ways to change an organization's culture are to: (1) develop a clear strategic vision; (2) gain commitment from top management; (3) use symbolic leadership; (4) support organizational change; and (5) select and socialize newcomers.

Successful organizational cultures in the future will, according to Handy, emphasize federalism, develop a sense of community, emphasize contractual work, obliterate divisions between managers and workers, and reduce middle management's role.

REFERENCES

Carroll, D. I. (1983). A disappointing search for excellence. *Harvard Business Review*, Nov.–Dec., 24–27.

Deal, T. E., & Kennedy, A. A. (1982). *Corporate cultures: the rites and rituals of corporate life.* Reading, MA: Addison-Wesley.

Denison, D. R. (1984). Bringing corporate culture to the bottom line. *Organizational Dynamics*, Autumn, 5–22.

Department of Health and Social Security (1989). *Caring for people.* London: DoH.

Department of Health and Social Security (1989). *Working for patients: the health service; caring for the 1990s.* London: DoH (Cm 555).

Geertz, C. (1973). *The interpretation of cultures.* New York: Basic Books.

Handy, C. B. (1985a). *The gods of management.* London: Pan Books.

Handy, C. B. (1985b). *Understanding organizations.* London: Penguin Books.

Harrison, R. (1972). Understanding your organization's character. *Harvard Business Review*, May–June.

Hofstede, G. (1980). *Culture's consequences: international differences in world-related values.* Beverly Hills, CA: Sage.

Huse, E. F., & Cummings, T. G. (1985). *Organization development and change.* St. Paul, MN: West Publishing Co.

Kroeber, A. L., & Kluckhohn, C. (1952). *Culture: a critical review of concepts and definitions.* Cambridge, MA: Harvard University Press.

Levi-Strauss, C. (1958). *Anthropologie structurale.* Paris: Librairie Plon.

Lynn Meek, V. (1988). Organizational culture: origins and weaknesses. *Organization Studies, 9*(4), 453–473.

Malinowski, B. (1944). *A scientific theory of culture and other essays.* New York: Galaxy Books.

Managing Health Services (1990). Book 8, Open University, Walton Hall. Milton Keynes: Open University.

Martin, J., & Siehl, C. (1983). Organizational culture and counterculture: an uneasy symbiosis. *Organizational Dynamics,* Autumn, 52–64.

NHS Management Inquiry (1983). *Letter to the Secretary of State and recommendations for action* (The Griffiths Report). London: DHSS.

Nord, W. R. (1985). Can organizational cultures be managed? In P. J. Frost, L. F. Moore, M. R. Louis, C. C. Lundberg and J. Martin (eds.). *Organizational culture.* Beverly Hills, CA: Sage.

Nordstrom, R. D., & Allen, B. H. (1987). Culture change versus behavioral change. *Health Care Management Review, 12,* Spring, 43–49.

Ouchi, W. G. (1981). *Theory Z: how American business can meet the Japanese challenge.* Reading, MA: Addison-Wesley.

Pascale, R. (1985). The paradox of "corporate culture": reconciling ourselves to socialization. *California Management Review,* Winter, 27.

Pascale, R. T., & Athos, A. G. (1982). *The art of Japanese management.* London: Penguin.

Peters, T. J., & Austin, N. A. (1985). *A passion for excellence.* New York: Random House.

Peters, T. J., & Waterman, R. H. Jr. (1982). *In search of excellence: lessons from America's best run companies.* New York: Harper & Row.

Radcliffe-Brown, A. R. (1952). *Structure and function in primitive society.* London: Oxford University Press.

Sathe, V. (1983). Implications of corporate culture: a manager's guide to action. *Organizational Dynamics,* Autumn, 5–23.

Schein, E. H. (1983). The role of the founder in creating organizational culture. *Organizational Dynamics,* Summer, 13–28.

Schein, E. H. (1985). *Organizational culture and leadership.* San Francisco: Jossey–Bass.

Schwartz, H., & Davis, S. (1981). Matching corporate culture and business strategy. *Organizational Dynamics,* Summer, 30–48.

Sullivan, J. J. (1983). A critique of Theory Z. *Academy of Management Review, 8,* 132–142.

Utall, B. (1983). The corporate culture vultures. *Fortune,* 17 October, 66–72.

Van Maanen, J., & Barley, S. R. (1984). Occupational culture and control in organizations. In B. M. Staw (Ed.). *Research in Occupational Behavior,* Vol. 6. Greenwich, CT: JAI Press, 287–365.

Epilogue

For Learners . . .   No matter what you do, make it your best.
Leave nothing undone.

Be sensitive to your own way of growing,
And

Have clear goals for youself.
Be strict in your journey
Toward their fulfillment.

Learn to know and to feel with yourself.
Only then will you be free to know and
To feel with others.

Set high goals and then
Put your mind on reaching them.

In all, only hold on to the positive and
Illuminate it.
Life can then be full of sunshine;
Life can then be successful
At every moment. . . .

Elaine Lynne La Monica

Appendix: Selected Bibliography on Experiential Learning

Benne, K., Bradford, L., Gibb, J., & Lippitt, R. (Eds.). (1975). *Laboratory method of changing and learning: Theory and application.* Palo Alto, CA: Science and Behavior Books.

Brill, N. (1976). *Teamwork: Working together in human services.* Philadelphia: Lippincott.

Burton, A., (Ed.). (1969). *Encounter.* San Francisco: Jossey-Bass.

Corey, G., & Corey, M. (1982). *Groups: Process and practice* (2nd ed.). Monterey, CA: Brooks/Cole.

Dyer, W. (Ed.). (1972). *Modern theory & method in group training.* New York: Van Nostrand Reinhold.

Egan, G. (1970). *Encounter: Group processes for interpersonal growth.* Belmont, CA: Brooks/Cole.

Egan, G. (1973). *Face to face: The small-group experience and interpersonal growth.* Monterey, CA: Brooks/Cole.

Gazda, G., Asbury, F., Balzer, F., Childers, W., Desselle, R., & Walters, R. (1973). *Human relations development: A manual for educators.* Boston: Allyn & Bacon.

Gazda, G., Asbury, F., Balzer, F., Childers, W., & Walters, R. (1977). *Human relations development: A manual for educators.* (2nd ed.). Boston: Allyn & Bacon.

Gazda, G., Asbury, F., Balzer, F., Childers, W., & Walters, R. (1983). *Human relations development: A manual for educators* (3rd ed.). Boston: Allyn & Bacon.

Golembiewski, R., & Blumberg, A. (Eds.). (1970). *Sensitivity training and the laboratory approach: Readings about concepts and applications.* Itasca, IL: Peacock.

Golembiewski, R., & Blumberg, A. (Eds.). (1973). *Sensitivity training and the laboratory approach: Readings about concepts and applications.* (2nd ed.). Itasca, IL: Peacock.

Golembiewski, R. & Blumberg, A. (Eds.). (1977). *Sensitivity training and the laboratory approach: Readings about concepts and applications.* (3rd ed.). Itasca, IL: Peacock.

Goodstein, L., Pfeiffer, J. (Eds.). (1983). *The 1983 annual for facilitators, trainers, and consultants.* San Diego: University Associates.

Grove, I. (1976). *Experiences in interpersonal communication.* Englewood Cliffs, NJ: Prentice-Hall.

Harvard Business Reviews on human relations. (1979). New York: Harper & Row.

Johnson, D. (1986). *Reaching out: Interpersonal effectiveness and self-actualization* (3rd ed.). Englewood Cliffs, NJ: Prentice-Hall.

Johnson, D., & Johnson, F. (1987). *Joining together: Group theory & group skills* (3rd ed.). Englewood Cliffs, NJ: Prentice-Hall.

Jones, J., & Pfeiffer, J. (Eds.). (1975). *The 1975 annual handbook for group facilitators.* La Jolla, CA: University Associates.

Jones, J., & Pfeiffer, J. (Eds.). (1977). *The 1977 annual handbook for group facilitators.* La Jolla, CA: University Associates.

Jones, J., & Pfeiffer, J. (Eds.). (1979). *The 1979 annual handbook for group facilitators.* La Jolla, CA: University Associates.

Jones, J., & Pfeiffer, J. (Eds.). (1981). *The 1981 annual handbook for group facilitators.* San Diego: University Associates.

Kolb, D., Rubin, I., & McIntyre, J. (1979). *Organizational psychology: An experiential approach* (3rd ed.). Englewood Cliffs, NJ: Prentice-Hall.

Lieberman, M., Yalom, I., & Miles, M. (1973). *Encounter groups: First facts.* New York: Basic Books.

Luft, J. (1970). *Group processes: An introduction to group dynamics* (2nd ed.). Palo Alto, CA: National Press Books.

Maier, N., Solem, A., & Maier, A. (1975). *The role-play technique: A handbook for management & leadership practice.* La Jolla, CA: University Associates.

Morris, K., & Cinnamon, K. (1974). *A handbook of verbal group exercises.* San Diego: University Associates.

Morris, K., & Cinnamon, K. (1975). *A handbook of non-verbal group exercises.* San Diego: University Associates.

Napier, R., & Gershenfeld, M. (1985). *Groups: Theory & experience* (3rd ed.). Boston: Houghton Mifflin.

O'Banion, T., & O'Connell, A. (1970). *The shared journey: An introduction to encounter.* Englewood Cliffs, NJ: Prentice-Hall.

Pfeiffer, J. (Ed.) (1987–88). *The annual series for group facilitators.* San Diego: University Associates.

Pfeiffer, J., & Goodstein, L. (Eds.). (1982–1986). *The annual series for facilitators, trainers, and consultants.* San Diego: University Associates.

Pfeiffer, J. & Jones, J. (Eds.). (1972–81). *The annual series for group facilitators.* La Jolla, CA: University Associates.

Pfeiffer, J. & Jones, J. (Eds.). (1974–85). *A handbook of structured experiences for human relations training* (Vols I–X). La Jolla, CA: University Associates.

Saulnier, L., & Simard, T. (1973). *Personal growth & interpersonal relations.* Englewood Cliffs, NJ: Prentice-Hall.

Schein, E. (1969). *Process consultation: Its role in organization development.* Reading, MA: Addison-Wesley.

Schein, E., & Bennis, W. (1965). *Personal and organizational change through group methods: The laboratory approach.* New York: Wiley.

Additional Bibliography for the Macmillan Adaption

Beatty, R. W., & Schneier, C. E. (1982). *Personnel administration: an experiential skill building approach* (2nd ed.). Reading, MA: Addison-Wesley Publishing Co.

Finch, F. E., Halsey, R. J., & Litterer, J. A. (1976). *Managing for organizational effectiveness: an experiential approach.* New York: McGraw-Hill Book Co.

Hall, D. T., Bowen, D. D., Lewicki, R. L., & Hall, F. S. (1982). *Experiences in management and organizational behavior* (2nd ed.). New York: John Wiley & Sons.

Kast, F. E., & Rosenzweig, J. E. (1976). *Experiential exercises and cases in management.* New York: McGraw-Hill Book Co.

Lau, J. B. (1979). *Behavior in organizations: an experiential approach* (revised ed.). Homewood, IL: Richard D. Irwin.

Author Index

Subject Index